Membrane Fluidity in Biology

Volume 1

Concepts of Membrane Structure

Membrane Fluidity in Biology

Volume 1
Concepts of Membrane Structure

EDITED BY

ROLAND C. ALOIA

Departments of Anesthesiology and Biochemistry
Loma Linda University
School of Medicine
and
Anesthesia Service
Pettis Memorial Veterans Hospital
Loma Linda, California

1983

ACADEMIC PRESS

A Subsidiary of Harcourt Brace Jovanovich, Publishers

New York   London
Paris   San Diego   San Francisco   São Paulo   Sydney   Tokyo   Toronto

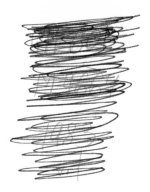

ACADEMIC PRESS, INC.
111 Fifth Avenue, New York, New York 10003

United Kingdom Edition published by
ACADEMIC PRESS, INC. (LONDON) LTD.
24/28 Oval Road, London NW1 7DX

Library of Congress Cataloging in Publication Data

Main entry under title:

Membrane fluidity in biology.

    Bibliography: p.
    Includes index.
    Contents: v. 1. Concepts of membrane struc-
ture --
    1. Membranes (Biology)--2. Membranes (Biology)--
Mechanical properties. 1. Aloia, Roland C.
QH601.M4664   1982   574.87'5   82-11535
ISBN 0-12-053001-5

PRINTED IN THE UNITED STATES OF AMERICA

83 84 85 86   9 8 7 6 5 4 3 2 1

Contents

Contributors   *ix*

Preface   *xi*

1. Nonrandom Lateral Organization in Bilayers and Biomembranes

Mahendra Kumar Jain

Introduction   2
Domains of One Phase in Single Component Bilayers   4
Coexistence of Solid and Liquid Phases at the Main Transition   10
Domains of Monotectic and Eutectic Phases
in Multicomponent Bilayers   14
Induction of Isothermal Phase Change   21
Lateral Organization in Biomembranes   23
Patching and Capping of Cell Surface Receptors in Response
to Ligand Binding   28
Epilog   30
References   33

2. Structural Properties of Lipids and Their Functional Roles in Biological Membranes

P. R. Cullis, B. de Kruijff, M. J. Hope, A. J. Verkleij, R. Nayar, S. B. Farren, C. Tilcock, T. D. Madden, and M. B. Bally

Introduction   40
Structural Preferences of Membrane Lipids   43
Isothermal Modulation of Membrane Lipid Structure   52
Potential Roles of Nonbilayer Lipid Structure in Membranes   60
A Rationale for Lipid Diversity—The Shape Concept   71
Closing Remarks   77
References   79

v

3. *Diversity in the Observed Structure of Cellular Membranes*

Fritiof S. Sjöstrand

Introduction   84
The Approach and the Methods   84
The Crista Membrane in Mitochondria   93
Surface Membranes in Mitochondria   116
Mitochondrial Membranes: Conclusions   121
Outer Segment Disks in Photoreceptor Cells   122
Plasma Membrane of the Outer Segment   134
Outer Segment of Photoreceptor Cells: Conclusions   138
References   140

4. *Correlation of Membrane Models with Transmission Electron Microscopic Images*

Ronald B. Luftig and Paul N. McMillan

Introduction: The Unit Membrane Model and the Unit Membrane
Image   143
Problems of Adequate Fixation for Erythrocyte Ghosts   146
Fixation in Other Membrane Systems   163
New Techniques   165
References   168

5. *Negative Images and the Interpretation of Membrane Structure*

K. A. Platt-Aloia and W. W. Thomson

Introduction   171
Preparative Procedures Which Result in a Negative Membrane
Image   176
Negative Images in Chloroplast Granal Membranes   192
Conclusions   195
References   197

6. Interactions of Cytochrome P-450 with Phospholipids and Proteins in the Endoplasmic Reticulum

James R. Trudell and Bernhard Bösterling

Protein–Lipid Interactions of Intrinsic Membrane Proteins   201
Lipid–Protein Interactions of Cytochrome *P*-450 in Reconstituted Vesicles   207
References   232

7. Membrane Composition, Structure, and Function

George Rouser

Introduction   236
Steps in the Derivation of Membrane Structure and Packing Principles   238
Graphic Analysis and Membrane Structure   252
Packing of Cholesterol, Gangliosides, and Ceramide Polyhexosides in Membranes   283
References   285

8. Mechanoelastic Properties of Biological Membranes

J. D. Brailsford

Introduction   291
Special Problems of Biconcave Membranes   292
Calculation of Elastic Strain Energy   311
Conclusion   317
References   318

Index   321

Contributors

Numbers in parentheses indicate the pages on which the authors' contributions begin.

M. B. Bally (39), Department of Biochemistry, University of British Columbia, Vancouver, British Columbia V6T 1W5, Canada

Bernhard Bösterling (201), Department of Anesthesiology, Stanford University School of Medicine, Stanford, California 94305

J. D. Brailsford (291), School of Allied Health Professions, Loma Linda University, Loma Linda, California 92354

P. R. Cullis (39), Department of Biochemistry, University of British Columbia, Vancouver, British Columbia V6T 1W5, Canada

B. de Kruijff (39), Department of Molecular Biology, Rijksuniversiteit te Utrecht, Utrecht, The Netherlands

S. B. Farren (39), Department of Biochemistry, University of British Columbia, Vancouver, British Columbia V6T 1W5, Canada

M. J. Hope (39), Department of Biochemistry, University of British Columbia, Vancouver, British Columbia V6T 1W5, Canada

Mahendra Kumar Jain (1), Department of Chemistry, University of Delaware, Newark, Delaware 19711

Ronald B. Luftig (143), Department of Microbiology and Immunology, University of South Carolina, School of Medicine, Columbia, South Carolina 29208

T. D. Madden (39), Department of Biochemistry, University of British Columbia, Vancouver, British Columbia V6T 1W5, Canada

Paul N. McMillan (143), Rhode Island Hospital, Providence, Rhode Island 02902

R. Nayar (39), Department of Biochemistry, University of British Columbia, Vancouver, British Columbia V6T 1W5, Canada

K. A. Platt-Aloia (171), Department of Botany and Plant Sciences, University of California, Riverside, California 92521

George Rouser (235), City of Hope Research Institute, Duarte, California 91010

Fritiof S. Sjöstrand (83), Department of Biology, and Molecular Biology Institute, University of California, Los Angeles, California 90024

W. W. Thomson (171), Department of Botany and Plant Sciences, University of California, Riverside, California 92521

C. Tilcock (39), Department of Biochemistry, University of British Columbia, Vancouver, British Columbia V6T 1W5, Canada

James R. Trudell (201), Department of Anesthesiology, Stanford University School of Medicine, Stanford, California 94305

A. J. Verkleij (39), Department of Molecular Biology, Rijksuniversiteit te Utrecht, Utrecht, The Netherlands

Preface

Over the past several years, hundreds of books have been published on many facets of cell and membrane function. However, only a few of these have contained discussions of the various aspects of membrane fluidity and membrane structure–function relationships. Throughout the past decade it has become increasingly clear that alterations in membrane lipid composition and membrane fluidity can be influenced by diet, environmental factors, exogenous agents to which the cell membranes are exposed (e.g., ions, pH, drugs, hormones), and various pathological states. Furthermore, such alterations in membrane composition and fluidity have been shown to influence important cellular functions such as the transport of substances across the cell membrane, immunological recognition, protein–membrane binding, the activity of key membrane-bound enzymes, and the number and affinity of cell receptors. For example, the modulations of integral membrane enzymes such as Na^+/K^+-ATPases, adenylate cyclase, and Ca^{2+}/Mg^{2+}-ATPase, and peripheral enzymes such as acetylcholinesterase have been correlated with alterations in membrane lipid composition and fluidity. Alterations in membrane fluidity have been shown to influence a myriad of cell surface-related phenomena and, hence, to modify cellular and organ function. Conversely, alterations of metabolic state in various physiological processes such as cellular development are reflected in alterations in membrane fluidity.

Although the extensive relationship of membrane fluidity to membrane and cellular function has been documented in numerous journal publications, there has been no published treatise to review the tenets of membrane fluidity and to analyze and evaluate critically the relationship of fluidity to cellular activity. This set of volumes entitled *Membrane Fluidity in Biology* is intended to provide that function. The contributors to these volumes will examine the many membrane properties influenced by alterations in membrane lipid compositions and/or other organizational parameters that are encompassed by the term fluidity. This treatise will serve as a comprehensive source within which the precepts of membrane fluidity are elaborated and the significance of fluidity changes in both normal and pathological cellular functions is discussed. Each volume will represent a state-of-the-art review and should be a valuable reference source and a springboard for future research.

The present volume, entitled *Membrane Fluidity in Biology: Concepts of Membrane Structure*, is the first volume in this series. I am beginning the series with a work on membrane structure because our perception and understanding of membrane fluidity are ultimately based on our understanding of membrane architecture and organization. I have selected authors who present many new ideas about membrane structural organization and who provide unique and challenging ways to think about the composition and arrangement of the molecular components of cell membranes. Although sometimes controversial, the concepts presented are elaborated with detail and clarity. The authors provide a lucid account of recent evidence, a re-evaluation of older evidence, and a discussion of new perspectives in our understanding of the diversity and complexity of membrane lipids and structure–function relationships. They elaborate structural principles that should provide a sound conceptual framework for evaluating the facets of membrane fluidity discussed briefly in this volume and more extensively in subsequent volumes. Perhaps more importantly, the authors provide new insight into membrane packing principles and constraints that may herald a new era of questioning the architectural basis governing current, popular membrane models. This volume should be valuable and essential reading for all scientists and researchers concerned with an understanding of the molecular principles of cell function.

Volume 2 will cover such topics as phase transitions, hydrophobic and electrostatic effects of proteins, lateral phase separations, phospholipid transfer proteins, calcium and magnesium ion effects, sphingolipids, and cell-associated water. Volume 3 will examine the relationship of membrane fluidity to disease processes. Thus, the entire treatise should serve as a primary source for research scientists and teachers interested in cellular membrane fluidity phenomena.

I wish to express my sincerest thanks to the Department of Anesthesiology at Loma Linda University and the Anesthesiology Service at the Pettis Memorial Veterans Hospital for allowing me the time to devote to this effort. I am also indebted to Drs. George Rouser, Gene Kritchevsky, and William Thomson for kindling my interest in membranes and for their continued support, and to Darla Leeper, Gizete Babcock, Hilda McClure, Julie Porter, and Helen Mayfield for their dedicated and patient secretarial assistance.

Chapter 1

Nonrandom Lateral Organization in Bilayers and Biomembranes

Mahendra Kumar Jain

"The question is" said Alice, "whether you can make words mean so many different things."

"The question is which is to be master, that's all." Humpty Dumpty continued in a scornful tone, "when I use a word, it means just what I choose it to mean . . . neither more nor less."

"Contrariwise," said Tweedledee, "if it was so, it might be; and if it were so, it would be; but as it isn't, it ain't. That's logic."

"Tut, tut, child," said the Duchess. "Everything has got a moral if only you can find it."

Taken somewhat out of context from
Through the Looking Glass

Introduction. 2
Domains of One Phase in Single Component Bilayers. 4
Coexistence of Solid and Liquid Phases at the Main Transition. 10
Domains of Monotectic and Eutectic Phases in Multicomponent Bilayers 14
Induction of Isothermal Phase Change. 21
Lateral Organization in Biomembranes. 23
Patching and Capping of Cell Surface Receptors in Response to Ligand
    Binding. 28
Epilog. 30
References. 33

Membrane Fluidity in Biology, Vol. 1
Concepts of Membrane Structure

1

Introduction

Considerable progress in our understanding of biomembrane structure and function has resulted from structural generalizations invoked and articulated in the various models proposed over the last 50 years (Jain and White, 1977). Admittedly, models are meant to articulate consensus, to consolidate and formalize collective thinking, and to polarize the dialectics. Thus the generalizations implicit in various membrane models do provide a framework within which we can generate structural correlates of membrane function. The following structural and organizational generalizations are inherent in the various models in the literature and incorporated into the *plate-tectonics* model of membrane organization presented elsewhere (Jain and White, 1977).

Organization of phospholipids and proteins is in a two-dimensional matrix that arises from a bilayer arrangement of phospholipids. In this matrix the various components are held together by noncovalent forces; formation and stability of the matrix is due to hydrophobic effects arising from the amphipathic nature of the membrane components whereby the free energy gain is 750–800 cal/mole for the transfer of a methylene residue from the aqueous phase to bilayers; energetic contribution from polar groups is minimum; however, their shape and size determines the polymorphic behavior of the aggregate. It follows that the concentration of the membrane components in the surrounding aqueous medium is negligibly low (less than 10^{-10} M for phospholipids), and therefore the uncatalyzed or nonmediated exchange and transfer of components between different membranes is rather slow for phospholipids (half-time more than several hours). Proteins in membranes interrupt bilayer organization; however, factors governing the state of proteins in bilayers are not understood. It is generally agreed that membrane proteins contain segments of hydrophobic residues that dip into or protrude across the bilayer; the aqueous phase concentration and the intermembrane exchange rate of these proteins is immeasurably low; and the phase properties of bilayers influence properties of membrane proteins.

Molecular motions (rotational, segmental) of methylene chains of phospholipids give rise to a gradient of motional freedom ("fluidity") across the thickness of a phospholipid bilayer. Flexing of the acyl chains (segmental motion) increases the "disorder" from the aqueous phase to the center of the bilayer. Similarly, the dielectric constant (a bulk property) is expected to be 2 in the center of the bilayer and 80 in the aqueous phase. Thus both the disorder and the polarity do not necessarily change abruptly at the interface. One of the consequences of such gradients is existence of activation energy barriers for partitioning and diffusion of solutes in and across the bilayer.

Biomembranes exhibit functional and compositional asymmetry (Op den Kamp, 1979; Van Deenen, 1981). The phospholipid composition of the two monolayer halves are generally quite different; some proteins are exposed only on one side, or different parts of the same protein are exposed on the two sides, thus giving rise to a characteristic orientation to membrane proteins; asymmetric distribution of proteins is absolute and that of the phospholipids is relative, that is only a quantitative difference between the phospholipid composition of the two monolayer halves is noted; glycolipids and the carbohydrate conjugates of glycoproteins are always exposed to the outside surface of the plasma membrane. Existence of asymmetry implies that the exchange of the components between the two halves of a bilayer is very slow (half-time of several hours) or nonexistent.

The ability of phospholipids in aqueous media to adopt a variety of organized forms (bilayer, micelle, hexagonal) has been used to explain membrane functions such as endocytosis, secretion, fusion, and transbilayer exchange ("flip-flop"). Although such polymorphs are not widely recognized to be present in biomembranes, it is becoming increasingly obvious that the nonbilayer polymorphs such as hexagonal and micellar phases can be generated under physiological conditions (Cullis and DeKruijff, 1979; Verkleij and DeGier, 1981). The role of nonbilayer polymorphs in the lateral organization of biomembranes is not considered in this chapter, but their potential importance in certain membrane processes deserves serious consideration. Constraints of molecular geometry that may lead to the generation of one polymorph over the others have been discussed (Israelachvilli *et al.*, 1977). Generally speaking relative cross-sectional areas of the polar group and the acyl chain are important. A cylindrical molecule would favor a planar bilayer type of organization, whereas a wedge or cone shaped molecule would give rise to polymorphs with a highly curved lipid–water interface as seen in hexagonal and micellar phases. Obviously effective sizes of polar and nonpolar groups are determined not only by their structure, but also by temperature, the state of ionization, ion binding, and association with other membrane components.

Selective ordering and segregation of components in the plane of a membrane can lead to a nonrandom organization (Jain and White, 1977). Such ordering arises from favorable constraints of packing and specific interactions between membrane conponents. Nonrandom lateral organization gives rise to phase separation, patching, phase boundaries, multiple relaxations, and anomalous temperature dependence of membrane processes. Such aspects of lateral organization in bilayers and biomembranes are considered in this chapter.

Domains of One Phase in Single Component Bilayers

Intuitively, all the apparent and emergent properties of materials are governed by the spatiotemporal patterns generated by the components. The role of spatial heterogeneity and coexistence of discrete iso- and polymorphic clusters and domains in apparently homogeneous systems is crucial to our understanding of a wide variety of aggregate systems. According to the third law of thermodynamics a perfect crystal cannot exist at temperatures above absolute zero. Thus, in analogy with any organized structure, the bilayer lattice of single phospholipid species would have its organization interrupted with defects and imperfections. Such imperfections locally disturb the regular arrangement of the atoms and molecules, and they accommodate trace impurities and other constraints of organization and thermal motion. The phenomenon of lattice defects and imperfections is exhibited by all types of crystals, metals, magnetic materials, and even liquid crystals and amorphous glassy solids (Adams, 1974; Hull, 1975). Segregation into domains is facilitated not only by specific interactions within domains, but also by the fact that the strain (thermal and geometrical) can be relieved by "plating-out" of the impurities and by creation of defect regions (dislocations, defects, voids, cluster–cluster interfaces).[1] A visual demonstration of such a phenomenon is presented in Fig. 1, where spontaneous close packing of identical steel ball bearings under the force of gravity into a two-dimensional lattice always leads to the formation of domains of close-packed hexagonal lattice interrupted by point, line, and nodal defects, as well as the grain boundaries. *Point defects* arise from a vacancy in the lattice, and at all temperatures above absolute zero there is a thermodynamically stable number of vacancies. *Line defects* or dislocations or subgrain boundaries arise primarily due to plastic deformation, and they describe the registry of atoms or molecules across a line. Dislocation lines can end in closed loops, or branch into other dislocations, or terminate in grain boundaries. Two or more line dislocations can meet at a point or a node. Crystalline solids consist of ordered

---

[1] Several types of imperfections in organization are described in the literature (see Hull, 1975; Lee, 1975). One of the interesting analogies may be found in the "polymorphic" structure and consequent imperfections in the organization of human society, where segregation into nations, communities and clans results from economic and social factors (interests, ties, affiliations, inequalities and webs of countless other trivia of everyday life that separates or brings us together!). The "biological advantage" of such patches and their imperfections are that the individuals exploit the local environment and resources, facilitate competition and predation, and relieve internal strains and external pressures often at the cost of some patches (see Levin and Paine, 1974).

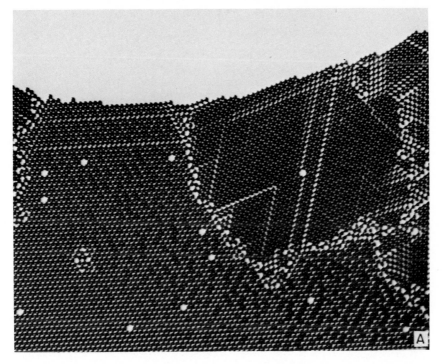

Fig. 1. Photograph of back illuminated panel of a randomly organized "monolayer" of identical ball bearings (between two lucite sheets) close packed under the force of gravity. Although the same arrangement cannot be reproduced by shaking the ball bearings, one always observes several types of defects that interrupt the hexagonally close-packed lattice. The most common types of defects are: *point defects* that appear as white dots; *line defects* which appear as sharp straight lines; *grain boundaries* that appear as diffuse regions between hexagonally close-packed domains. These terms for the various types of defects are used in the same general sense as they are used to describe defects in three-dimensional solid crystals.

domains (grains) separated by grain boundaries where such order does not exist. Each domain is a single close-packed lattice that is separated from other domains by defects. Random orientation of molecules at *grain boundaries* gives rise to disordered regions that are several molecules wide.

The existence of imperfections in bilayers of a single phospholipid species is indicated by a variety of techniques. The organization of bilayers is largely a consequence of acyl chain interactions, and the conformation of acyl chains is determined by temperature. Therefore, the temperature-dependent changes in the organization of bilayers are of considerable interest. Probably the most important thermotropic change in acyl chain conformation is due to rotation around C—C bonds which gives rise to two energetically favorable

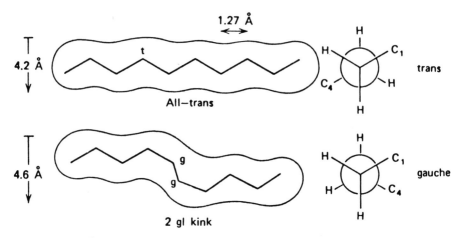

Fig. 2. Alkyl chains in an all-trans(t) and mixed trans–gauche(g) conformation. The Newman projections for the trans and gauche conformations are also shown. The dihedral angle (C_1—C_4) is 180° for the trans conformation and 120° or 240° for the gauche conformation. A kink is formed by rotating one C—C bond by an angle of 120° and then rotating either of the two next-nearest neighboring bonds by −120°.

states (Fig. 2): trans (continuous rotation angle $\theta = 0°$), and gauche ($\theta = \pm 120°$). The free energy change associated with such a change is about 0.3 to 0.5 kcal/mole in the favor of trans conformation and the activation energy is about 3 kcal/mole. Therefore at 25°C one gauche conformer is expected to be present for every five trans conformers in the acyl chain. The all-trans acyl chains can pack closely. Introduction of gauche conformers bends acyl chains (Fig. 2) so that they cannot close-pack unless two or more gauche conformers form a kink which mainimizes the bend of the acyl chain. The kinked chains, however, introduce some disorder in an otherwise close-packed bilayer. The acyl chains containing gauche conformers and kinks can plate out and collate into grain boundaries, and the all-trans chains can form close-packed two-dimensional domains (grains). Thus a conformational disorder of acyl chains can be translated into an organizational imperfection or defect. The thermodynamic and geometrical constraints of such an ensemble containing localized disorder would show up in the sizes and life times of the ordered domains. Other types of imperfections (point and line defects) could still exist in such ordered close-packed domains separated by the grain boundaries.

Diacylphospholipid bilayers exhibit thermotropic transitions. With phosphatidylcholines three transitions have been reported: (*a*) the main transition due to increased disorder resulting from increased gauche conformers in acyl chains; (*b*) the pretransition arising probably from a change in the orientation of acyl chains; and *(c)* the subtransition at a still lower temperature whose origin is yet unknown (Chen *et al.*, 1980).

Bilayers of pure phospholipids below their main transition are said to be in "solid," "gel," or "ordered" phase; and in "liquid," "fluid," "disordered," or "liquid-crystalline" phase above their main transition. Although all these terms have some historical or mechanistic significance, in this review I shall use only solid and liquid phase to characterize bilayers below and above their main transition. The terms are not meant to imply any similarity to the bulk solid and liquid phases. The bilayers between the pre- and main transitions are said to be in Pβ′ phase. All the three types of transitions exhibit a hysteresis in the heating and cooling cycles. The subtransition has been reported only in the first heating cycle of bilayers stored for several days at 0°C. The pretransition is seen in the heating cycles only when the sample is preequilibrated at low temperature for more than 15 min. The main transition is seen both in the heating and in the cooling cycles, however the exact shape and the transition temperature is not the same for the heating and the cooling cycles. These transitions also exhibit a finite width, that is the phase transition occurs over a finite temperature range. Both the finite width and hysteresis of transitions are most probably due to structural imperfections in bilayers. It should be noted that there is a tendency among the theoreticians to assume that the main transition is first order, and it is argued that the width and hysteresis are probably due to trace impurities that cause imperfections in the solid phase and influence nucleation in the liquid phase. It is also possible that the heating and cooling rates may be too fast to attain an equilibrium during the scan for a transition profile.

The presence of imperfections or organizational disorders in bilayers can be demonstrated by freeze-fracture electron microscopic studies. Bilayers quenched from the solid or the liquid phase exhibit a characteristically smooth fracture face, whereas, the bilayers quenched from the Pβ′ phase exhibit a characteristically rippled pattern (Fig. 3). The periodicity of these ripples probably arises from internal strain in the bilayer organization induced by a change in the orientation of phospholipid molecules. The linearity of the ridge of the ripple probably arises from a distortion of the symmetry properties in one dimension (singularly oriented strain in an array). The cumulative strain of domains with rippled patterns could give rise to secondary ripples of larger periodicity of the type seen in mixed lipid systems (see Fig. 4 and the discussion in the next section).

The rippled bands in such fracture faces of bilayers in Pβ′ phase are seldom, if ever, uniform over the whole bilayer surface. In fact such disorders in the long range organization of bilayers can be introduced simply by manipulating the history of the sample. The freeze-fracture electron micrographs of ditetradecylphosphatidylcholine (the ether analog of dimyristoyl-

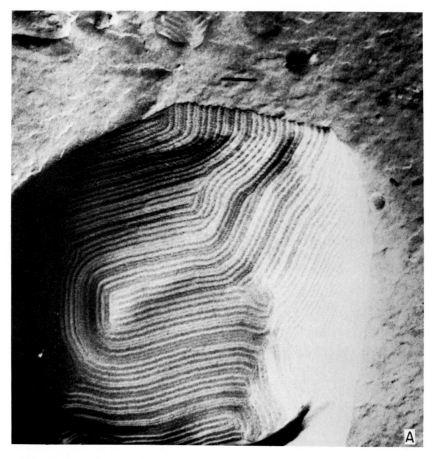

Fig. 3. Freeze-fracture electron micrographs of aqueous dispersions of ditetradecyl-phosphatidylcholine quenched at 21°C. The main transition temperature is 18°C. Sample for **A** was annealed at 30°C for 1 h, whereas the dispersions for **B** were not allowed to go above 21°C (unannealed). The freeze-fracture study was done by Mrs. J. Leunissen-Byvelt of the State University of Utrecht. Bar = 100 nm.

phosphatidylcholine) bilayers prepared under a variety of conditions and quenched from Pβ′ phase are shown in Fig. 3. An explanation for such a large difference in the rippled structure of fracture faces is not offered here, however a change in the long range order induced by the history of the bilayer is indicated by these electron micrographs. If one assumes that the termination of rippled domains represents domain boundaries, it follows that such domain boundaries predominate in unannealed bilayers. Such struc-

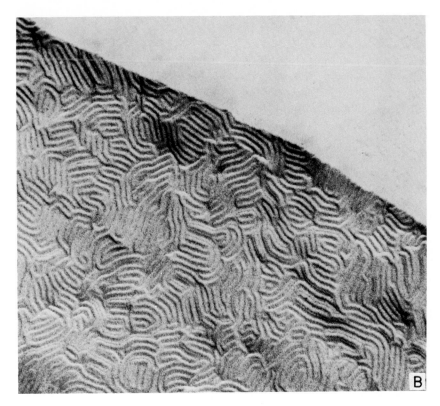

Fig. 3. Continued.

tural faults could persist in the solid phase well below pretransition. This is demonstrated by selective decoration of such defects (Stewart and Hui, 1979).

A loss of long range order in bilayer organization means an increase in disordered regions or grain boundaries between the ordered domains (grains). A high proportion of disordered regions persist in "unannealed" bilayers below their main phase transition temperature (Lawaczeck *et al.*, 1976). Thus phospholipid samples kept below the main phase transition temperature during hydration yield bilayers that have a relatively high proportion of their molecules in a mobile (on the proton NMR time scale) state. The molecules are presumably in the defect regions. If bilayers are incubated above their phase transition temperature for several hours (that is, "annealed") the resulting bilayers contain only a small fraction of molecules in the mobile state. Even in properly annealed bilayers some imperfections in organization should persist in order to accommodate thermal and geometrical constraints of packing. In freeze-fracture electron micrographs (Fig. 3) these regions appear as discontinuities in ripple patterns. The molecules in such discontinuities may be more mobile. This is indicated by physicochemical data. In NMR studies a few sharp peaks of low intensity are seen on a broad line (Salsbury and Chapman, 1968). Grain boundaries of ~400 Å width are consistent with X-ray data on dipalmitolyphosphatidylcholine bilayers in solid phase (Levine, quoted in Lee, 1975). Similarly, Raman studies suggest that two gauche conformers are present for each molecule in dipalmitoylphosphatidylcholine bilayers in solid phase (Yellin and Levin, 1977). These are probably restricted to the molecules present in defect regions. Susceptibility of bilayers to phospholipase A_2 is considerably enhanced not only near the phase transition temperature but also for unannealed bilayers (Upreti and Jain, 1980). At this stage it is very difficult to evaluate and quantitate the type, density, lifetime, and the fraction of molecules in defect regions or grain boundaries of an otherwise ordered close-packed bilayer lattice in the solid phase. It appears that in pure phospholipid bilayers such domains are large (see Hui and Parsons, 1975), and the fraction of molecules in the vicinity of defects may be about 0.1% in the annealed gel phase of dipalmitoylphosphatidylcholine bilayers. It is very difficult to control the level of trace impurities in phospholipids, and such impurities could give rise to and stabilize the defects which otherwise may be transient (flickering).

To summarize, the preceding discussion is an attempt to elaborate a general theme for lateral organization of molecules in bilayers in the solid phase. The observations presented above suggest that the organization of phospholipids in bilayers in the solid phase is in domains of uniform organization, and such domains are separated by disordered regions similar to the grain boundaries in crystals. Such ordered domains, however small, could persist as clusters even in a loosely packed bilayer matrix in the liquid phase (see Lee *et al.*, 1974; Baldassare *et al.*, 1976).

Coexistence of Solid and Liquid Phases at the Main Transition

The main transition of phospholipid bilayers is endothermic and is characterized by a phase transition temperature (strictly speaking, the onset of the transition is defined as transition temperature, however, we have used the midpoint of transition, T_m) and the enthalpy of transition (ΔH). The main transition is approximated as first order, that is the associated change in free energy approaches zero and at least one of the thermodynamic properties of the system undergoes an abrupt change. These thermodynamic criteria are applied to the bilayer phase only as extrapolations from the phase transition properties of bulk phases where medium is absent and it is assumed that the anisotropy of organization is not as crucial.

Several features of this thermotropic event in bilayers are noteworthy (see Chapman, 1975; Nagle, 1980 for reviews). The transition temperature increases with the acyl chain length; decreases with unsaturation and branching; cis double bonds lower the T_m more than the trans double bonds; a double bond in the middle of the chain lowers the T_m more than those closer to either ends of the chain; T_m for asymmetric phospholipids, for example 1-short, 2-long-, and 1-long, 2-short-phosphatidylcholines, are not identical and neither are they at the mean T_m for the mixture of phospholipids containing only the short and the long chains; the transition is accompanied by an increase in the average area (from 42 to 55 Å^2) per molecule, a decrease in thickness (about 6 Å), and an increase ($\sim$3%) in volume (all these values are for DPPC bilayers); interactions between lamellae do not appear to be important for phase transition; the lowered T_m and a broad transition exhibited by sonicated vesicles is due to constraints of packing. T_m also depends upon the nature of the head group as well as on all the factors that influence its state of ionization; both T_m and ΔH of a bilayer are modified by the presence of other solutes (lipids, proteins, hydrophobic solutes like anesthetics) in bilayers. Such observations suggest that the main transition manifests a change in the state of acyl chains, and all the factors that influence the conformation of acyl chains also influence the main transition. Intermolecular hydrogen bond formation (regulated by the pH of the medium since the protonated species may undergo such interactions) and ionic repulsion due to net surface charge also appear to modulate phase transition temperatures (Boggs, 1980).

The characteristics of the main solid to liquid phase transition in bilayers strongly suggest that this phase change is accompanied by a change in the conformation of acyl chains and that the role of the head group is largely through modulation of acyl chain interactions. A precise quantitative description of the molecular events accompanying the solid-to-liquid transition is not available. It has been demonstrated that the transition is accompanied by an increase in the rotational, conformational, and translational disorder, however the thermodynamic parameters of the solid-to-liquid transition in bilayers are not the same as those for the melting of solid hydrocarbons. The available data suggests that the transition in bilayers is accompanied by an increase in gauche conformation in methylene chains, which presumably gives rise to several conformational states of acyl chains including kinks (see Fig. 2). The solid phase domains which contain close packed all-trans chains of phospholipids are probably disrupted by the introduction of gauche conformation, thus creating new defects.

The solid-to-liquid transition in bilayers is rather sharp, suggesting that the underlying molecular event is highly cooperative. Like all thermodynamic parameters, the molecular interpretation of cooperativity is subject to certain arbitrary or axiomatic assumptions. Cooperativity arises from the tendency of neighboring lipid molecules to stay in isoenergetic states and to plate-out conformational disorder and impurities in grain boundaries. Thus depending upon the assumptions one feels comfortable with and the approximations one wishes to make (see Marsh *et al.*, 1977; Kanehisa and Tsong, 1978; also references in Nagle, 1980), one can generate a thermodynamic parameter—cluster or cooperative unit size. From the calorimetric data the cooperative unit size for diacylphosphatidylcholines has been computed to be several hundred. This alone argues against a strictly first-order phase transition for which the size of the cooperative unit should be infinite corresponding to the melting of perfect crystals. However the experimental values of the size of the cooperative unit are subject to considerable variation depending upon trace impurities in the sample, as well as on the history (temperature and duration of storage which induce annealing) and hysteresis behavior of the sample (see Copeland and McConnell, 1980; Albon and Sturtevant, 1978).

The state of molecules in bilayers during the course of phase transition is intriguing since in the phase transition range the molecules in both the solid and liquid phases must coexist in the bilayer lattice. Thus properties of such a phase would be determined not only by the proportion of molecules in these two phases, but also by the molecules in the (boundary) regions between the two phases. This has provoked considerable speculation. The following observations that bear on the properties of such a mixed phase bilayer may be noted:

1. Permeability across bilayers for sparingly permeable solutes shows a maximum at T_m; for example, for potassium ions (Blok *et al.*, 1975), sodium ions (Papahadjopoulos *et al.*, 1973), ANS (Tsong, 1975), glucose (Singer, 1981), TEMPO choline (Marsh *et al.*, 1976). Such effects are also modulated by the presence of solutes that modify the phase transition properties of bilayers (Singer and Jain, 1980).

2. Freeze-fracture electron microscopy of bilayers quenched from different temperatures demonstrates a change in the organization of the fracture plane (Verkleij and DeGier, 1981). As shown in Fig. 3, in the Pβ' phase one observes a banded structure which is not present in either the solid or the liquid phase.

3. An anomalously high susceptibility of pure phospholipid dispersions to phospholipase A_2 from pig pancreas (Op den Kamp *et al.*, 1977) and bee venom (Upreti and Jain, 1980) has been observed at T_m and in unannealed bilayers. However this effect is not wholly due to an increased binding or incorporation of the enzyme into bilayers containing both the solid and liquid phases at T_m (Jain *et al.*, 1982). Binding of the enzyme to bilayers at or below or above T_m is quite insignificant. The enzyme binds to bilayers only in the presence of both the products of hydrolysis, and the redistribution of the products in the bilayer is facilitated at T_m. Thus the formation of product induced binding sites is considerably facilitated at T_m.

4. Spontaneous phospholipid exchange, vesicle fusion and enlargment of vesicles is accelerated in the range of the phase transition temperatures, especially in the presence of fatty acids and negatively charged phospholipids (Massari *et al.*, 1980; Liao and Prestegard, 1980; and references therein).

The characteristics of the main transition suggest that pure phospholipid bilayers at or near their solid to liquid transition have features that are not dominant in the pure solid or the liquid phases. This is taken to imply that the anomalous properties of bilayers in the transition range are due to the "phase boundaries" or "regions of mismatch" that exist between the coexisting solid and liquid phases. It is also possible that in this temperature range the "critical fluctuations" and "lateral compressability" are maximized (see Marsh *et al.*, 1976; Marcelja and Wolfe, 1979). The major difficulty in resolving these alternatives (which are not necessarily mutually exculsive) arises from a lack of understanding of the nature of molecular events accompanying the phase transition. The solid and liquid phases of a bilayer have different packing constraints arising from different conformational states of acyl chains in the two states, and from the thermodynamic constraints of temperature that determine the energy of molecules and of the organized states in the bilayer. Introduction of gauche conformers reduces the length of acyl chains about 1.27 Å for each kink formed from two gauche conformers. The shortened chains cannot pack closely with all-trans acyl chains, thus the mixed bilayers containing randomly distributed chains would have internal strain. This would influence lateral organization of the bilayer. A high cooperativity of transition does not stipulate any specific arrangement of the molecules undergoing the phase transition except that they should be in an isoenergetic state. It may be intuitively or mathematically convenient, but probably incorrect, to assume that the "cooperative unit" is a two-dimensional domain, that the bilayer is made up of such cooperative domains, and that all the molecules within each domain undergo the transition simultaneously.

An alternative mechanism postulating a one-dimensional cooperative unit has been presented (Jain *et al.*, 1980) and is qualitatively elaborated in sequel. According to this suggestion, only the molecules at the grain boundaries of solid domain or at the line defects in solid phase domains constitute a cooperative unit. The thermodynamic state of molecules in such regions is quite different than the state of molecules within a solid phase domain or in grain boundaries. This situation is analogous to the isoenergetic state manifested in the fugacity (escaping tendency) of molecules at the surface of a bulk liquid. Thus the model postulating a one-dimensional cooperative unit invokes that: (*a*) the molecules along the defect regions of a solid phase domain are isoenergetic; (*b*) these molecules have different energies and degrees of freedom compared to those of the molecules within the domains of the solid phase which are more restricted; and (*c*) the molecules along the defect regions (grain boundaries or line defects) undergo a conformational change simultaneously.

The cooperative unit is postulated to be linear, however its shape is not stipulated; it may be straight or tortuous. Introduction of a new line defect or a grain boundary would be analogous (but not necessarily identical) to the thermotropic transition of a cooperative unit. The size of the cooperative unit would be the number of isoenergetic molecules that simultaneously undergo a change of state along a line defect or a grain boundary, or those perturbed by the introduction of a defect to release internal strain within a close-packed domain. Defect structures can be isothermally introduced by incorporating "impurities" into bilayers, therefore the average length of a line defect and the average distance between two different line defects would be effectively reduced. Both of these factors would decrease the average size of the cooperative unit. Indeed the introduction of impurities into bilayers in the gel phase decreases the sharpness of the transition (amounting to a decrease in cooperativity) in a concentration dependent fashion (Jain and Wu, 1977). Such a view of a one-dimensional cooperative unit is further necessitated by the observed phase transition of dipalmitoylphosphatidylcholesterol bilayers (Jain *et al.*, 1980) as discussed later in this chapter.

In summary: the changes in the lateral organization of a bilayer during its main thermotropic transition can be described in terms of a cooperative change in the state of the molecules along the grain boundaries or line defects in the solid phase.

Domains of Monotectic and Eutectic Phases in Multicomponent Bilayers

The role of a large variety of phospholipid species present in biomembranes has not been satisfactorily explained. A functional significance is implied not only by the remarkably fixed lipid composition of a given membrane, but also by a change in the lipid composition of membranes on changing diet, growth environment, and the pathological state of the organism. On a gross macroscopic level it is taken to be due to a change in a membrane phase property such as fluidity or "microviscosity." This is substantially based on the assumption that the lipid molecules are randomly distributed in mixed lipid membranes. However, recent studies on multicomponent phospholipid bilayers have demonstrated that the phase properties of such bilayers arise from nonideal mixing or phase separation of components in the bilayer. Phase separation leading to domain formation in bilayers is a consequence of anisotropy of organization of phospholipid molecules. In bulk phases such anisotropy is not present, therefore caution must be exercised in extrapolating the phase rules of bulk systems to bilayers.

In bilayers prepared from a mixture of phospholipids, the transition is not a single sharp change, but covers a rather broad temperature range. An interpretation of such transition profiles requires analysis of their phase diagrams (Fig. 4) which are essentially relationships of thermodynamic variables such as temperature, pressure, and composition (Lee, 1977a,b). Typically, the onset and completion of the phase transition are plotted against bilayer composition (generally taken to be the same as the composition of the lipid mixture from which the bilayers are prepared). The data can be generated from a temperature-dependent parameter of the bilayer or of a probe localized in bilayers of varying composition. Through phase diagrams one establishes the temperature and the concentration range over which the components are present in one or both phases. Ideal mixing of components in all three states (gel, gel and fluid, fluid) of a bilayer is indicated by the phase diagram of the type shown in Fig. 4a. Immiscibility in one or both phases is indicated by phase diagrams of the type shown in Fig. 4b and 4c. A list of mixed lipid bilayer systems exhibiting nonideal mixing is presented in Table I.

These observations suggest that an ideal mixing of phospholipids in bilayers is rather rare; it is seen over a wide range of composition only when the component phospholipids have the same head group and the acyl chains differ by about two methylene residues. Under almost all other conditions, phase separation is seen over a broad range of the mole fraction of components. Phase separation is frequently observed when at least one of the components is the gel phase (solid–solid or solid–liquid immiscibility), however liquid–liquid phase separation has been seen only in a few cases. Some generalizations for eutectic and monotectic behavior of lipids in mixed bilayers are outlined by Untracht and Shipley (1977).

The driving force for phase separation and for formation of eutectic mixtures in bilayers is not understood; however, the minimization of free energy would be achieved by any organizational feature that minimizes void spaces in the bilayer and maximizes interchain interactions. Free energy minimiza-

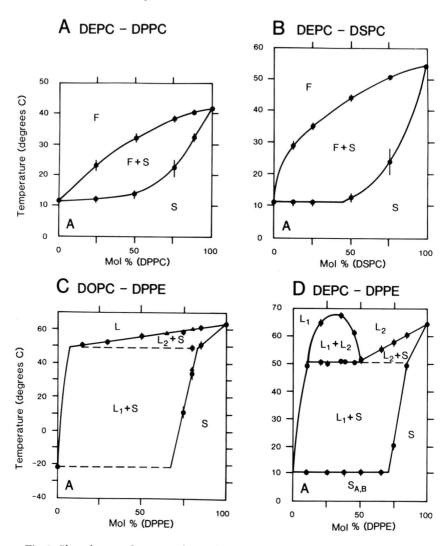

Fig. 4. Phase diagrams for aqueous binary dispersions of (**A**) dielaidoylphosphatidylcholine + dipalmitoylphosphatidylcholine; (**B**) dielaidoylphosphatidylcholine + distearoylphosphatidylcholine; (**C**) dioleoylphosphatidylcholine + dipalmitoylphosphatidylethanolamine; and (**D**) dielaidoylphosphatidylcholine and dipalmitoylphosphatidylethanolamine. The regions of the phase diagram containing solid (S), liquid (L), and solid + liquid (S+L) phases are shown. The data is derived from measurement of the Tempo spectral parameter, f, as a function of temperature. Reprinted with permission from Wu and McConnell (1975). Copyright (1975) American Chemical Society.

TABLE I

Some Mixed Phospholipid Bilayers That Exhibit Phase Separation

Lipids	References
Phosphatidylcholines of varying chain lengths	Van Dijck et al. (1977); Grant et al. (1974); Gent and HØ (1977); Bashfold et al. (1976); Andrich and Vanderkooi (1976)
Phosphatidylethanolamines	Lee (1978)
Phosphatidylcholine + fatty acid	Hauser et al. (1979)
Phosphatidylcholine + lysophosphatidylcholine	Van Echteld et al. (1980)
Phosphatidylcholine + lysophosphatidylcholine + fatty acid	Jain and DeHaas (1981)
Phosphatidylcholine + cholesterol	Verkleij et al. (1974); Shimshick and Mc-Connell (1973); Copeland and McConnell (1980) and references therein; Cherry et al. (1980)
Phosphatidylcholine + sphingomyelin	Untracht and Shipley (1977)
Phosphatidylcholine + phosphatidyl-ethanolamine	Wu and McConnell (1975); Lee (1978)
Phosphatidylcholine + phosphatidic acid or cardiolipin (+ cations)	Galla and Sackman (1975a,b); Gebhardt et al. (1977); Hartman et al. (1977); Massari and Pascolini (1977)
Phosphatidylcholine + phosphatidylserine	Luna and McConnell (1977); Stewart et al. (1979); Tokutomi et al. (1980)
Phosphatidylcholine + cerebroside	Pascher (1976)
Galactosylceramide + phosphatidylserine	Sharom and Grant, 1975
Cardiolipin + sterol	Birrell and Griffith (1976)

tion can also be achieved by minimizing interaction of acyl chains with the aqueous phase by plating the randomly distributed defects, by specific molecular associations that give rise to phases of different symmetry, and by minimizing a gauche:trans ratio for the molecules in a domain. Also, non-equivalence of the two acyl chains in phospholipids leads to a tilt of the phospholipid molecule in the solid phase of the bilayer, whereby the methyl ends of the chains are close packed. The bilayers containing phospholipids of different tilt and/or different lengths are more likely to be phase separated such that the defects are plated at the domain boundaries. An attempt to quantitate the factors governing phase separation in bilayers has been reported (Gebhardt et al., 1975).

Evidence for phase separation in mixed lipid bilayers comes from a variety of techniques as summarized below:

1. Broad phase transition profiles showing strong asymmetry or multiple transitions indicate coexisting multiple phases which may not necessarily

exist in the same bilayer. A somewhat stronger indication (not necessarily a proof) of nonideal mixing in bilayers can be obtained by constructing the phase diagrams (Lee, 1977b) of the type shown in Fig. 4. The phase transition ranges for bilayers of phospholipid mixtures of known composition are used to generate such diagrams. The experimental points can be fitted for the theroetically derived phase diagram to ascertain ideal mixing or phase separation (Lee, 1977a,b). It should also be noted that there are occasional inconsistencies between the probe and differential scanning calorimetric data (e.g. Van Dijck *et al.*, 1977). Solid–solid and solid–liquid immiscibilities are quite common, however, liquid–liquid immiscibility has been observed in dioleoylphosphatidylcholine and dipalmitoylphosphatidylethanolamine mixtures (Wu and McConnell, 1975) and a few other systems (see Melchior and Steim, 1979, for a review).

2. Direct visualization of separate domains coexisting in bilayers has been achieved by electron microscopic techniques (Krbecek *et al.*, 1979). Just below the phase transition temperature, pure phospholipids appear as distinct corrugated, rippled, or spiral structures manifesting the packing constraints of individual phospholipids. Above the phase transition temperature most bilayers exhibit a flat, smooth-textured fracture surface. As expected such studies have shown that the size and shape of domains depend upon the temperature and the composition. The results obtained from electron microscopic studies are quantitatively consistent with those obtained from other studies (Hui, 1981). In general the domains in mixed lipid bilayers are smaller (diam. 0.1–1 μm) than those in pure phospholipid bilayers (1–10 μm). The drift velocity of domains has been estimated as 10^{-5}–10^{-6} cm/sec (Hui, 1976a).

An interesting example of phase separation visualized by freeze-fracture electron microscopy is shown in Fig. 5. In aqueous dispersions of dipalmitoylphosphatidylcholine and beef brain phosphatidylserine mixtures, the Pβ' phase of phosphatidylcholine appears as banded domains, and phos-

---

Fig. 5. Freeze-fracture micrographs of multilamellar vesicles quenched from 34°C. The composition of the vesicles is 33 mol% bovine phosphatidylserine in dipalmitoylphosphatidylcholine. The textures displayed on the fracture faces of the vesicles indicate the coexistence of solid (P$_{B'}$) and fluid (L$_{\alpha}$) phases. The separation of rippled phosphatidylcholine domains from smooth phosphatidylserine domains in a fracture plane is shown by such micrographs. The rippled domains are apparently divided into subdomains where the ripples take sharp turns, presumably at dislocations. Ripples of larger periodicity appear as bright and shadowed areas reflecting internal strain. Particularly intriguing are ridges that "peel" off from the boundaries of rippled domains. These could reflect the regions that undergo phase change cooperatively. Bar = 500 nm. Micrographs contributed by Dr. Thomas P. Stewart, Department of Biophysics, Rosell Park Memorial Institute, Buffalo, New York; see also Stewart *et al.*, 1979.

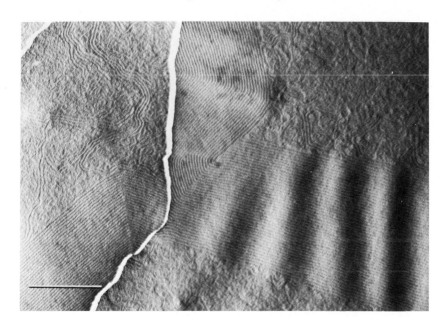

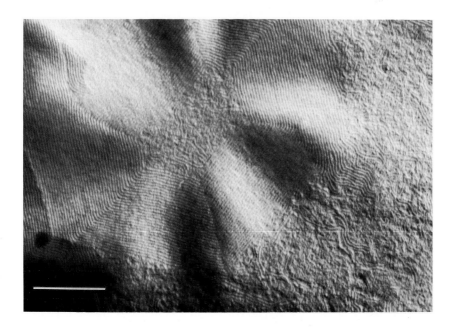

phatidylserine in liquid phase appears as a smooth surface. A particularly striking feature is seen at the boundaries of smooth and banded domains where individual bands appear to "peel off" from the banded domains. It is tempting to suggest that such peeling at the phase boundaries has something to do with a linear arrangement of molecules undergoing the transition (cf. the preceding section).

3. Dyes and other probes have been used to monitor self-association of lipids in bilayers. For example, dioleoylphosphatidylcholine appears to cluster about 50° above its phase transition temperature (Lee, 1975). Similarly, the degree of association of different acidic lipids at neutral pH appears to be phosphatidylinositol > phosphatidic acid > phosphatidylserine > phosphatidylcholine in mixed bilayers (Massari *et al.*, 1978). Such studies suffer from an inherent problem of probe induced reorganization. However these results do provide a method for detection of clustering and self association in liquid phase, and such indications may be used for corroboration with other techniques.

4. In phase-separated systems one would expect a difference in the ability of the various solutes to partition in different phases. This is manifested not only in the ability of the various solutes to modify the phase transition characteristics of bilayers (Jain and Wu, 1977) but also in the spectral properties of these solutes. Cation-induced phase separation in mixed dipalmitoylphosphatidylcholine and dipalmitoylphosphatidic acid bilayers has been demonstrated by using fluorescent probes (Galla and Sackman, 1975a,b). Fluorescent probes that partition differently in the various phases have been developed. For example, diacyl-3,3′-indocarbocyanine type of dyes experience a large difference in lateral diffusion coefficients ($D < 10^{-10}$ cm²/sec in the solid phase versus $D \sim 10^{-8}$ cm²/sec in the liquid phase), and in mixed-phase multilayers they show mobile fractions which reflect their phase-partition preference (Klausner and Wolf, 1980). Such a lifetime heterogeneity is also expected in rotational and vibrational modes.

5. Photoactivable phospholipid derivatives that react only with phospholipids in liquid phase provide chemical evidence for phase separation (Curatolo *et al.*, 1981). This approach is potentially useful for detecting phase separation in biomembranes.

In summary: solid–solid and solid–liquid phase separation in mixed lipid bilayers can be demonstrated by a variety of techniques. The domain size in such laterally phase separated systems appears to be very large, and the resulting phase boundaries are manifested in permeability of ions and other polar solutes, in binding and action of pig pancreatic phospholipase A$_2$, and in fusion of vesicles. However, such effects are manifested under different conditions. The phase boundaries present under different conditions may represent different spatiotemporal manifestations of statistical density fluctuations in the organization of components in two-dimensional domains. In a single-component bilayer such fluctuations would occur with equal probability at all points. The resulting defects would therefore be very short-lived (<1 psec) on a time averaged basis. Such defects are probably responsible for a very low but measurable permeability of ions, which cannot be accounted for in terms of their solubility in bilayers. At the phase transition temperature the fluctuations are expected to have a somewhat longer lifetime (<1 μsec) because conformations of several hundred molecules must be correlated for the thermotropic change. The resulting defects are manifested in the anomalously high permeability of polar solutes at T_m. In bilayers containing immisicle lipids or solutes, the geometrical constraints of packing and a finite rate of lateral diffusion of additives would tend to localize the defects. Under these conditions the localized defects may be considerably long lived (<1 msec). Such defects are probably best manifested in the enhanced fusion of vesicles or binding of pig pancreatic phospholipase A_2 to bilayers at the T_m in the presence of certain additives. These considerations provide a basis for understanding a variety of interactions ranging from permeability of ions to fusion of membranes.

Induction of Isothermal Phase Change

A phase change can be induced at constant temperature by a variety of factors that modulate the packing of acyl chains in bilayers, such as perturbation of the ionic environment by altering pH, salt, and divalent ion concentration; incorporation of lipid soluble agents such as anesthetics and detergents; and incorporation of other lipids including cholesterol and fatty acid plus lysophosphatidylcholine (Jain and DeHaas, 1981). The physiological importance of such perturbations can hardly be overemphasized and the role of isothermal phase changes in the regulation of membrane function has far reaching implications. In this context the role of cholesterol as an isothermal inducer of phase separation in bilayers is particularly interesting, and is discussed below.

   Cholesterol is a major component of mammalian plasma membranes. Early observations on the role of cholesterol in bilayers and biological membranes are reviewed elsewhere (Jain, 1975; Damel and DeKruyff, 1976). Recent studies are directed at understanding the lateral distribution of cholesterol in phospholipid bilayers. Differential scanning calorimetric studies on phospholipid + cholesterol mixtures (Melchior *et al.*, 1980 and references therein) suggest phase separation of cholesterol-containing domains from cholesterol-free phospholipid domains in bilayers containing less than 20% cholesterol. The freeze-fracture studies of Copeland and McConnell (1980) show that bilayers containing less than 20% cholesterol consist of banded domains of pure phospholipid separated by smooth domains of cholesterol + phospholipid (probably 1:4 mole ratio) phase. Such a phase separation would imply that the phase boundaries are at their maximum at about 10% cholesterol. This is consistent with an anomalous maximum in water permeability (Jain *et al.*, 1973) and lateral diffusion coefficient (Kuo and Wade, 1979) at 10 mol% cholesterol in phosphatidylcholine bilayers. Such a cholesterol induced phase separation may be responsible for the activation of reconstituted adenylate cyclase (Hebdon *et al.*, 1981).

Cholesterol appears to have different affinities for different phospholipids in bilayers in the order (Van Dijck, 1979): sphingomyelin $\gg$ phosphatidylserine and -glycerol $>$ phosphatidylcholine $\gg$ phosphatidylethanolamine, regardless of the transition temperature of the preferred lipid. Such associations would suggest that the lateral distribution of cholesterol in biomembranes is nonrandom. Interactions giving rise to such affinities do not involve hydrogen bonding between the hydroxyl group of sterol and carbonyl groups of phospholipids (Bittman *et al.*, 1981). Monolayer studies suggest that such interactions are probably due to constraints of packing (Cadenhead and Muller-Landau, 1979). Close packing of cholesterol + diacylphospholipids (1:1) requires extensive cholesterol–cholesterol interaction. Indeed, self-quenching of fluorescence of cholestatrienol in phosphatidylcholine bilayers is very strong at $>5\%$ sterol (Rogers *et al.*, 1979). The properties of bilayers and biomembranes containing cholesterol or cholestatrienol are not noticeably different. It means that the cholesterol– cholesterol interaction is extensive even at a low mole fraction of cholesterol. This is consistent with the suggestion that cholesterol + phospholipid domains separate from free phospholipid domains. The composition of these cholesterol-containing domains remains to be established. The X-ray diffraction work of Hui (1976a) shows the presence of arrays of acyl chains in bilayers containing equimolar phosphatidylcholine and cholesterol. Such a long range ordering of acyl chains is also required to explain the thermotropic phase transition characteristics of diacylphosphatidylcholesterol— the phosphate ester of cholesterol with diacylphosphatidic acid (Jain *et al.*, 1980, Noggle *et al.*, 1983). The monolayer studies of Cadenhead *et al.*, (1979) also point to possible arrays of acyl chains. In all these cases arrays of acyl chains are linear (that is, one dimensional) as articulated in the model outlined in Fig. 6.

The model postulating a linear array of cholesterol in bilayers also invokes a linear array of acyl chains. Such a long range order is probably manifested in the phase transition properties of diacylphosphatidylcholesterol in the

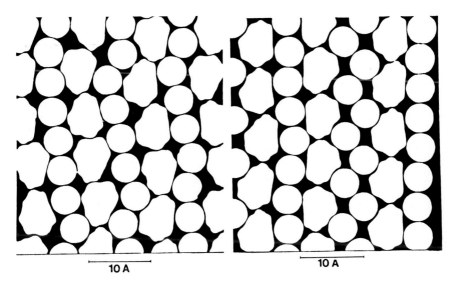

Fig. 6. Two possible models for a phospholipid–cholesterol mixed phase (1:1 molar ratio) viewed perpendicular to the plane of the lamellar phase. The circles represent the acyl chains and the irregular shapes represent cholesterol molecules as projected down their long axes. From Rogers *et al.* (1979), with permission.

presence of divalent ions (Jain *et al.*, 1980). The role of the divalent ions would be to bridge the neighboring molecules of the linear array. Such a bridging by divalent ions is not possible with equimolar mixtures of phospholipids and cholesterol, and therefore the transition of acyl chains is not manifested as a cooperative event. This does not mean that the acyl chains are not in an essentially all-trans state in cholesterol + phospholipid (1:1) bilayers. Indeed, Raman studies have demonstrated that the incorporation of cholesterol into phospholipid bilayers does not introduce any new gauche conformers (Levin, 1980).

To recapitulate, the role of cholesterol as an inducer of isothermal lateral phase separation in biomembranes deserves a serious consideration while evaluating its physiological role.

Lateral Organization in Biomembranes

Segregation of lipids and proteins of biomembranes into patches and domains appears to be universal, and such a process appears to be modulated by a variety of environmental factors that regulate membrane functions. A nonrandom distribution of components in biomembranes has been suggested by observations such as ease of removal of certain membrane components with detergents and organic solvents (Michel *et al.*, 1980), cross-linking of lipids to other lipids and to proteins (Marinetti and Love, 1974), isolation of membrane fragments that are rich in certain components (Horst *et al.*, 1980, and references therein), multiple relaxation processes (rotational, translational, and conformational), and direct visualization of patches by fluorescence and electron microscopic techniques. Some of the examples where a nonrandom distribution of membrane components has been reported, are given in Table II.

Electron micrographs of freeze-fractured biomembranes consist of a patchwork of diverse textural domains. Three types of domains are readily distinguishable:

1. A regular, almost crystalline, array of particles in a variety of cell types, where they are identified with functional specialization such as junctions (gap, synaptic, intercellular), light-harvesting complexes (chloroplasts, purple membranes, green algae), and mitochondria. These patches tend to be flat.

2. Regions of high particle density which appear in a variety of shapes and sizes.

3. Regions of curvature of varying particle density which sometimes appear almost completely devoid of any intramembrane particles.

Particle-free regions in freeze-fracture electron micrographs apparently arise from solid lipid phases, which "squeeze" out most proteins. However this appears to be characteristic only for certain membrane proteins (see Chapman *et al.*, 1977, and references therein). The existence of solid lipid domains in membranes can be demonstrated by differential scanning calorimetry. Bilayers in several bacterial membranes show a broad (20–30°C) asymmetric solid–liquid thermotropic phase transition (reviewed by Melchior and Steim, 1979). Generally two transitions are seen: a lower temperature peak due to lipids, and a higher temperature (50–80°C) peak due to denaturation of proteins. More than 90% of the lipid in bacterial membranes is in bilayer form, and the enthalpy of the intact membrane is 10–20% less than the enthalpy of the extracted lipid from the same sample. This suggests that 10–20% of the lipid is presumably bound to proteins, and it does not exhibit the transition. The lipid transition is reversible and its peak is generally asymmetric with a gradual onset and a more abrupt completion; it depends upon fatty acid composition which can be modulated by the growth temperature and the fatty acid supplements; the transition is similar in whole cells, isolated membranes, and extracted lipids; whole cells

TABLE II

Lateral Domains in Biomembranes

Cells	Method (Reference)
Smooth muscle cell	Filipin-sterol complex (Montesano, 1979)
Rat liver units	IMP[a] (Hackenbrock et al., 1976)
E. coli	Lipopolysaccharide, membrane isolation, chemical analysis (Leive, 1977)
	IMP (Kleeman and McConnell, 1974)
Rat mesenteric lymph node cells	Fluorescein-labelled cholera-toxin (Craig and Cuatrecases, 1975)
Tetrahymena pyriformis	IMP and lipid clustering by several techniques (Wunderlich et al., 1977)
Red blood cells	IMP/cholesterol (Hui et al., 1980)
Spleenic lymphocytes	Klausner et al. (1980a,b)
Red blood cells	Acyl chain transition (Cullis (1976) and references therein)
Muscle cells	Acetylcholine receptors (Yee et al., 1978)
See urchin egg	Probe (Wolf et al., 1981)
Mouse egg	Probe (Wolf et al., 1981)
Chloroplasts and photosynthetic bacteria and green alga	EM[b] (McDonnell and Staehelin, 1980; Staehelin et al., 1980; Giddings et al., 1980)
Red blood cell ghosts	EM (Moll, 1975; Pearson, 1979)
Clostridium spp.	EM (Sleytr, 1975)
Purple membranes of halobacterium spp.	X-ray (Henderson, 1977)
Guinea pig spermatozoa	EM (Bearer and Friend, 1980)

[a] IMP = intramembrane particles
[b] EM = electron microscopy

remain viable after calorimetry; and removal or proteolytic digestion of membrane proteins has little effect on the lipid transition.

The effects of lipid phase change in membranes are observed on the distribution of intramembrane particles, as well as on the conformation (Fourcans and Jain, 1974; also see below) and the vertical displacement (Borochov and Shinitzky, 1976; Armond and Staehelin, 1979; see however Amar et al., 1979) of the proteins. Unfortunately, no generalizations can be made at this stage (see Chapman et al., 1977; Melchior and Steim, 1979). The growth temperatures of organisms generally fall in the envelope of their lipid transition, however it is not certain if the transitions are necessary for viability, survival, or the physiological well-being of an organism. Indeed, meaningful biochemical criteria to evaluate the role of membrane transitions in the life of a cell are yet to be established. The usual criteria of cell growth are at best a qualitative index of the end result of all the changes that may be induced by altering membrane composition.

Correlation of the phase properties of lipids with the molecular properties of membrane proteins is probably most obvious in the discontinuities in Arrhenius plots. It is extensively documented that altering the fatty acid composition of membranes can profoundly alter the shapes of Arrhenius plots of functions of certain membrane proteins. Such discontinuities appear either as a sharp break or as a change in slope at a characteristic temperature (see Fourcans and Jain, 1974; Aloia, 1979; Melchior and Steim, 1979 for reviews). These anomalies are generally interpreted to suggest that the discontinuities manifest a change in the phase properties of lipids. Often multiple transitions are seen for the same process in the same membrane, or different processes in the same membrane exhibit different transitions. Similarly a break in the Arrhenius plot does not always correspond to a transition in the bulk lipid, although correlations between breaks in Arrhenius plots and the transitions reported by probes are more frequent. Although these observations suggest that homogeneous phases are not being sampled, the origin of such inhomogeneities remains obscure. One of the possibilities is that these membranes contain proteins in different microenvironments which arise from the formation of transient clusters or are due to segregation of lipid domains. The paucity of any meaningful generalization is amply demonstrated by the ongoing debate on the existence of boundary lipids, which could provide a mechanism for segregated lipid domains in membranes containing proteins.

A difference in the organization and/or composition of the lipid phase in the vicinity of membrane proteins, compared to that of the membrane as a whole, is implied in the postulate of "boundary" or "annulus" lipids. Such a segregated population of lipids can be detected by differential scanning calorimetry, Raman spectroscopy, and ESR; however "immobilization" of this lipid population is not seen by NMR (see Chapman *et al.*, 1979 for a review). Binding proteins to bilayers increases their phase transition temperature and lowers the cooperativity of transition as indicated by broad phase transition profiles which are also shifted towards higher temperatures. This suggests an increase in trans to gauche conformer ratio over a certain temperature range, which is confirmed by Raman spectroscopy (Curatolo *et al.*, 1978; Chapman *et al.*, 1977; Lavaille *et al.*, 1980; Jain *et al.*, 1982). Such an increase in trans to gauche ratio could form a basis for a novel interpretation of the interaction of proteins with defect sites which have a higher gauche to trans ratio compared to the average for the bilayer as a whole.

Let us examine the consequences of the binding of a protein to defect sites in bilayers. Macroscopically, conditions that favor phase separation in bilayers would favor enhanced protein binding and accommodate the resulting lateral compression by gauche to trans change at the phase boundaries. Thus, the binding of proteins to bilayers would increase the transition temperature without significantly altering the rotational and translational motional parameters of the lipid.

Thermodynamic parameters for the binding of proteins to defect sites in lipid bilayers can be measured. Since the number of such "binding sites" for proteins in bilayers is constant, the binding equilibrium can be described as:

$$\text{Protein} + \text{Site} \rightleftharpoons \text{Complex}$$

The binding sites in bilayers may be assumed to be discrete, independent, and made up of n lipid molecules. The incorporation of protein into bilayers is viewed not as the partitioning of a "solute" in a hydrophobic medium, but as a saturable equilibrium binding process (Jain *et al.*, 1982). The resulting binding isotherm can be experimentally measured, and the binding parameters (both n and the true binding constant) calculated readily for water-soluble proteins which exhibit little tendency to aggregate in the aqueous phase, although they readily bind to bilayers. The true (not apparent) binding constant in such a saturable binding process is for the binding of one protein molecule to a site consititued of n lipid molecules.

One can develop a thermodynamic interpretation of the binding constant in terms of gauche to trans conformational change in $2n$ acyl chains from n diacylphospholipids. The standard free energy change associated with a gauche to trans conformational change in polymethylene chains is about -0.2 to -0.5 kcal/mol. One gauche to trans change per chain in 50 moles of acyl chains ($n = 25$) on the binding of one mole of protein could provide -10 to -25 kcal of binding energy. Obviously several approximations and assumptions are made to arrive at this value. However the magnitude of the dissociation constant ($<10^{-6}$ M) for a lipid·protein complex suggests that, indeed, most of the binding energy could come from gauche to trans conformational change in acyl chains on binding the protein to a defect site.

Thus, according to this model numerous low energy changes provide the driving force for lipid–protein interaction, a feature that is often seen in macromolecular assemblies in biological systems. The binding sites for proteins are postualted to be the defect regions containing a high local concentration of gauche conformers in acyl chains. The binding of protein to the defect sites increases the trans to gauche ratio, and thus provides the binding energy. It should be emphasized that additional binding energy could come from the hydrophobic effect associated with the transfer of amino acid residues. However, such contributions are expected to be small since the hydrophobic residues of proteins in the aqueous phase tend to be buried away from the aqueous phase, and therefore their transfer from the aqueous phase to bilayers provides little thermodynamic force for the binding of a protein to bilayers.

Patching and Capping of Cell Surface Receptors in Response to Ligand Binding

The aggregation of membrane proteins has been associated with a variety of cellular processes such as endocytosis, viral budding, and fusion (see Chapman *et al.*, 1977 for references). The binding of a variety of ligands (toxins, hormones, transmitters, lectins, and antibodies) to cell surfaces induces a redistribution of their receptors (Table III). The sequence of events appears to be binding → aggregation → patching → capping → internalization. Not all of these events are exhibited by most ligand–surface receptor systems, however it is becoming increasingly apparent that such events may be related to functional aspects of ligand–receptor interaction such as ligand specificity, multiple binding constants, multiple relaxations, hormone degradation, down regulation, and negative cooperativity.

The redistribution of ligand–receptor complexes has been measured by a variety of techniques ranging from freeze-fracture electron microscopy to photobleach recovery of fluorescent probe-labeled cell surfaces. Such studies demonstrate that the free receptors are generally distributed over a wide area of cell surface. A fraction of both the free and bound receptor populations appear to have multiple rotational and translational mobilities. Based on the lateral mobility of lipids and lipid-localized probes ($D \sim 10^{-8}$ cm²/sec) the lateral diffusion constant of proteins (MW 10^5) is expected to be about 10^{-9} cm²/sec. However, depending upon the cell type and the protein probes used, a significant proportion (ranging from 10 to 90%) of the receptors exhibit one or more lateral diffusion constants in the range of 10^{-11} to 10^{-13} cm²/sec. It appears that other proteins and a majority of lipids are not immobilized by such ligand-induced patching. The ligand-induced patching and consequent immobilization of receptors could arise from one of the following mechanisms:

1. Ligand binding could lead to the formation of large cross-linked patches (see Dragsten *et al.*, 1979) which move *en masse* as a plate on the cell surface.

TABLE III

Ligand Induced Redistribution of Surface Receptors

Cell Type (Ref.)	Receptor/Ligand	Remarks
Mouse lymphocyte (Dragsten *et al.*, 1979)	Surface immunoglobulin Thy-1 antigen Lipid	— $D \approx 10^{-10}$ (0.5–0.9) $D \simeq 10^{-8}$ (>0.9)
3T3 Fibroblasts (Schlessinger *et al.*, 1978)	Glycoprotein/con A	$D < 10^{-12}$
3T3 Fibroblasts (Maxfield *et al.*, 1979)	Insulin Epidermal growth factor α_2-macroglobulin	Patching and internalization
Erythrocyte (Golan and Veatch, 1980; see also Nigg and Cherry, 1980)	Band 3	$D \simeq 10^{-11}$ (10–90)
Cultured muscle cells (Yee *et al.*, 1978)	Acetylcholine receptors	Patches of 10 μm diameter
Neuroblastoma cells (Hazum *et al.*, 1980)	Opiate receptors	Agonist and antagonist induced patching
Neutrophils (Weinbaum *et al.*, 1980)	Con A receptor	The receptors cluster at the front of polarized neutrophils, and the complex moves to the tail.
Lymphocyte (Klausner *et al.*, 1980a,b)	Free fatty acids	Capping and multiple relaxation for DPH
Fibroblasts (Schlessinger *et al.*, 1978)	Insulin	The complex patches and becomes immobilized and internalized
Lymphocyte (Curtain *et al.*, 1980)	Glycosphingolipid/con A	

2. The attachment of receptors or a receptor–ligand complex to cytoskeletal elements (such as microtubules or microfilaments) or to an actin–myosin type matrix of membrane proteins (Nicholson, 1976; Bourguignon and Singer, 1977) would immobilize one or more of the membrane-localized receptors. Such interactions may require energy (ATP, pH, or ionic gradient), a phosphorylation–dephosphorylation cycle, and the aggregation of filaments, and these events may be interrupted by inhibitors such as cytochalain B, colchicin, azide, or uncouplers.

3. The free and occupied receptors may be located in different lipid environments, and the aggregated species, which is "plated-out" into regions between lipid domains, would exhibit an apparently low diffusion coefficient because diffusion through such canalized regions is much more tortuous than

the free stochastic lateral movement that is assumed in the calculation of lateral diffusion coefficient.

4. Lateral electrophoresis (Jaffe, 1977), or membrane streaming (Bretcher, 1976), or recyling (Harris, 1976), could modulate the motion of membrane components by modulating the membrane surface charge distribution or electrical double layer.

Obviously a choice of mechanisms based on the available data is difficult (for example compare Klausner *et al.*, 1980a,b with Corps *et al.*, 1980; see also discussion in Dragsten *et al.*, 1979). It is possible that different mechanisms may predominate in different cell types under different perturbations, and that more than one mechanism may operate in parallel.

Several possible physiological roles for phase separation leading to the formation of local domains and clusters in cell membranes have been suggested. They provide a distinct microenvironment needed for the various physicochemical processes including modulation of the protein functions, such as catalytic and transport functions, immunological recognition and sensitization (Ruysschaert *et al.*, 1977) and procoagulant activity (Tans *et al.*, 1979). The coexistence of solid and liquid phases gives rise to lateral compressibility that may be required for the incorporation of proteins (Phillips *et al.*, 1975). Dislocations in cell walls and membranes have been suggested as possible growth centers (Harris and Scriven, 1970). Organization defects in lipid bilayers of biomembranes could be the site of phospholipase A_2 activity (Upreti and Jain, 1980) which ultimately regulates prostaglandin synthesis. The recycling of receptors and receptor bound ligands could occur by capping and internalization (Harris, 1976). Relatively rigid lateral distirbution of the monovalent antigens in the plane of the membrane could facilitate complement fixation (Humphries and McConnell, 1975). In short, correlation of domain structure and dynamics with biological functions is strongly suggested by such observations.

Epilog

Carl Jung wrote "fantasy is just as much feeling as thinking, as much intuition as sensation. Sometimes it appears in primordial form, sometimes it is the boldest product of all the faculties combined. Fantasy, therefore, is preeminently the creative activity from which the answers to all answerable questions come; it is the mother of all possibilities."

The use of terms such as clusters, patches, and domains is all too frequent now in the context of cell membranes. Although attempts to elaborate the lateral organization of biomembranes continue, several techniques have emerged to provide different windows to examine this phenomenon. Thus, differential scanning calorimetry, freeze-fracture electron microscopy, and fluorescence probes have been successfully used to provide information about the lateral organization and translational motion properties of the components in bilayers. Under favorable conditions it is possible to visualize domains of lipids and patches of proteins, and it is possible to demonstrate multiple relaxations for a given probe in bilayers. Still the most exciting period lies ahead where the progress in the available technology and the conceptual advancement in the various disciplines could lead to a quantitative description of the lateral organization of biomembranes.

Probably the most widely studied system is the solid (gel) phase of phosphatidylcholine and other synthetic phospholipids. Although several theoretical suggestions have been made to account for its thermotropic transition properties, few are consistent with most of the experimental observations. In order to elaborate a coherent description of order and disorder in bilayers, some heuristic suggestions have been outlined, all of which are applicable within the constraints of bilayer organization. Specific postulates that are proposed in the various sections of this chapter are:

1. The order in bilayers arising from the trans conformation of acyl chains is interrupted by the introduction of gauche conformers. The resulting disorder is "plated out" in the form of organizational imperfections, such as point defects (vacancies), line defects, and grain boundaries. The shape, size and lifetime of the domains separated by such imperfections depends upon the history of the sample, temperature, and the presence of other components. Such factors would therefore regulate the defect density, and would manifest in hysteresis and impurity effects, strain ripples, and related features of organization.

2. During the thermotropic transition the molecules along an existing or potential line defect or grain boundary undergo trans to gauche change. Thus, the cooperative unit is visualized as an isoenergetic linear array of molecules in the solid (gel) phase but along the defects.

3. Proteins, lipids, and drugs incorporated into bilayers would influence the lateral organization by two possible mechanisms: partitioning driven by hydrophobic effect, and binding on defect sites driven by lateral compressibility. Solutes that partition into bilayers could create new defects or modify and stabilize the existing defects. Such a process would be governed by a partitioning type of equilibrium. The driving force for the creation of new defects (trans to gauche) must come from the hydrophobic effect. In contrast, a modification of existing defects (gauche to trans) is energetically

favorable. Such a process would be governed by a saturable binding type of equilibrium. This is offered as a possible explanation for the existence of the so called boundary lipid.

The physiological relevance of order and disorder in the solid phase of lipid bilayers has been questioned on the grounds that a cooperative ther-motropic phase transition is not seen under physiological conditions (Melchior and Steim, 1979). Indeed, such transitions cannot be seen by the differential scanning calorimetry of natural membranes. The difficulty may be with the technique, which requires certain organizational constraints. A lack of thermotropic cooperativity cannot be construed to conclude that the acyl chains do not exist in an ordered state in bilayers. Indeed, there is ample circumstantial evidence suggesting the existence of a solid-like phase and of phase separation and microdomains in biomembranes. The distribu-tion of lipids in domains and clusters has been inferred from freeze-fracture electron microscopy of membranes treated with filipin which interacts with cholesterol (Elias *et al.*, 1979), and those treated with polymyxin B which interacts with anionic lipids (Bearer and Friend, 1980). Acyl chains in erythrocytes also appear to undergo a phase change (Cullis, 1976; Galla and Luisetti, 1980), suggesting a heterogeneous lipid distribution. Similarly, phase changes may occur in dioleoylphosphatidylcholine bilayers (Lee *et al.*, 1974; Baldeassare *et al.*, 1976), in *Tetrahymena pyriformis* (Wunderlich *et al.*, 1975), in *E. coli* (Baldassare *et al.*, 1976), in the sarcoplasmic reticulum (Davis *et al.*, 1975), in *Bacillus stearothermophilus* (McElhaney and Souza, 1976), and in mitochondria (Raison, 1972; Lee and Geer, 1974). None of these transitions correspond to the thermal transitions observed by DSC, however in some cases such transitions are detectable with probe tech-niques.

To account for such behavior we have postulated the plate-tectonics model (Jain and White, 1977) for the lateral organization of biomembranes. In analogy with the strained mixed-cluster state of· organization in glasses (Goodman, 1975), biomembranes are postulated to contain a mixed-cluster lattice which results in a persistent, consistent, interacting network leaving many of the domain boundaries separated by more disordered, liquid-like regions. Such a system, as a whole, would behave like a "locked-up" solid, and would have a "memory." Such a continuous network of clusters would have low cooperativity and high lateral compressibility, would be able to accommodate a variety of phospholipids which do not mix ideally, and could lead to yet another transition wherein all the clusters have melted. It would appear that these clusters are small and short-lived compared to the critical size and lifetime required for nucleation to form a long-lived, large domain. In contrast the "supercooled glassy liquid state" for biomembrane organization postulated by Melchior and Steim (1979) lacks such features and would lead to a uniformity of lateral organization through the membrane phase.

Acknowledgment

I wish to thank Dr. Michael Singer for a critical reading and helpful comments.

References

Adams, N. G.(1974). "Inorganic Solids," Chapter 9. Wiley, New York.
Albon, N., and Sturtevant, J. M. (1978). *Proc. Nat. Acad. Sci. USA* **75**, 2258–2260.
Aloia, R. C. (1979). *Chem. Zool.* **11** 49–75.
Amar, A., Rottem, S., and Razin, S. (1979). *Biochim. Biophys. Acta* **552**, 457–467.
Andrich, M. P., and Vanderkooi, J. M. (1976). *Biochemistry* **15**, 1257–1261.
Armond, P. A., and Staehelin, L. A. (1979). *Proc. Nat. Acad. Sci. USA* **76**, 1901–1905.
Baldassare, J. J., Rhinehart, K. B., and Silbert, D. F. (1976). *Biochemistry* **15**, 2989–2994.
Bashford, C. L., Morgan, C. G., and Radda, G. K. (1976). *Biochim. Biophys. Acta* **426**, 157–172.
Bearer, E. L., and Friend, D. S. (1980). *Proc. Nat. Acad. Sci. USA* **77**, 6601–6605.
Birrell, G. B., and Griffith, O. H. (1976). *Biochemistry* **15**, 2925–2929.
Bittman, R., Clejan, S., Jain, M. K., Deroo, P. W., and Rosenthal, A. F. (1981). *Biochemistry* **20**, 2790–2795.
Blok, M. C., van der Neut-Kok, E. C. M., van Dennen, L. L. M., and Degier, J. (1975). *Biochim. Biphys. Acta* **406**, 187–196.
Boggs, J. M. (1980). *Can. J. Biochem.* **58**, 755–770.
Borochov, H., and Shinitzky, M. (1976). *Proc. Nat. Acad. Sci. USA* **73**, 4526–2530.
Bourguignon, L. Y. W., and Singer, S. J. (1977). *Proc. Nat. Acad. Sci. USA* **74**, 5031–5035.
Bretscher, M. S. (1976). *Nature (London)* **260**, 21–23.
Cadenhead, D. A., Kellner, B. M. H., and Phillips, M. C. (1976). *J. Colloid Interface Sci.* **57**, 224–230.
Cadenhead, D. A., Müller-Landau, F., and Kellner, B. M. J. (1980). *In* "Ordering in Two Dimensions" (A. Sinha, ed.) pp. 73–81. Elsevier, Amsterdam/New York.
Chapman, D. (1975). *Q. Rev. Biophys.* **8**, 185–235.
Chapman, D., Cornell, B. A., Eliasz, A. W., and Perry A. (1977). *J. Mol. Biol.* **113**, 517–533.
Chapman, D., Cornell, B. A., and Quinn, P. J. (1977). *In* "Biochemistry of Membrane Transport" (G. Semenza and E. Carafoli, eds.) pp. 72–85. Springer, New York and Berlin.
Chapman, D., Gomez-Fernandez, G. C., and Goni, F. M. (1979). *FEBS Lett.* **98**, 211–223.
Chen, S. C., Sturtevant, J. M., and Gaffney, B. J. (1980). *Proc. Nat. Acad. Sci. USA* **77**, 5060–5063.
Cherry R. J., Muller, U., Holenstein, C., and Heyn, M. P. (1980a). *Biochim. Biophys. Acta* **596**, 145–151.

Cherry R. J., Nigg, E. A., and Beddard, G. S. (1980b). *Proc. Nat. Acad. Sci. USA* **77**, 5899–5903.

Copeland, B. R., and McConnell, H. M. (1980). *Biochim. Biophys. Acta* **599**, 95–109.

Corps, A. N., Pozzan, T., Hasketh, T. R., and Metcalfe, J. C. (1980). *J. Biol. Chem.* **255**, 10566–10568.

Craig, S. W., and Cuatrecasas, P. (1975). *Proc. Nat. Acad. Sci. USA* **72**, 3844–3848.

Cullis, P. R. (1976). *FEBS Lett.* **68**, 173–177.

Cullis, P. R., and DeKruyff, B. (1979). *Biochim. Biophys. Acta* **559**, 399–420.

Curatolo, W., Verma, S. P., Sakura, J. D., Small, D. M., Shipley, G. G., and Wallach, D. F. H. (1978). *Biochemistry* **17**, 1802–1807.

Curatolo, W., Radhakrishnan, R., Gupta, C. M., and Khorana, H. G. (1981). *Biochemistry* **20**, 1374–1378.

Curtain, C. C., Looney, F. D., and Smelstorium, J. A. (1980). *Biochim. Biophys. Acta* **596**, 43–56.

Damel, R. A., and DeKruyff, B. (1976). *Biochem. Biophys. Acta* **457**, 109–132.

Dragsten, P., Henkart, P., Blumenthal, R., Weinstein, J., and Schlessinger, J. (1979). *Proc. Nat. Acad. Sci. USA* **76**, 5163–5167.

Elias, P., Friend, D. S., and Goerke, J. (1979). *J. Histochem. Cytochem.* **27**, 1247–1262.

Fourcans, B., and Jain, M. K. (1974). *Adv. Lipid Res.* **12**, 147–226.

Galla, H., and Luisetti, J. (1980). *Biochim. Biophys. Acta* **596**, 108–117.

Galla, H. J., and Sackman, E. (1975a). *Biochim. Biophys. Acta* **401**, 509–529.

Galla, H. J., and Sackman, E. (1975b). *J. Am. Chem. Soc.*, 97, 4114–4120.

Gebhardt, C., Gruler, H., and Sackman, E. (1977). *Z. Naturforsch.* **32C**, 581–596.

Gent, M. P. N., and Ho, C. (1977). *Biochemistry* **17**, 3023–3038.

Giddings, T. H., Brower, D. L., and Staehelin, L. A. (1980). *J. Cell. Biol.* **84**, 327–339.

Golan, D. E., and Veatch, W. (1980). *Proc. Nat. Acad. Sci. USA* **77**, 2537–2541.

Goodman, C. H. L. (1975). *Nature (London)* **257**, 370–372.

Grant, C. W. M., Wu, S. H., and McConnell, H. M. (1974). *Biochim. Biophys. Acta* **363**, 151–158.

Hackenbrock, C. R., Hochli, M., and Chau, R. M. (1976). *Biochim. Biophys. Acta* **455**, 466–484.

Harris, A. K. (1976). *Nature (London)* **263**, 781–783.

Hartmann, W., Galla, A. J., and Sackmann, E. (1977). *FEBS Lett.* **78**, 169–172.

Hauser, H., Guyer, W., and Howell, K. (1979). *Biochemistry* **18**, 3285–3291.

Hazum, E., Chang, K., and Cuatrecasas, P. (1980). *Proc. Nat. Acad. Sci. USA* **77**, 3038–3041.

Hebdon, G. M., LeVine, H., Sahyoun, N. E., Schmitges, C. J., and Cuatrecases, P. (1981). *Proc Nat Acad. Sci. USA* **78**, 120–123.

Henderson, R. (1977). *Ann. Rev. Biophys. Bioeng.* **6**, 87–109.

Hoover, R. L., Bhalla, D. K., Yanovich, S., Inbar, M., and Karnovsky, M. J. (1980). *J. Cell. Physiol.* **103**, 399–406.

Horst, M. N., Baumbach, G. A., Olympio, M. A., and Roberts, R. M. (1980). *Biochim. Biophys Acta* **600**, 48–61.

Hui, S. W. (1976a) *In* "Membranes and Neoplasia: New Approaches and Strategies," pp. 159–170. Alan R. Liss Inc., New York.

Hui, S. W. (1976b). *Proc. Eur. Congr. Electron Microsc.*, 6th, Jerusalem (Y. Ben Shaul, ed.), Vol. 11, pp. 73–78.

Hui, S. W. (1981). Biophys. J. **34**, 383–95.

Hui, S. W., and Parsons, D. F. (1975). *Science* **190**, 383–384.

Hui, S. W., Stewart, C. M., Carpenter, M. P., and Stewart, T. P. (1980). *J. Cell. Biol.* **85**, 283–291.

Hull, D. (1975). "Introduction to Dislocations," 2nd ed. Pergamon, Oxford.

Israelachvilli, J. N., Mitchell, D. J., and Ninham, B. W. (1977). *Biochim. Biophys. Acta* **470**, 185–201.

Jaffe, L. F. (1977). *Nature (London)* **265**, 600–602.

Jain, M. K. (1975). *Curr. Top. Membrane Trans.* **6**, 1–51.

Jain, M. K., and DeHaas, G. H. (1981). *Biochim. Biophys. Acta* **642**, 203–211.

Jain, M. K., and White, H. B. (1977). *Adv. Lipid Res.* **15**, 1–60.

Jain, M. K., and Wu, N. M. (1977). *Biochem. Biophys. Res. Commun.* **81**, 1412–1417.

Jain, M. K., Toussaint, D. G., and Cordes, E. H. (1973). *J. Membrane Biol.* **14**, 1–16.

Jain, M. K., Egmond, M. R., Verheij, H. M., Apitz-Castro, R., Dijkman, R., and DeHaas, G. (1982). *Biochim. Biophys. Acta.* **688**, 341–348.

Jain, M. K., Ramirez, F., McCaffrey, T. M., Ioannou, P. V., Marecek, J. F., and Leunissen-Bijvelt, J. (1980). *Biochim. Biophys. Acta* **600**, 678–688.

Kanehisa, M. I., and T. Y. Tsong (1978). *J. Am. Chem. Soc.* **100**, 424–432.

Kapitza, H. G., and Sackman, E. (1980). *Biochim. Biophys. Acta* **596**, 56–64.

Kawato, S., Sigel, E., Carafoli, E., and Cherry, R. J. (1980). *J. Biol. Chem.* **255**, 5508–5510.

Klausner, R. D., and Wolf, D. E. (1980). *Biochemistry* **19**, 6199–6203.

Klausner, R. D., Bhalla, D. K., Dragsten, P., Hoover, R. L., and Karnovsky, M. J. (1980a). *Proc. Nat. Acad. Sci. USA* **77**, 437–441.

Klausner, R. D., Kleinfeld, A. M., Hoover, R. L., and Karnovsky, M. J. (1980b). *J. Biol. Chem.* **255**, 1286–1295.

Kleeman, W., and McConnell, H. M. (1974). *Biochim. Biophys. Acta* **345**, 220–230.

Korten, K., Sommer, T. J., and Miller, K. W. (1980). *Biochim. Biophys. Acta* **599**, 271–279.

Krbecek, R., Gebhardt, C., Gruler, H., and Sackman, E. (1979). *Biochim. Biophys. Acta* **554**, 1–22.

Kuo, A.-L., and Wade C. (1979). *Chem. Phys. Lipids* **25**, 135–139, and personal communication.

Lavaille, F., Levin, I. W., and Mollay, C. (1980). *Biochim. Biophys. Acta* **600**, 62–71.

Lawaczeck, R., Kainosho, M., and Chan, S. I. (1976). *Biochim. Biophys. Acta* **443**, 313–330.

Lee, A. G. (1975). *Prog. Biophys. Mol. Biol.* **29**, 3–56.

Lee, A. G. (1977a). *Biochim. Biophys. Acta* **472**, 237–281, 285–344.

Lee, A. G. (1977b). *Biochemistry* **16**, 835–841.

Lee, A. G. (1978). *Biochim. Biophys. Acta* **507**, 433–444.

Lee, A. G., Birdsall, N. J. M., Metcalfe, J. C., Toon, P. A., and Warren, G. B. (1974). *Biochemistry* **13**, 3699–3705.

Lee, M. P., and Gear, A. R. L. (1974). *J. Biol. Chem.* **249**, 7541–7549.

Leive, L. (1977). *Proc. Nat. Acad. Sci. USA* **74**, 5065–5068.

Levin, S. A., and Paine, R. T. (1974). *Proc. Nat. Acad. Sci. USA* **71**, 2744–2747.

Liao, M., and Prestegard, J. H. (1980). *Biochim Biophys. Acta* **599**, 81–94.

Luna, E. J., and McConnell, H. M. (1977). *Biochim. Biophys. Acta* **470**, 303–316.

Mabrey, S., and Sturtevant, J. M. (1976). *Proc. Nat. Acad. Sci. USA* **73**, 3862–3866.

Marcelja, S., and Wolfe, J. (1979). *Biochim. Biophys. Acta* **557**, 24–31.

Marinetti, G. V., and Love, R. (1974). *Biochem. Biophys. Res. Commun.* **61**, 30–37.

Marsh, D., Watts, A., and Knowles, P. F. (1976). *Biochemistry* **15**, 3570–3578.

Marsh, D., Watts, A., and Knowles, P. F. (1977). *Biochim. Biophys. Acta* **465**, 500–514.

Massari, S., and Pascolini, D. (1977). *Biochemistry* **16**, 1189–1194.

Massari, S., Pascolini, D., and Gradenigo, G. (1978). *Biochemistry* **17**, 4465–4469.

Massari, S., Arslan, P., Nicolussi, A., and Colonna, R. (1980). *Biochim. Biophys. Acta* **599**, 118–126.

Maxfield, F. R., Schlessinger, J., Schechter, Y., Pastan, I., and Willingham, M. C. (1978). *Cell* **14**, 805–810.

McDonnell, A., and Staehelin, L. A. (1980). *J. Cell. Biol.* **84**, 40–56.

McElhaney, R. N., and Souza, K. A. (1976). *Biochim. Biophys. Acta* **443**, 348–359.

Melchior, D. L., and Steim, J. (1979). *Prog. Surf. Sci.* **13**, 211–296.

Melchior, D. L., Scavitto, F. J., and Steim, J. M. (1980). *Biochimistry* **19**, 4828–4834.

Michel, H., Oesterhelt, D., and Henderson, R. (1980). *Proc. Nat. Acad. Sci. USA* **77**, 338–343.

Moll, G. (1975). *Bioenergetics* **6**, 41–44.

Montesano, R. (1979). *Nature (London)* **280**, 328–329.

Nagle, J. F. (1980). *Ann. Rev. Phys. Chem.* **31**, 157–95.

Nicholson, G. L. (1976). *Biochim. Biophys. Acta* **457**, 57–108.

Nigg. E. A., and Cherry, R. J. (1980). *Proc. Nat. Acad. Sci. USA* **77**, 4702–4706.

Noggle, J. H., Merecek, J. F., Mandal, S. B., van Vanetie, R., Rogers, J., Jain, M. K., and Ramirez, F. (1983). *Biochim. Biophys. Acta*. In press.

Op den Kamp, J. A. F. (1979). *Ann. Rev. Biochem.* **48**, 47–71.

Op den Kamp, J. A. F., Kauertz, M. T., and Van Deenen, L. L. M. (1975). *Biochim. Biophys. Acta* **406**, 169–177.

Papahadjopoulos, D., Jacobson, K., Nir, S., and Isac, T. (1973). *Biochim. Biophys. Acta* **311**, 330–348.

Pascher, I. (1976). *Biochim. Biophys. Acta* **455**, 433–451.

Pearson, R. P., Hui, S. W., and Stewart, T. P. (1979). *Biochim. Biophys. Acta* **557**, 265–282.

Phillips, M. C., and Finer, E. G. (1974). *Biochim. Biophys. Acta* **356**, 199–206.

Raison, J. K. (1972). *Bioenergetics* **4**, 285–309.

Rogers, J., Lee, A. G., and Wilton, D. C. (1979). *Biochim. Biophys. Acta* **552**, 23–37.

Ruysschaert, J. M., Tenenbaum, A., Berliner, C., and Delmelle, M. (1977). *FEBS Lett.* **81**, 406–409.

Salsbury, N. J., and Chapman, D. (1968). *Biochim. Biophys. Acta* **163**, 314–320.

Schlessinger, J., Barak, L. S., Hammes, G. G., Yamada, K. M., Pastan, I., Webb, W. W., and Elson, E. L. (1977a). *Proc. Nat. Acad. Sci. USA* **74**, 2909–2913.

Schlessinger, J., Elson, E. L., Webb, W. W., Yahara, I., Rutishauser, V., and Edelman, G. M. (1977b). *Proc. Nat. Acad. Sci. USA* **74**, 1110–1114.

Schlessinger, J., Shechter, Y., Willingham, M. C., and Pastan, I. (1978). *Proc. Nat. Acad. Sci. USA* **75**, 2659–2663.

Sharom, F. J., and Grant, C. W. M. (1975). *Biochem. Biophys. Res. Commun.* **67**, 1501–1507.

Shimshick, E. J., and McConnell, H. M. (1973). *Biochemistry* **12**, 2351–2360.

Singer, M. A. (1981). *Chem. Phys. Lipids* **28**, 253–267.

Singer, M. A., and Jain, M. K. (1980). *Can. J. Biochem.* **58**, 815–821.

Sleytr, U. B. (1975). *Nature (London)* **257**, 400–402.

Staehelin, L. A., and Hull, B. E. (1978). *Sci. Am.* **238**(5), 140–152.

Staehalin, L. A., Golecki, G. R., and Drews, G. (1980). *Biochim. Biophys. Acta* **589**, 30–45.

Stewart, T. P., and Hui, S. W. (1979). *Biochim. Biophys. Acta* **558**, 353–357.

Stewart, T. P., Hui, S. W., Portis, A. R., and Papahadjopoulos, D. (1979). *Biochim. Biophys. Acta* **556**, 1–16.

Tans, G., Van Zutphen, H., Comfurius, P., Hemker, H. C., and Zwaal, R. F. A. (1979). *Eur. J. Biochem.* **95**, 449–457.

Tokutomi, S., Ohki, K., and Ohnishi, S. I. (1980). *Biochim. Biophys. Acta*, **596**, 192–200.

Tsong, T. Y. (1975). *Biochemistry* **14**, 5409–5414.

Untracht, S. H., and Shipley, G. G. (1977). *J. Biol. Chem.* **252**, 4449–4457.

Upreti, G. C., and Jain, M. K. (1980). *J. Membrane Biol.* **55**, 113–123.

Van Deenen, L. L. M. (1981). *FEBS Lett.* **123**, 3–15.

Van Dijck, P. W. M. (1979). *Biochem. Biophys. Acta* **555**, 89–101.

Van Dijck, P. W. M., De Kruijeff, B., Van Deenen, L. L. M., De Gier, J., and Demel, R. A. (1976). *Biochim. Biophys. Acta* **455**, 576–587.

Van Dijck, P. W. M., Kaper, A. J., Oonk, H. A. J., and De Gier, J. (1977). *Biochim. Biophys. Acta* **470**, 58–69.

Van Dijck, P. W. M., De Kruijf, B., Verkleij, A. J., van Deenen, L. L. M., and De Gier, J. (1978). *Biochim. Biophys. Acta* **512**, 84–96.

Van Echteld, C. J. A., De Kruijff, B., and De Gier, J. (1980). *Biochim. Biophys. Acta* **595**, 71–81.

Verkleij, A. J., and De Gier, J. (1981). In press.

Verkleij, A. J., Ververgaert, P. H. J., deKruyff, B., and Van Deenen, L. L. M. (1974). *Biochim. Biophys. Acta* **373**, 495–501.

Weinbaum, D. L., Sullivan, J. A., and Mandell, G. L. (1980). *Nature (London)* **286**, 725–727.

Wolf, D. E., Kinsey, W., Lennarz, W., and Edidin, M. (1981). *Dev. Biol.* **81**, 133–138.

Wu, S. H., and McConnell, H. M. (1975). *Biochemistry* **14**, 847–854.

Wunderlich, F., Ronai, A., Speth, V., Seelig, J., and Blume, A. (1975). *Biochemistry* **14**, 3730–3734.

Yee, A. G., Fischbach, G. D., and Karnovsky, M. J. (1978). *Proc. Nat. Acad. Sci.* **75**, 3004–3008.

Yellin, N., and Levin, I. W. (1977). *Biochemistry* **16**, 642–647.

Chapter *2*

Structural Properties of Lipids and Their Functional Roles in Biological Membranes[1]

P. R. Cullis[2], B. de Kruijff, M. J. Hope, A. J. Verkleij,
R. Nayar, S. B. Farren, C. Tilcock[3], T. D. Madden[3], and
M. B. Bally

Introduction. 40
Structural Preferences of Membrane Lipids. 43
   Introduction. 43
   Techniques for Visualizing Lipid Organization. 44
   Phase Preferences of Lipids. 45
Isothermal Modulation of Membrane Lipid Structure. 52
   Influence of Divalent Cations and pH. 52
   Influence of Protein on Membrane Lipid Structure 58
Potential Roles of Nonbilayer Lipid Structures in Membranes. 60
   Membrane Fusion. 60
   Exocytosis. 65
   Transbilayer Transport. 66
   Intermembrane Communication. 70
A Rationale for Lipid Diversity—The Shape Concept. 71
Closing Remarks. 77
References. 79

[1]The research presented here was supported by the MRC (Canada), the Canadian Heart Foundation (B.C. chapter), and the B.C. Health Care Research Foundation.
[2]Scholar of the MRC (Canada).
[3]MRC (Canada) Postdoctoral Fellow.

Introduction

It is commonly assumed that lipids in biological membranes play rather inert structural roles, serving to maintain a permeability barrier between external and internal environments as well as providing a matrix with which functional membrane proteins are associated. However the sheer diversity of membrane lipids, as indicated in Fig. 1 for phospholipids, suggests that this does not provide a complete picture. A single phospholipid species such as phosphatidylcholine could maintain the required liquid crystalline bilayer envelope, immediately leading to questions concerning the functional roles of the many other lipid species present.

The nature of the problem can be more clearly indicated from the ^{31}P nuclear magnetic resonance (NMR) spectra presented in Fig. 2. As explained in slightly more detail in the next section, the observation of broad asymmetric ^{31}P-NMR signals with a low field shoulder and high field peak from large (diameter > 2000 Å) phospholipid systems indicates the presence of phospholipids in a bilayer arrangement. Thus Fig. 2 shows that phospholipids of the human erythrocyte membrane experience a bilayer organization (reflecting the behavior of over 97% of the endogeneous phospholipids [1]), as do dispersions of the total lipids extracted from the erythrocyte membrane. These results are consistent with the view that the lipid component provides the basic bilayer structure of biomembranes, since

PHOSPHOLIPIDS

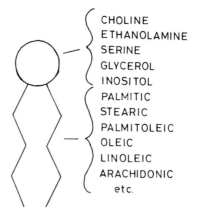

CHOLINE
ETHANOLAMINE
SERINE
GLYCEROL
INOSITOL
PALMITIC
STEARIC
PALMITOLEIC
OLEIC
LINOLEIC
ARACHIDONIC
etc.

Fig. 1. Chemical diversity in the headgroup and acyl chain regions of phospholipids.

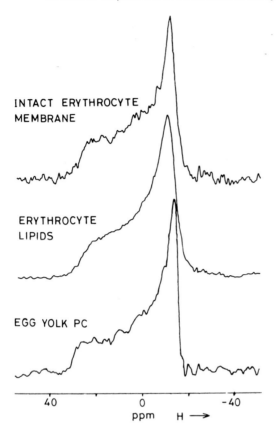

INTACT ERYTHROCYTE
MEMBRANE

ERYTHROCYTE
LIPIDS

EGG YOLK PC

40   0   -40
ppm   H ⟶

Fig. 2. ^{31}P-NMR spectra (81.0 MHz) at 37°C of human erythrocyte ghost preparations (100 mg dry wt. ghosts), total extracted rehydrated lipids of the erythrocyte (100 mg), and hydrated egg PC (100 mg). All preparations were hydrated in 1 ml of a 100 mM NaCl, 10 mM Tris-acetic acid (pH = 7.4) buffer containing 10% D_2O by vortex mixing. Spectra were collected from 1000 transients employing a 0.8 sec interpulse time, an 11 μsec 90° r.f. pulse and high power broadband proton decoupling. An exponential filter corresponding to 50 Hz line broadening was applied prior to Fourier transformation.

such structure is maintained in the absence of protein. The problems concerning lipid diversity are implicitly posed by the bilayer ^{31}P-NMR spectrum obtained from egg yolk phosphatidylcholine (PC) (see Fig. 2) suggesting that this PC (as well as PC with a single species of acyl chain substituent—see Fig. 5) could satisfy this structural demand. In the particular case of the erythrocyte membrane, the question is then, What are the functional roles of major phospholipids such as phosphatidylethanolamine (PE), phosphatidylserine (PS), and sphingomyelin (SPM) which respectively make up 30, 15, and 25 mol% of the total membrane phospholipid? Indeed, this is a great oversimplification of the problem, which must also include questions about the reasons for acyl chain diversity and location, the roles of cholesterol, the reasons why phospholipids are asymmetrically distributed across the membrane, and the roles of a host of minority lipid species found in this single membrane.

Previous attempts to rationalize lipid diversity have emphasized a hypothetical need for proteins to experience local regions of differing "fluidity" (as provided by local regions of varying lipid composition) for regulation of function, or a need of individual proteins for specific lipids for activity. As we have indicated elsewhere (see introduction of Cullis and de Kruijff [2]), the evidence supporting such a rationale for lipid diversity remains unconvincing. In spite of intensive effort there is little evidence to support the possibility that modulation of fluidity in the region of membrane protein plays an important regulatory role *in vivo*. Reasons for this situation include the fact that gel state lipids, which can modulate (inhibit) the activity of integral proteins in model reconstituted lipid–protein systems (see Warren, *et al.* [3] for example) do not appear to exist in most biological systems. They are notably absent from eukaryotic cell membranes. Further, the ability of physiologically relevant factors (such as pH, ionic strength, divalent cation concentration or even membrane protein) to isothermally modulate membrane fluidity to gain the necessary regulation in appropriate lipid mixtures is far from established.

In this work we review and develop recent work showing that the structural properties of lipids, as indicated by the macroscopic structures they adopt on hydration, are strongly dependent on the type of polar headgroup and acyl chain composition. Further, it is shown that these structural preferences are sensitive to and can be modulated by pH, Ca^{2+} and membrane protein among other factors. This leads to the possibility that some functional roles of lipids in membranes may be dictated by their ability to adopt bilayer or nonbilayer configurations. Evidence suggesting a role of nonbilayer lipid structures in processes such as membrane fusion is reviewed. Subsequently it is noted that the structural preferences of lipids appear to reflect, at least in part, the molecular shape of the lipid molecule, and this shape factor alone may play structural roles related to optimum biomembrane packing and sealing. In turn, this suggests a possible rationale for lipid diversity in terms of the molecular shapes of various components, allowing the formation of bilayer or nonbilayer structures as well as allowing local architectural roles at the lipid–protein interface.

Structural Preferences of Membrane Lipids

INTRODUCTION

In the presence of excess water and at concentrations above the "critical micellar concentration" (CMC) lipids form a variety of macromolecular organizations (the most common of these are indicated in Fig. 3). As we shall indicate momentarily, major membrane lipids generally assume the bilayer

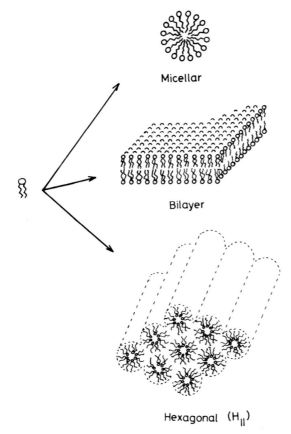

Micellar

Bilayer

Hexagonal (H_{II})

Fig. 3. Structural preferences of lipids at aqueous concentrations above the critical micellar concentration (c.m.c.).

or hexagonal (H_{II}) organization when hydrated. Lipids that assume micellar structures (e.g., lysophospholipids) are normally minority components of biomembranes. This is not the case for lipids preferring the hexagonal (H_{II}) phase in isolation, however, which often constitute up to 30% of the membrane lipid. The structure of this phase as elucidated by X-ray techniques [4] contrasts dramatically with the familiar bilayer organization, and two points must be emphasized. First, the H_{II} phase is basically a liquid crystalline hydrocarbon matrix penetrated by hexagonally packed aqueous channels (of approximately 20 Å diameter [4]) toward which the polar groups of the lipid are oriented (see Fig. 3). Second, lipids in the H_{II} phase cannot provide a permeability barrier between internal and external environments, and it is not clear that they can help to maintain a stable bilayer organization These functions are commonly thought to constitute the major role of membrane lipids. The observation that such lipids are major components of biological membranes immediately raises questions about the other functional properties of membranes they may satisfy, and such considerations have provided the major impetus for many of the studies summarized in this chapter.

TECHNIQUES FOR VISUALIZING LIPID ORGANIZATION

There are several techniques available to investigate the structural properties of hydrated lipids, namely X-ray diffraction [4], freeze-fracture [5, 6], and NMR [2, 7]. X-ray diffraction techniques are clearly the classical procedures allowing unambiguous determinations of the structure of hydrated lipid aggregates, provided that these structures are present in some regular array. Freeze-fracture electron microscopy procedures, on the other hand, provide a local visualization of the macromolecular lipid structures present, rather than averaged information arising simultaneously from many sites. Structures that can be detected include not only the ordered lamellar and hexagonal (H_{II}) phases [5], but also local intermediary structures [7] which may not be organized in a regular pattern. Finally, NMR techniques, particularly ^{31}P NMR for phospholipids [2], provide a valuable diagnostic procedure for determining lipid organization in large (diameter > 2000 Å) bilayer systems or cylindrical structures such as the H_{II} phase. However, NMR techniques do not provide unambiguous structural information for phospholipids in smaller systems where isotropic motional averaging (due to tumbling or lateral diffusion) occurs. Some of the advantages and disadvantages of the ^{31}P NMR-technique have been discussed elsewhere [2].

The ^{31}P-NMR and freeze-fracture characteristics of phospholipids in bilayer, H_{II} phase, and alternative structures are summarized in Fig. 4. Briefly, phospholipids in lamellar arrangements give rise to broad, asymmetric ^{31}P NMR spectra with a low field shoulder and high field peak separated by approximately 40 ppm, whereas freeze-fracture micrographs show large sheets which may be occasionally interrupted by ridges which appear to represent jumps of the fracture plane from the interior of one bilayer to an adjacent one. Phospholipids organized in the hexagonal (H_{II}) phase, on the other hand, give rise to asymmetric ^{31}P-NMR spectra which have reversed asymmetry compared to the bilayer spectrum and are narrower by a factor of two. This structure is visualized by freeze-fracture as a regular striated pattern created as the fracture plane fractures at all angles between the hexagonally packed cylinders (see Deamer *et al.* [5], Verkleij and Ververgaert [6], Verkleij and deGier [7], and Cullis *et al.* [8]). Finally, as mentioned previously, lipids in a variety of other structures allowing isotropic motional averaging give rise to narrow, symmetric ^{31}P-NMR spectra. Freeze-fracture representations can give less ambiguous assessments of the structures present, as shown for sonicated vesicles and "lipidic particle" structures (see next section).

PHASE PREFERENCES OF LIPIDS

In order to understand the behavior and organization of complex lipid mixtures such as those obtained in biomembranes, it is necessary to understand the structural preferences of the individual lipid species themselves. As indicated in Fig. 2, egg PC assumes a bilayer organization when hydrated, and similar behavior is observed for synthetic $18:1_c/18:1_c$ (DOPC) PC and bovine brain SPM as shown in Fig. 5. Such bilayer ^{31}P-NMR spectra are also observed in the presence of equimolar cholesterol. These results are consistent with extensive X-ray investigations of long chain PCs [9] and SPM [10], and suggest that a primary functional role of PC and SPM is to maintain the bilayer organization of biological membranes. A similar function may be ascribed to glycolipids such as diglucosyl and digalactosyl diglycerides, which also assume a lamellar organization upon hydration [11, 12]. This contrasts strongly with the behavior of naturally occurring PEs, which adopt either the bilayer or hexagonal (H_{II}) phase depending on the temperature [13, 14]. The ^{31}P-NMR behavior of a variety of PEs is illustrated in Fig. 6, where bilayer to H_{II} transitions are observed as the temperature is increased through ~8°C for erythrocyte PE, ~3°C for rat liver endoplasmic reticulum

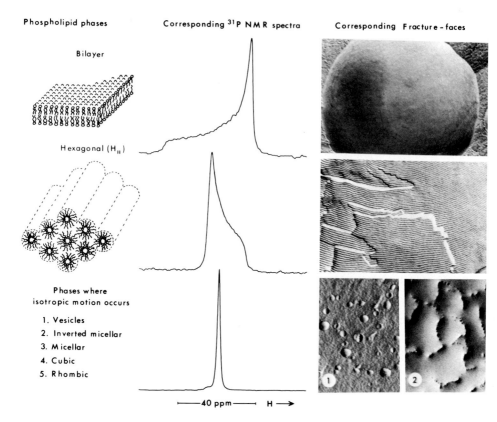

Phospholipid phases   Corresponding ³¹P NMR spectra   Corresponding Fracture-faces

Bilayer

Hexagonal (H$_{II}$)

Phases where
isotropic motion occurs

1. Vesicles
2. Inverted micellar
3. Micellar
4. Cubic
5. Rhombic

⊢——40 ppm——⊣   H ⟶

Fig. 4. ³¹P-NMR and freeze-fracture characteristics of phospholipids in various phases. The bilayer spectrum was obtained from aqueous dispersions of egg yolk phosphatidylcholine, and the hexagonal (H$_{II}$) phase spectrum from phosphatidylethanolamine prepared from soya bean phosphatidylcholine employing the head group exchange capacity of phospholipase D. The ³¹P-NMR spectrum representing isotropic motion was obtained from a mixture of 70 mol% soya phosphatidylethanolamine and 30% egg yolk phosphatidylcholine. All preparations were hydrated in 10 mM Tris-acetic acid (pH 7.0) containing 100 mM NaCl and spectra recorded at 30°C in the presence of proton decoupling. The freeze-fracture micrographs represent typical fracture faces obtained. The bilayer configuration (total erythrocyte lipids) gives rise to a smooth fracture face whereas the hexagonal (H$_{II}$) configuration is characterized by ridges displaying a periodicity of 6–15 nm. Two common conformations that give rise to isotropic motion are represented in the bottom micrograph (**1**) small bilayer vesicles (sonicated PS–PE [1:4] vesicles) (< 200 nm diam.) and (**2**) large lipid structures containing lipidic particles (PI–PE containing 15 Mol% PI: Ca^{2+}:PI = 1:2).

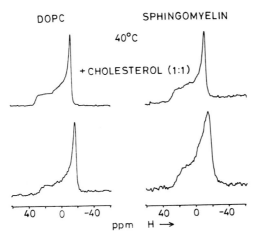

Fig. 5. 81.0 MHz ^{31}P-NMR spectra at 37°C arising from aqueous dispersions of 18:1$_c$/18:1$_c$ PC (DOPC) and bovine brain sphingomyelin (SPM) in the presence and absence of equimolar cholesterol. The cholesterol-containing samples were prepared from appropriate mixtures of DOPC and SPM in chloroform, which was subsequently evaporated under a stream of nitrogen and subsequent high vacuum (1 hr). The lipid film was then hydrated by vortex mixing in the aqueous buffer described in the legend of Fig. 2. All other conditions same as for Fig. 2.

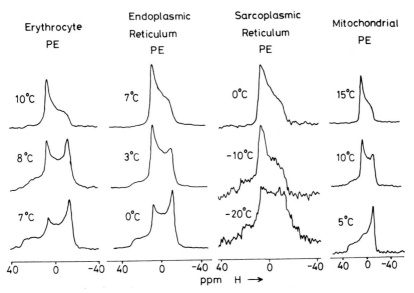

Fig. 6. ^{31}P-NMR spectra at selected temperatures illustrating bilayer to H$_{II}$ transitions for various species of naturally occuring phosphatidylethanolamines hydrated in excess aqueous buffer. For experimental conditions and other details on erythrocyte PE, see Cullis and deKruijff [85] endoplasmic reticulum PE, see deKruijff *et al.* [86]; and mitochondrial PE, see Cullis *et al.* [91]. Sarcoplasmic reticulum PE was isolated from rabbit muscle sarcoplasmic reticulum.

PE, $\sim -10°C$ for rabbit muscle sarcoplasmic reticulum PE, and $\sim 10°C$ for rat liver mitochondrial PE. Thus all these PEs prefer the H_{II} organization at physiological temperatures. Similarly, hydrated monoglucosyl and mono-galactosyl diglycerides from different sources prefer the hexagonal phase at growth temperatures [11, 12]. It is intriguing that there appears to be a relationship between the occurrence of these glycolipids and PE in bacterial membranes [15], despite their chemical disparity, suggesting a regulated requirement for lipids favoring the H_{II} organization.

The behavior of acidic (negatively charged) phospholipids is of particular interest because they experience strong interactions with divalent cations, thus the macroscopic structures assumed after hydration may be modulated by the presence or absence of Ca^{2+}, for example. The structural preferences of hydrated beef heart cardiolipin (CL), egg PS, egg phosphatidylglycerol (PG), and beef brain phosphatidylinositol (PI) in the presence and absence of Ca^{2+} are indicated in Fig. 7. Two points are apparent. First, in the absence of Ca^{2+}, all these negatively charged phospholipids adopt the bilayer orga-nization as indicated by ^{31}P NMR. Second, the addition of Ca^{2+} can have a variety of effects depending on the lipid species involved. These cation-dependent effects are discussed in greater detail in the next section dealing with isothermal regulation of lipid structure.

In mixed lipid systems, phospholipids preferring a bilayer organization in isolation (such as PC, SPM, and the acidic phospholipids) would be expected to stabilize a bilayer arrangement when mixed with an H_{II} phase lipid such as an unsaturated PE. This is the case for DOPC, as equimolar mixtures of this lipid with $18:1_c/18:1_c$ PE (DOPE) (which adopts the H_{II} phase above 15°C [16]) exhibit bilayer ^{31}P-NMR spectra (Fig. 8(a)). It is difficult to pre-dict a priori, however, the influence of a lipid such as cholesterol, which adopts neither the bilayer nor the H_{II} phase when hydrated but remains in a crystalline form. In mixtures with bilayer lipids cholesterol produces a state of intermediate fluidity, consistent with an ability to condense PC bilayers [17], and decrease the permeability of such systems. This may suggest a bilayer-stabilizing role, and the action of cholesterol in PC and SPM bilayers (Fig. 5) in no way contradicts this. However the presence of cholesterol in mixed unsaturated PE–PC systems produces a strong bilayer destabilization effect, inducing the hexagonal H_{II} phase at equimolar cholesterol to phos-pholipid concentrations (see Fig. 8(d)).

An interesting feature of the cholesterol titration of Fig. 8 is the ap-pearance of a narrow spectral feature indicating the presence of phospholipid in structures allowing isotropic motional averaging. Similar components are observed in unsaturated PE–PC systems at PC concentrations below those required to achieve full bilayer stabilization (see Cullis and de Kruijff [18], Cullis *et al.* [19]). As noted earlier, ^{31}P NMR does not provide an unam-

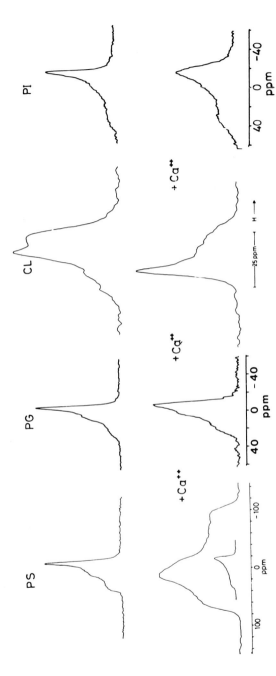

Fig. 7. ^{31}P-NMR spectra obtained for various species of acidic phospholipids (sodium salt) in the absence and presence of equimolar (with respect to charge) Ca^{2+}. For full details of sample preparation and signal accumulation procedures for cardiolipin (CL), see Cullis et al. [8], for phosphatidylserine (egg PS), see Hope and Cullis [29], for phosphatidylglycerol (egg PG), see Farren and Cullis [33], and for phosphatidylinositol (soya PI), see Nayer et al. [34]. The small insert on the PS + Ca^{2+} spectrum indicates the influence of Mg^{2+}. All previously published spectra reproduced with permission.

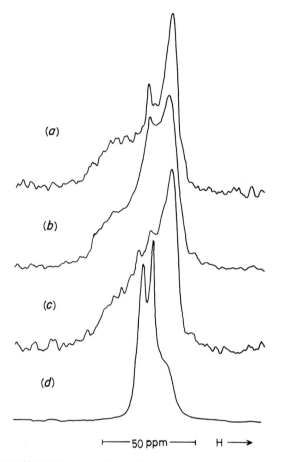

Fig. 8. 36.4 MHz ^{31}P-NMR spectra obtained at 30°C from equimolar mixtures of DOPE with DOPC in the presence of (a) 0 mol%; (b) 15 mol%; (c) 30 mol%; and (d) 50 mol% cholesterol. All dispersions contained 10 mM Tris-acetic acid (pH = 7.0) and 2 mM EDTA. Reproduced with permission from Cullis *et al.* [19].

biguous determination of the structures present in such situations. However the freeze-fracture results obtained from systems composed of mixtures of bilayer and H_{II} preferring lipids are most intriguing because small "lipidic particles" [20] are visible on the fracture face (Fig. 9). Although alternative possibilities have been proposed [23, 24], available evidence strongly suggests that these uniformly sized particles correspond to intrabilayer inverted micelles as illustrated in Fig. 9(b) [21, 22]. These inverted lipid micelles can occur as an intermediate structure between the bilayer and H_{II} organizations [25]. An important aspect of such a structure is that if nonbilayer lipid organizations are present in biomembranes, inverted micelles are more at-

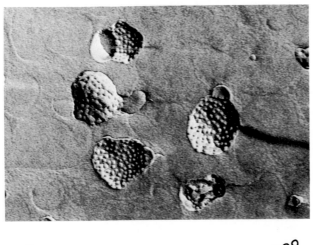

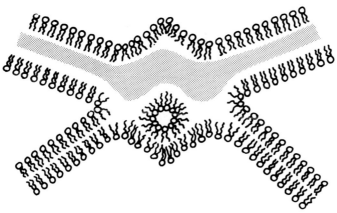

Fig. 9. Freeze-fracture micrograph of lipidic particles induced by Ca^{2+} in a lipid system consisting of cardiolipin and soya phosphatidylethanolamine in the molar ratio of 1:4 (magnification 80,000). A model of the lipidic particle as an inverted micelle is depicted below the micrograph. The shaded area represents the fracture region.

tractive candidates than the long inverted cylinders characteristic of the H_{II} phase. Reasons for this include the obvious fact that biomembranes are mixed lipid systems and thus would be mimicked more closely by the model systems composed of bilayer and H_{II} phase lipids, as well as the fact that a membrane containing an intrabilayer inverted micelle can conceivably maintain a permeability barrier. Further, inverted micelles can be generated at discrete locales as required, in contrast to a long inverted cylinder. However, such cylinders may play roles in "arrested fusion" situations such as tight junctions [92].

Isothermal Modulation of Membrane Lipid Structure

INFLUENCE OF DIVALENT CATIONS AND pH

It is clear that in order for nonbilayer lipid structures such as inverted micelles or extended inverted cylinders to be of some functional use in biomembranes mechanisms must exist for their isothermal regulation and control. Logical agents for such control include the local pH, ionic strength, divalent cation concentration, and membrane protein. In this section we point out that the pH and the divalent cation concentration (particularly Ca^{2+}) can strongly influence the structural preferences of membrane phospholipids under conditions that are within physiological bounds.

The ability of Ca^{2+} to modulate the structures formed by acidic (negatively charged) phospholipids is clearly illustrated in Fig. 7. In the case of beef heart CL, Ca^{2+} triggers a bilayer to H_{II} phase transition (see Cullis *et al.*, [8] for background detail) in agreement with previous X-ray results [26]. Similar behavior is observed for PA at pH 6 [28], results supported by freeze-fracture [27] and ^{2}H-NMR [28] techniques. It may be noted that other divalent cations such as Mg^{2+} and Ba^{2+} are able to trigger H_{II} phase formation for CL [26], as can Mg^{2+} and Mn^{2+} for PA at pH 6 [27, 28]. In the case of PS, the addition of Ca^{2+} results in a much broader ^{31}P-NMR spectrum (see Hope and Cullis [29] for details) which corresponds to a "rigid lattice" (no motion) situation commonly observed for anhydrous phospholipids. This appears to be characteristic of the "cochleate" Ca^{2+}–PS structure identified by Papahadjopoulos and co-workers [30]. A specificity of the divalent cation—PS interaction is indicated by the fact that Mg^{2+} is not able to produce similar effects (PS remains in the liquid crystalline lamellar organization in the presence of Mg^{2+}, see Fig. 7). Much different behavior is exhibited by egg PG and soya PI. In common with the other acidic phospholipids they precipitate on addition of Ca^{2+}, but remain in lamellar structures as indicated by ^{31}P NMR.

The ability of Ca^{2+} and other divalent cations to influence the structural preferences of acidic phospholipids (particularly CL, PA, and PS) is clearly of fundamental interest. However it is difficult to extrapolate this behavior to biological membranes where these phospholipids are not majority components. We have therefore examined the influence of Ca^{2+} on systems that may be expected to be both more representative of biomembrane lipid mixtures as well as more sensitive to the presence of divalent cations. Particularly interesting combinations are those containing acidic phospholipids with a PE species which prefers the H_{II} organization in isolation. In such systems situations can be achieved where the acidic phospholipid is barely stabilizing a bilayer configuration, and the net structure may thus be expected to be very sensitive to factors affecting the distribution and/or net charge on the negatively charged species.

The ability of representative acidic phospholipids to stabilize the bilayer in the presence of a polyunsaturated (soya) H_{II} phase PE at 30 mol% concentrations is illustrated in Fig. 10. Also illustrated is the ability of Ca^{2+} in all these systems to trigger a bilayer to H_{II} phase transition. It is interesting to

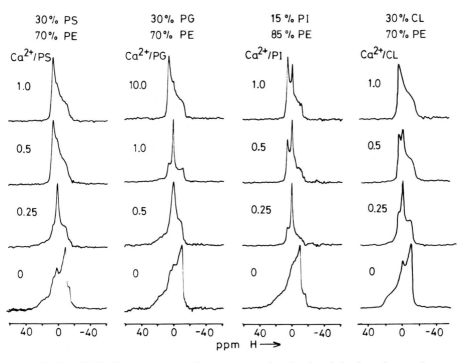

Fig. 10. ^{31}P-NMR spectra arising from mixtures of acidic phospholipids with soya phosphatidylethanolamine (a polyunsaturated PE derived from soya PC employing the base exchange reaction catalyzed by phospholipase D—see Comfurius and Zwaal [88] and Cullis and Hope [89] for further detail on PE preparation) in the presence of the various molar ratios of Ca^{2+}. All samples were prepared from 50 μmol total phospholipid mixed in chloroform, from which the chloroform was removed, and the lipid then hydrated in 1 ml of the buffer employed for Fig. 2 by vortex mixing. The Ca^{2+} was added as aliquots from a 100 mM stock solution. For further details for (egg) PS–PE, see Tilcock and Cullis [32], (egg) PG–PE, see Farren and Cullis [33], (soya) PI–PE, see Nayar *et al.* [34], and for (beef heart) CL–PE, see deKruijff [31]. All previously published spectra reproduced with permission.

note that the detailed mechanism involved differs according to the acidic phospholipid species involved. In the case of CL, Ca^{2+} converts the CL to an H_{II}-preferring species, thus allowing the entire mixture to adopt the H_{II} phase (see deKruijff and Cullis [31]). Alternatively, in the case of PS, Ca^{2+} appears to induce a lateral segregation of PS into "cochleate" domains [32], allowing the PE to adopt the H_{II} configuration it prefers in isolation. This contrasts with the behavior of systems stabilized by PG, where the presence of Ca^{2+} appears to reduce the bilayer-stabilizing capacity of PG, and both the PG and PE enter the H_{II} configuration [33]. Conversely a Ca^{2+}-induced lateral segregation of PI into liquid crystalline lamellar domains is possible, although not yet proven, leaving the PE to revert to the H_{II} phase [34]. It may also be noted that the molar ratios of Ca^{2+}:acidic phospholipid required to induce H_{II} phase organization vary significantly, with the CL–PE and PS–PE systems being more sensitive to the presence of Ca^{2+} than the PI–PE and PG–PE systems. Systems stabilized by 30 mol% or more PI will not adopt the H_{II} phase even at very high (50 mM) Ca^{2+} concentrations.

The polymorphic phase preferences of acidic phospholipids would be expected to be most sensitive to pH changes in the region of the pK of ionizable groups. This is indeed the case for $18:1_c/18:1_c$ PS (DOPS) and DOPA, which have a pK in the region of 3.5 and 4 respectively, as illustrated in Fig. 11. Both these lipid species exhibit bilayer to H_{II} transitions as the pH is lowered so that the charge on the head group is neutralized. DOPA undergoes this transition at pH values above 3.5 due to the presence of 100 mM NaCl in the buffer, which acts to raise the pH at which the H_{II} phase is preferred. Following the reasoning indicated above, it may be expected that the polymorphism of PE systems stabilized by these acidic phospholipids would be particularly sensitive to a reduction of pH. This is indeed the case for soya PE systems stablized by egg PS, as shown in Fig. 12. It may be noted that systems in which bilayer structure is stabilized by low (15 mol%) PS concentrations exibit the strongest effects on lowering the pH, and components indicative of H_{II} phase structure are visible at pH values as high as 5.5. The mechanism involved would appear to correspond to the Ca^{2+} induced bilayer–H_{II} transitons in CL–PE systems (Fig. 10) because the PS is converted to an H_{II} lipid species as the pH is reduced.

A question that was not addressed for the Ca^{2+}-induced bilayer–H_{II} transitions in acidic phospholipid–PE systems concerns the absolute Ca^{2+} concentrations required. In the case of the PS–PE systems, for example, Ca^{2+} concentrations on the order of 2 mM or more (much higher than cytosol Ca^{2+} concentrations) are necessary to trigger such transitions [32]. Given the ability of cholesterol to destabilize PC–PE systems (Fig. 8), as well as the fact that cytosol levels of Mg^{2+} ($\sim$2 mM) can enhance the ability of Ca^{2+} to effect PE–PS bilayer–H_{II} transitions [35], it may be expected

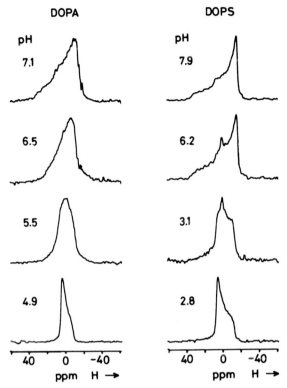

Fig. 11. 81.0 MHz ^{31}P-NMR spectra at 30°C arising from aqueous dispersions of DOPS and DOPA (sodium salt) at various pH values. The samples (50 μmol phospholipid) were hydrated in 1 ml of buffer containing 100 mM NaCl, 20 mM HEPES and the pH was adjusted by adding aliquots of 0.1M HCl. For further details, see Hope and Cullis [29] and Farren and Cullis [28].

that much lower Ca^{2+} concentrations are required to trigger these structural reorganizations in PE–PS–cholesterol systems in the presence of 2 mM Mg^{2+}. This is indeed the case as illustrated in Fig. 13, where Ca^{2+} concentrations in the region of 0.2 mM are sufficient to induce appreciable effects.

These types of investigations can be extended to lipid mixtures more closely representative of biological membranes. One such system is the inner monolayer of the erythrocyte, which is composed (on a molar basis) of 50% PE, 25% PS and 12.5% each of PC and SPM [36]. The polymorphism of systems composed of erythrocyte lipids reconstituted in these proportions (in the presence of equimolar cholesterol) is indeed sensitive to the presence of Ca^{2+} (see Fig. 14), where a Ca^{2+}:PS molar ratio of 0.5 induces an

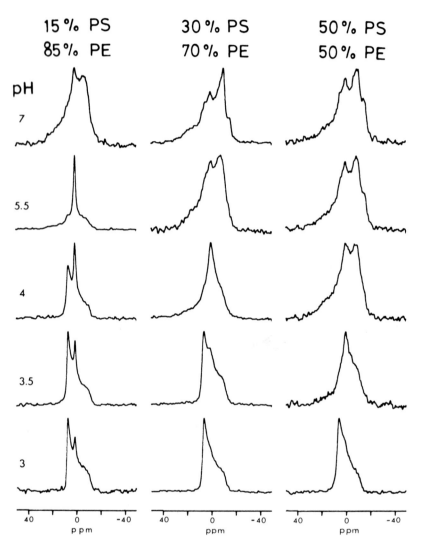

Fig. 12. 81.0 MHz ^{31}P-NMR spectra at 30°C obtained from aqueous dispersions of soya PE containing (a) 15% soya PS (b) 30% soya PS and (c) 50% soya PS at pH values 7.0, 5.5, 4, 3.5 and 3. The pH was adjusted as indicated in the legend of Fig. 11. Reproduced with permission from Tilcock and Cullis [32].

appreciable H_{II} phase component (see Hope and Cullis [37] for further details). These results suggest that when erythrocyte cytosol Ca^{2+} concentrations increase the inner monolayer will be unstable in the sense that a sizeable portion of the phospholipid would prefer nonbilayer structure. Such instability may be related to the fusion events involved in the "blebbing off"

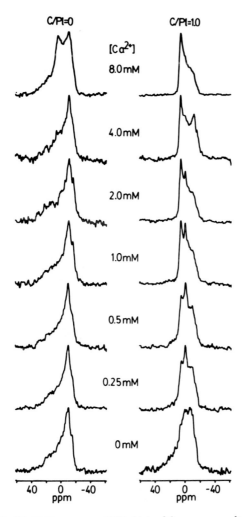

Fig. 13. 81.0 MHz ^{31}P-NMR spectra at 30°C obtained from aqueous dispersions of soya PE and soya PS (1:1) in the presence of 2 mM *mg*$^{2+}$, and dialyzed against various concentrations of Ca$_2$$^+$. The ratio C:PL refers to the molar ratio of cholesterol to phospholipid present. For full details of the dialysis procedure and other protocols, see Bally and Cullis [35].

processes [38] noted for erythrocytes upon ATP depletion, as discussed elsewhere [37]. These results also suggest a possible reason why the erythrocyte plasma membrane (and possibly other plasma membranes) exhibits lipid asymmetry. An outer monolayer of PC and SPM presents a rather inert permeability barrier to the extracellular environment, whereas an interior monolayer composed primarily of PE and PS will have structural

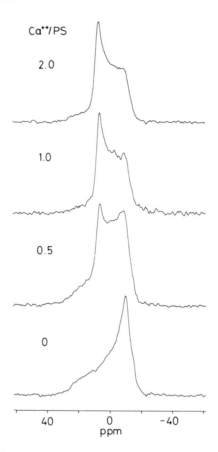

Fig. 14. 81.0 MHz ^{31}P-NMR spectra at 37°C arising from an aqueous dispersion of reconstituted "inner monolayer" lipid isolated from the human erythrocyte membrane. The lipid composition is PE:PS:PC:SPM (in the ratios 0.5:0.25:0.13:0.12) and containing equimolar cholesterol with respect to total phospholipid. The ratio Ca^{2+} = PS refers to the molar ratio Ca^{2+} to PS. Ca^{2+} was added as indicated in the legend to Fig. 10. Reproduced with permission from Hope and Cullis [37].

preferences which can be modulated locally. As we indicate in Section IVB such properties could play important roles in exocytotic events.

INFLUENCE OF PROTEIN ON MEMBRANE LIPID STRUCTURE

Most of the biochemical and physiological processes occurring in membranes are catalyzed or mediated by proteins which are often membrane bound. Given the fact that the majority of these proteins interact with lipids, this interaction is potentially of great functional importance. In particular, as indicated in Section IV, some of these membrane mediated processes may involve the participation of nonbilayer lipids and associated structures and it is therefore important to establish the effects of proteins on membrane lipid structure. That proteins can have a large effect on the structural preferences of lipids can be inferred from a comparison of the phase behavior of the lipids in a biomembrane and in model systems composed of the extracted lipids. For example, whereas the lipids in the *E. coli* inner membrane [39] and the rod outer segment membrane are (predominantly) organized in a bilayer, the hydrated total lipids prefer hexagonal and inverted micellar structures [40]. This suggests that membrane proteins such as rhodopsin stabilize the bilayer. Alternatively the total lipids of the liver microsomal membrane adopt a bilayer configuration upon hydration, whereas ^{31}P-NMR studies of the intact membrane at 37°C reveal a fraction of the phospholipid experiencing isotropic motional averaging, possibly indicating the transient occurrence of nonbilayer lipid structures [41, 42]. This has led to the suggestion that proteins in this membrane, particularly cytochrome *P*-450 [42] induce nonlamellar structure for the endogenous lipids.

More precise information on the influence of proteins on lipid polymorphism can be obtained in reconstituted model systems. Reconstitution of glycophorin, the major asialoglycoprotein from the human erythrocyte membrane, with unsaturated PE has a profound bilayer stabilization effect [43]. Bilayer structure is maintained 50°C above the bilayer–hexagonal H_{II} transition temperature of the PE. Removal of the large sugar- and sialic acid-containing section of the protein (by trypsin treatment) does not affect this bilayer-stabilizing ability, demonstrating that the hydrophobic membrane-spanning portion of the protein is responsible for this effect. However not all intrinsic polypeptides have the same effect, as shown by experiments with gramicidin. This peptide is commonly used as a model for an intrinsic membrane protein and can form (by dimerization) a helical membrane-spanning channel. Incorporation of gramicidin in PE-containing model membranes leads to a strong bilayer destabilization [44]. The hexagonal H_{II} phase-promoting ability of this peptide is so strong that H_{II} phase structure can be induced even in saturated phosphatidylcholine model systems [44]. These bilayer destabilization effects are strongly dependent on the length and nature of the acyl chains suggesting that in order to accommodate the peptide in a bilayer the thickness of the hydrophobic part of the molecule has to match the length of the gramicidin dimer [44].

Cytochrome *c* is another example of a protein that can induce nonbilayer structures in model membrane systems. This highly basic "extrinsic" protein from the inner mitochondrial membrane experiences strong interactions with many negatively charged phospholipids [31] where lamellar structure is maintained. Only in the case of cardiolipin (the major negatively charged inner mitochondrial membrane lipid) does this interaction result in the formation of the hexagonal H_{II} phase and structures which may be inverted micelles [31]. This observation is of interest for two reasons. First, it demonstrates specificity in lipid–protein interactions, and second, given the absolute requirement of cytochrome c oxidase for cardiolipin for activity [45] it can be suggested that nonbilayer structures formed by the cytochrome c–cardiolipin interactions may play a role in the functioning of the terminal part of the respiratory chain. This hypothesis is supported by the finding that the strongly cardiotoxic anticancer drug adriamycin specifically interacts with cardiolipin in model systems [46], blocks the formation of nonbilayer structures (47) and inhibits mitochondrial regulation [48].

Poly (L-lysine) is another highly basic polypeptide that has a pronounced effect on the structure of a cardiolipin dispersion. The strong electrostatic interaction of this polypeptide with cardiolipin leads to bilayer stabilization such that even in the presence of excess Ca^{2+}, cardiolipin remains organized in the lamellar phase [49]. Further, this polypeptide can induce phase separations in PE–CL mixed systems thereby triggering a bilayer– hexagonal H_{II} phase transition [49].

These preliminary studies demonstrate that lipid–protein interactions can isothermally modulate the phase preferences of lipids in a variety of ways consistent with the notion that nonbilayer structures may be of importance in biomembrane functioning. Other aspects of lipid–protein interactions in relation to lipid diversity will be discussed in section V.

Potential Roles of Nonbilayer Lipid Structures in Membranes

MEMBRANE FUSION

Membrane fusion is an important and ubiquitous event in cell biology, occuring in processes such as fertilization, formation of polykaryocytes, exo- and endocytosis and the intracellular turnover and delivery of membrane components to name but a few. The detailed mechanism involved is not well understood. As indicated in Fig. 15, two events are vital for fusion to proceed—close apposition, which is likely to be a protein-mediated event, and the fusion event itself. Our initial interest in a potential role of nonbilayer lipid structures as intermediates in the fusion event was stimulated by the

FUSION PROBLEMS

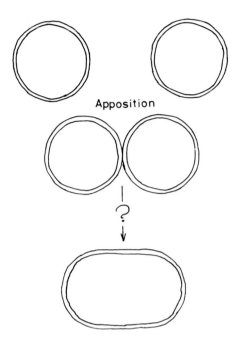

Fig. 15. Processes in membrane fusion phenomena.

observation that it is difficult (if not impossible) to imagine such an event occurring while bilayer lipid structure is maintained at the fusion interface. As a first approach to the problem, the properties of lipid-soluble fusogens (which enhance [50, 51] fusion between erythrocytes and other cells) were examined, with the precept in mind that these agents may enhance fusion by enabling endogenous lipids to adopt putative nonbilayer intermediates more easily.

The results obtained for the commonly employed fusogen glycerol monooleate (GMO) and the erythrocyte ghost membrane and model systems composed of the extracted lipids of the erythrocyte are illustrated in Figs. 16 and 17. Fig. 16 shows that the presence of equimolar (with respect to membrane phospholipid) or higher amounts of GMO associated with the intact erythrocyte (ghost) membrane results in appreciable formation of nonbilayer H_{II} phase phospholipid. Similar behavior is observed for reconstituted model systems of the erythrocyte phospholipids. In order for fusion to proceed between intact erythrocytes, equimolar or higher concentrations of membrane-associated GMO are required (see Fig. 17), and thus there is a

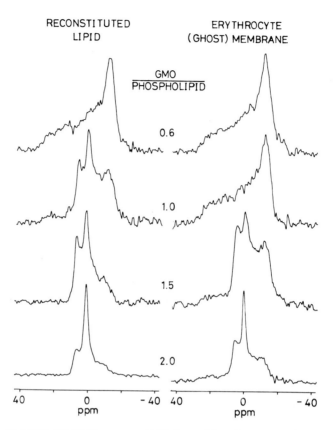

RECONSTITUTED   ERYTHROCYTE
LIPID   (GHOST) MEMBRANE

GMO
PHOSPHOLIPID

0.6

1.0

1.5

2.0

40   0   - 40   40   0   - 40
ppm   ppm

Fig. 16. 81.0 MHz ^{31}P-NMR spectra at 37°C obtained from (reconstituted) total erythrocyte lipid and erythrocyte (ghost) membrane in the presence of various concentrations of glycerol monoleate (GMO). For further details, see Hope and Cullis [51]. Reproduced with permission from Hope and Cullis [51].

strong correlation between the fusion event and the ability of endogeneous lipids to assume the nonbilayer (inverted cylinder) structure.

Although membrane-bound systems which undergo fusion *in vivo* do not contain equimolar (with respect to phospholipid) concentrations of fusogen, the fusogen results do suggest possible mechanisms of naturally occurring fusion. In particular they suggest that factors enhancing the ability of lipids to adopt inverted nonbilayer structures will also promote the fusion event. Given that Ca^{2+} is usually required for natural fusion [52], and that Ca^{2+} can trigger bilayer–H_{II} transitions in mixtures of acidic phospholipids with PE (Fig. 10), it is logical to suppose that the presence of Ca^{2+} allows the

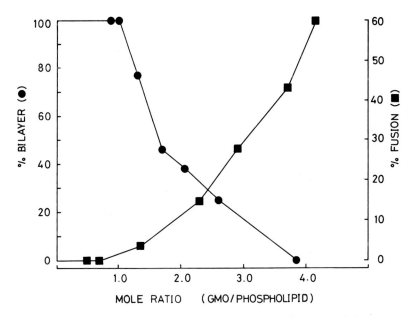

Fig. 17. A comparison of the extent of fusion between erythrocytes and the amount of phospholipid remaining in the bilayer phase in erythrocyte (ghost) membranes at various membrane concentrations of glycerol monoleate (GMO): ●—the percentage of membrane phospholipids in extended bilayers as indicated by ^{31}P-NMR; ■—the percentage fusion between erythrocytes following incubation for 2 hr with various concentrations of GMO which resulted in the indicated membrane-associated amounts of GMO. For further details, see Hope and Cullis [51]. Reproduced with permission from Hope and Cullis [51].

nonbilayer tendencies of endogenous lipid to be expressed, thus promoting the fusion event. Alternatively any other stimulus resulting in the same effect, such as lowering the pH in the case of systems containing PS and PA, should also promote fusion. These predictions appear to be justified, at least for model systems incubated in the presence of Ca^{2+}, as shown in the freeze-fracture micrographs of Fig. 18 (see also Verkleij *et al.* [25, 53]). These results, obtained for sonicated vesicle systems, composed of PE–PS [54], PE–PG [55], PE–PI [55], PE–CL [55], and PE–PA [55] illustrate two important points. First, in all cases the incubations result in the formation of larger structures, demonstrating that net fusion has occurred. Second, this fusion is accompanied by the observation of lipidic particles, and it is most interesting to note that these lipidic particles are often localized to regions corresponding to the fusion interface. This leads to the possibility that fusion proceeds via formation of intermediary inverted micellar structures; a possible model of this process is presented in Fig. 19.

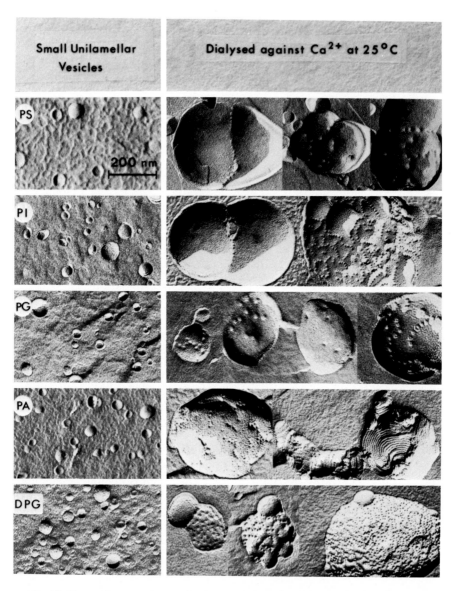

Fig. 18. Freeze-fracture micrographs showing Ca^{2+}-induced fusion of unilamellar vesicles consisting of soya phosphatidylethanolamine and a negatively charged phospholipid in the molar ratio of 4:1. Vesicles were prepared by sonication and subsequently dialysed at 25°C against buffer: 100 mM NaCl, 10 mM Hepes, pH 7.0 containing 10 mM Ca^{2+}. Samples were removed at various time intervals and frozen (in the presence of glycerol (25% v/v)) by plunging into a liquid–solid freon slush. Replicas were prepared employing standard procedures. The acidic phospholipids are: **PS** (egg phosphatidylserine), **PI** (soya phosphatidylinositol), **PG** (egg phosphatidylglycerol), **PA** (dioleoylphosphatidic acid) and **DPG** (beef heart cardiolipin).

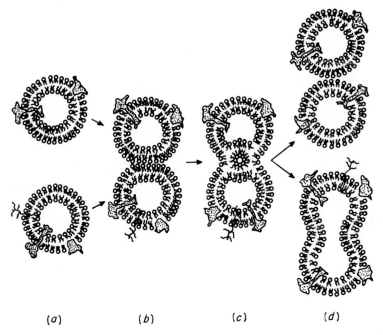

(a)   (b)   (c)   (d)

Fig. 19. Proposed mechanism of membrane fusion proceeding via an inverted cylinder or inverted micellar intermediate. The process whereby the membranes come into close apposition (a)–(b) is possibly protein mediated whereas the fusion event itself (b)–(c) is proposed to involve formation of an "inverted" lipid intermediate.

EXOCYTOSIS

An interesting expression of directed fusion *in vivo* is provided by the extracellular release of the contents of secretory granules, of which the Ca^{2+}-stimulated release of catecholamines from the chromaffin granules of adrenal medulla cells is particularly well characterized [56]. Our approach to studying the actual mechanism of exocytosis was based on the observation that release would be more efficient and controlled if Ca^{2+} stimulated granule–plasma membrane fusion rather than granule–granule fusion. Given our prejudice that nonbilayer lipid intermediates are required for fusion to proceed, it was reasoned that the inner monolayer lipids of the plasma membrane of the adrenal cells may play an active role. In particular, if this inner monolayer has a lipid composition approximately the same as that of the erythrocyte membrane, the influx of Ca^{2+} will destabilize this monolayer, enhancing the preference of the lipids for a nonlamellar organization. Such a reorganization appears to proceed as an *inter*bilayer event [57], hence the instability of the inner monolayer lipids could be relieved by formation of inverted micellar (lipidic particle) structures with the outer monolayer of closely opposed granules, thus initiating the fusion process.

The model system employed to test such speculation is shown in Fig. 20, and consists of chromaffin granules incubated with sonicated vesicles composed of lipids which undergo structural reorganization in the presence of Ca^{2+}. Ca^{2+} is added to this mixture subsequently, and the release of chromaffin granule contents assayed. As shown in Fig. 21, these protocols could result in immediate and total release of granule contents for Ca^{2+} concentrations well below those which produced no release by themselves. Thus lipid mixtures such as PE–PS (as well as mixtures approximating the erythrocyte inner monolayer [57, 58]) can act as adjuncts for the Ca^{2+}-stimulated release of granule contents. These and other considerations (see Nayar *et al.*, [58] for full detail) lead us to propose a model for the exocytotic event as shown in Fig. 22.

TRANSBILAYER TRANSPORT

The most important function of a membrane is to act as a selective permeability barrier between two aqueous compartments. It is generally as-

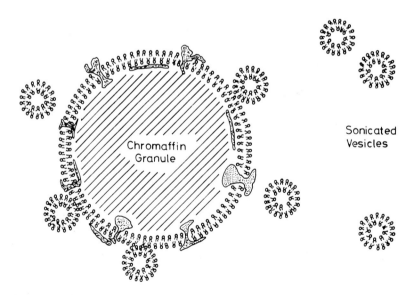

Fig. 20. Incubation procedure followed for incubation of chromaffin granules (large granule fraction) with sonicated vesicles. For further details, see Nayar *et al.* [58].

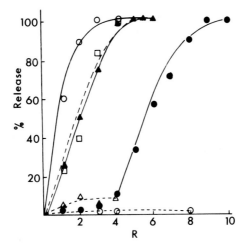

Fig. 21. Release of chromaffin granule contents after incubation (15 min) in the presence of increasing amounts of sonicated vesicles of varying composition, followed by the introduction of 5 mM Ca²⁺ after 10 min: ▲—soya PE:soya PS (3:1) vesicles; △—soya PC:soya PS (3:1) vesicles; □—egg PS vesicles; ◯—beef heart cardiolipin vesicles; ●—vesicles with the "inner mono-layer" lipid composition (PE:PS:PC:SPM in the ratios 0.5:0.25:0.13:0.12; equimolar cholesterol with respect to phospholipid); ◯---◯—vesicles with the "outer monolayer" composition. For details of experimental protocol, see Nayar *et al.* [58].

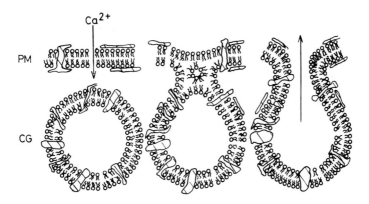

Fig. 22. Proposed mechanism of exocytotic release of chromaffin granule contents *in vivo*. PM refers to the chromaffin cell plasma membrane whereas CG denotes the chromaffin granule.

sumed that the lipid bilayer has an isolating function and only permits the free diffusion of small molecules and water. Specific permeability or translocation processes are thought to be mediated by proteins or polypeptides which may provide a pore or mobile carrier for particular substances. Although there is substantial experimental support for these hypotheses, the possibility that the lipids themselves may participate in translocation processes has not been seriously considered. This is because it is difficult to imagine how large polar molecules can move across a continuous lipid bilayer.

Nonbilayer lipids and the structures they can form give new possibilities however [57]. In particular lipids present in "inverted" structures such as the hexagonal H_{II} phase or inverted micellar structures can reside in a low energy configuration *within* a hydrophobic domain such as the interior of a lipid bilayer. Thus these structures with a hydrophilic interior and a hydrophobic exterior have some characteristics normally ascribed to a carrier molecule such as valinomycin. In Fig. 23 we depict a possible mechanism whereby the dynamic formation of inverted structures (inverted micelles) in a bilayer can act as a permeability pathway for both lipids and polar molecules within the aqueous compartment. Such transient events could be triggered by changes in the local concentrations of hexagonal H_{II} lipid species or by molecules which upon interaction with a lipid increase the tendency of that lipid to adopt an inverted structure.

An example of this latter process is the Ca^{2+} or cytochrome c interaction with cardiolipin which results in a transition from a lamellar to an inverted structure for a portion of the lipid. Two predictions can be made for systems displaying such behavior. First, transbilayer transport of lipids (flip–flop) which is usually a very slow process [59] should be greatly increased. Second, if the bilayer–nonbilayer transition is triggered by a modulator molecule, this molecule together with the lipid should be moved across the membrane via a carrier type of transport process. The first prediction has been tested in model systems containing unsaturated PE [60] and CL [61] where nonbilayer lipid structures have been induced by variations in temperature [60] and divalent cation concentrations [61]. Under both conditions phospholipid flip-flop was found to be greatly increased over that of control systems which did not contain "nonbilayer" lipid. Additional support comes from the observation that biological membranes in which phospholipid flip-flop is rapid (e.g., bacterial [59] and microsomal [62, 63] membranes) have a lipid composition and ^{31}P-NMR characteristics that are consistent with the presence of some nonbilayer lipid structures. Enhanced phospholipid flip-flop resulting from discontinuities in lipid packing around integral membrane proteins as well as at phase boundaries in mixed lipid systems is discussed elsewhere [2].

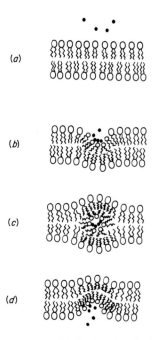

(a)

(b)

(c)

(d)

Fig. 23. A model of facilitated transport of Ca^{2+} (or other divalent cations) via formation of an intermediate intrabilayer inverted micellar cation—phospholipid complex—see part (c). The head-group of the charged phospholipid (e.g. CL or PA) interacting with the cation is depicted as being smaller in order to indicate a reduction in the area per phospholipid molecule in the headgroup region arising from reduced interheadgroup electrostatic repulsion in the presence of the cation. Reproduced with permission from Cullis *et al.* [57].

There is also evidence to support the prediction that nonbilayer lipid structures can act as carriers for molecules that trigger bilayer–nonbilayer transitions. For example, Mn^{2+} can induce the hexagonal H_{II} phase in pure cardiolipin dispersions [8] and rapidly permeates into mixed PC–CL liposomes, which also exhibit lipidic particle structure [61]. Furthermore, PA (which can undergo a bilayer to hexagonal transition upon interaction with divalent cations) can act as a carrier of cations across liposomal bilayers [64]. A further example concerns the addition of cytochrome *c* to multilayered cardiolipin liposomes resulting in the appearance of cytochrome *c* in the inner shells of the structure [31]. It has also been reported that phospholipids can form inverted micellar complexes which are soluble in organic solvents with a variety of polar compounds [65]. This is also consistent with carrier potential. The ability of a lipid to form such complexes with divalent cations has been related to the ability of the cation to induce the hexagonal H_{II} phase in an aqueous dispersion of that lipid [57]. In the case of biological membranes the possible involvement of nonbilayer lipids in divalent cation transport has been proposed for two systems. These include Ca^{2+} influx following hormone–receptor interactions (this has been suggested to be mediated by PA [66, 67]) and the possibility that cardiolipin might participate in the Ca^{2+} transport system in mitochondria. This latter proposal is supported by the observation that ruthenium red, the classical inhibitor of this transport system, effectively blocks the formation of inverted structures by Ca^{2+} in cardiolipin-containing model membranes and blocks Ca^{2+} uptake into organic solvents by cardiolipin [57].

INTERMEMBRANE COMMUNICATION

There are increasingly convincing indications that many different types of cell and organelle membranes are intimately connected with other membrane systems. Examples include the inner and outer membranes of *E. coli*, the inner and outer membranes of mitochondria, as well as continuities between the endoplasmic reticulum and the outer mictochondrial membrane, the nuclear membrane, and the Golgi [68, 69]. Such continuities could correspond to situations of arrested fusion (see Fig. 19(c)). Although

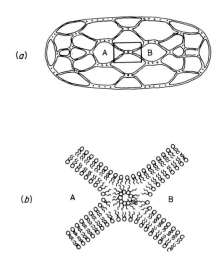

Fig. 24. A "honeycomb" structure compatible with ^{31}P-NMR, freeze-fracture and permeability results derived from systems containing mixtures of lipids which assume bilayer and hexagonal (H_{II}) phase structure in isolation. Compartmentalization within a continuous membrane structure is emphasized for compartments A and B in the expanded diagram of part (b).

direct evidence supporting such a conjecture is not available, freeze-fracture and ^{31}P NMR does suggest that lipidic particles (inverted micelles), formed between two closely opposed bilayers, can be long lived structures. In particular we have summarized evidence [57] indicating that multilamellar mixtures of bilayer and H_{II}-phase lipid can assume structures similar to that depicted in fig. 24. It is clear that such structures offer unique possibilities for maintaining compartmentalization within a continuous membrane structure.

A Rationale for Lipid Diversity—The Shape Concept

The ability of lipids to assume nonlamellar organizations offers new interpretations of the functional roles of lipids in biomembranes. In particular, lipids such as PC and SPM may be assigned functional roles related to maintenance of lamellar structure and an intact permeability barrier, whereas nonlamellar lipids such as PE allow formation of inverted micelles or cylinders which may play functional roles in fusion and related phenomena. Conversely, acidic phospholipids provide the possibility of isothermal transitions between lipid structures in appropriate lipid mixtures (as triggered by divalent cations or pH), thus providing mechanisms for isothermal regulation and control of membrane-mediated processes relying on nonbilayer intermediates. However there are a variety of factors that would suggest that this is not a complete story. First, the number of membrane functions potentially relying on nonlamellar lipid organization is not large (fusion, some transbilayer transport including flip-flop, and compartementalization within a continuous membrane structure) with membrane fusion being the only one for which relatively strong circumstantial evidence is available. Thus one is still left with the unsatisfactory situation indicated in the Introduction; the number of lipid species appears to vastly exceed the number of functional roles potentially involving expressions of nonlamellar lipid structure. Remaining questions that are not considered include the reasons for acyl chain diversity within a single phospholipid class, reasons why two or more lipid species preferring a bilayer organization are present in a single membrane (e.g. PC and SPM), questions concerning the role of cholesterol (which could play an adjunct role in fusion, but is not present in many membranes that undergo fusion), reasons why different acidic phospholipids are present in different membranes and so on. Although some of these differences could be caused by differences in metabolic pathways, it is difficult to imagine that the enormous lipid diversity would not serve other roles. In order to answer these questions one must examine basic molecular factors that lead to the phase structure preferred by individual lipid species.

Initially, it seems that the macromolecular structure assumed by lipids in hydration is sensitive to a balance between the cross-sectional areas subtended by the polar and apolar regions respectively [70]. In the case of PE and PC, for example, the smaller headgroup of PE and relatively limited hydration of this headgroup as compared to PC may be expected to lead to a more "cone" shaped molecule compatible with H_{II} phase organization (see Fig. 25). The effective cross-sectional area of the head-group would be expected to be sensitive to electrostatic repulsion, which is consistent with the protonation of PS inducing H_{II} phase structure and with Ca^{2+} triggering bilayer to H_{II} transitions in CL. Perhaps the clearest demonstration of the

Lipid	Phase	Molecular Shape
Lysophospholipids Detergents	Micellar	Inverted Cone
Phosphatidylcholine Sphingomyelin Phosphatidylserine Phosphatidylglycerol	Bilayer	Cylindrical
Phosphatidylethanol- amine (unsaturated) Cardiolipin – Ca^{2+} Phosphatidic acid – Ca^{2+}	Hexagonal (H_{II})	Cone

Fig. 25. Polymorphic phases and corresponding dynamic molecular shapes of component lipids. Reproduced with permission from Cullis and deKruijff [2].

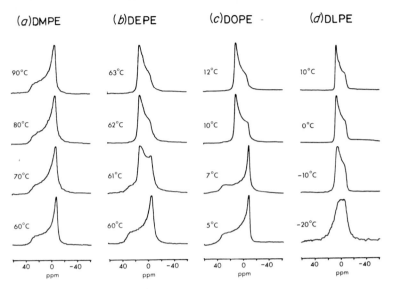

Fig. 26. 81.0 MHz ^{31}P-NMR spectra obtained from aqueous dispersions of different species of synthetic PE at various temperatures: (*a*) 14:0/14:0 PE (DMPE); (*b*) 18:1$_t$/18:1$_t$ PE (DEPE); (*c*) 18:1$_c$/18:1$_c$ PE (DOPE); (*d*) 18:2$_c$/18:2$_c$ PE (DLPE). For further details of phospholipid synthesis and other protocols, see Tilcock and Cullis [90].

shape of the lipid molecule dictating the phase assumed is given by the effects of increasing the acyl chain unsaturation for PE. As shown in Fig. 26, a saturated PE remains in a bilayer organization at temperatures up to 100°C, whereas 18:1$_t$/18:1$_t$ PE undergoes a bilayer to H$_{II}$ transition at T_{BH} = 60°C. This T_{BH} is lowered for 18:1$_c$/18:1$_c$ PE to 15°C and to ~ -15°C for 18:2$_c$/18:2$_c$ PE. This increased affinity for the H$_{II}$ organization as the acyl chain components assume a progressively larger cross-sectional area is most consistent with the shape hypothesis.

The proposal that the molecular shapes of lipids directly influence the structure formed is also supported by results obtained from mixed lipid systems. For example, from the simplistic divisions of Fig. 25 one may suggest that mixtures of cone (H$_{II}$ phase) lipid with inverted cone (micellar) lipid should exhibit bilayer structures at appropriate ratios. This is indeed the case [71], as illustrated in Fig. 27 for mixtures of egg PE with several detergents commonly employed for membrane solubilization. Such behavior may be rationalized according to the shape hypothesis as shown in Fig. 28.

There are other examples of mixed systems composed of nonbilayer components which can assume a net bilayer structure in a manner consistent with the shape concept. These include mixtures of lyso-PC (LPC) with cho-

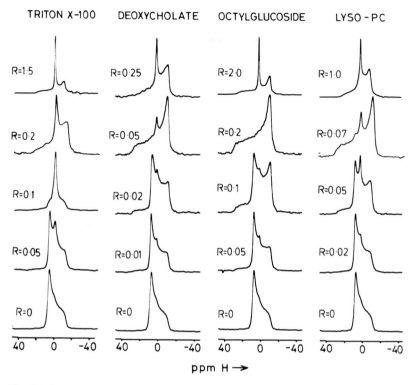

Fig. 27. 81.0 MHz ^{31}P-NMR spectra of egg yolk PE at 37°C in the presence of increasing amounts of various detergents. The detergent was added in appropriate amounts to the phospholipid in chloroform. Subsequently, the chloroform was evaporated and the lipid hydrated in 1 ml of standard buffer (see legend to Fig. 2). For details of protocol, see Madden and Cullis [71].

lesterol [72, 73] and fatty acids [74]. Again this behavior may be rationalized as resulting from complementarity between the inverted cone shape of LPC and cone-shaped cholesterol and fatty acids. That both cholesterol and fatty acids exhibit a net cone shape is suggested by the observation that both these agents can induce H_{II} phase structure in previously bilayer systems [18, 19, 50]. A further example is given by representative anaesthetics which can also stabilize the bilayer for unsaturated (egg) PE [75].

From the point of view of rationalizing lipid diversity in membranes, it is apparent that the shape concept offers some new possibilities for the functional roles of lipids. In particular, as originally proposed by Israelachvili and co-workers [39], it is likely that integral membrane proteins have somewhat irregular shapes within the bilayer. As indicated in Fig. 29, the availability of lipids with diverse geometry could provide possibilities for optimal packing

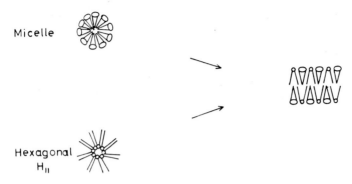

Fig. 28. Combination of "cone" shaped (H$_{II}$ phase) lipids with "inverted cone" (micellar) lipids to produce a net bilayer structure.

and sealing at the protein interface. Such conjectures are consistent with investigations of transbilayer transport in reconstituted glycophorin–lipid model systems. Incorporation of glycophorin in DOPC bilayers results in increased phospholipid flip-flop [76, 77] and permeability to shift reagents [78]. However incorporation of small amounts of cone or inverted cone shaped lipid (e.g., PE or LPC) [78] or reconstitution of the protein with total

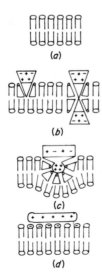

Fig. 29. Potential roles of lipid as a result of shape and/or charge in maintaining the architecture of (bilayer) lipid–protein membrane systems: (*a*) maintenance of bilayer structure, PC, SPM; (*b*) sealing at lipid–protein interface, PE, MGDG; (*c*) penetration (anchoring) of polar protein, CL, PA; (*d*) association of basic protein, PS, PG, PI.

(a) Solubilization

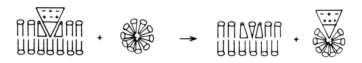

(b) Protein Distribution

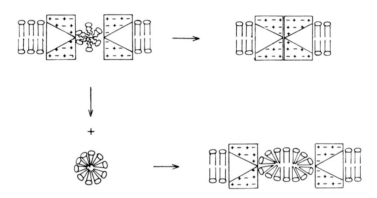

Fig. 30. Modulation of protein–protein interactions by the availability of lipids of various shapes: (*a*) dimer formation as a result of distribution of polar and apolar residues (see Israelachvili [84]) (*b*) production of stable monomers due to the availability of "inverted cone" (micellar) lipids.

erythrocyte lipids [79] results in sealed systems. Such observations give a rather different perspective on boundary or annular lipids than is currently in vogue. Alternative roles of lipids within the context of maintaining a stable semipermeable bilayer protein–lipid membrane are indicated in Fig. 29.

These and previous observations suggest that biological membranes regulate their lipid composition so as to obtain a variety of lipids with an appropriate distribution of various shapes. This proposal is consistent with the elegant experiments of Wieslander *et al.* [80] and Silvius *et al.* [81] on the *Acholeplasma laidlawii* membrane. Further, it may be noted that alterations in the lipid composition of *E. coli* [82] and other systems according to growth temperature, which have previously been interpreted as reflecting a need to conserve a certain membrane "fluidity", can equally well be taken to support the notion that lipid shape is the conserved quantity.

Before closing this section on the potential roles of lipids with varying molecular shapes, it is interesting to note that biomembranes usually contain only two major varieties—namely, those with cylindrical shapes (bilayer) and those with cone shapes (H_{II} phase). In this context, detergent lipids are members of a general class of amphiphilic molecules commonly designated as anesthetics [83]. Low membrane levels of such agents have many remarkable, and as yet inexplicable, effects on membranes and their mechanism of action poses a major problem in membrane biology. This is because a large body of evidence suggests that the anesthetic potency of a given compound is directly related to its solubility (partition coefficient) in a hydrocarbon environment [83], whereas the result of its presence clearly is to affect the ability of some membrane proteins (e.g., the Na^+ channel or other facilitated transport proteins) to function. Thus one is led to believe that the Na^+ channel, for example, exists as a lipid–protein complex, and anesthetics somehow disrupt or replace the lipid participating in that complex. The observation that anesthetics have, as a general property, shapes different than other membrane components leads to the possibility that they may affect membrane function by virtue of that shape. An example among many possibilities is given in Fig. 30, which is an extension of a model due to Israelachvilli [84] who suggested that membrane protein aggregation may result from an appropriate distribution of polar and apolar residues. In Fig. 30 we suggest that anesthetic type lipids could affect such oligomer formation by virtue of these shapes, thus modulating protein function.

Closing Remarks

In closing, the spirit in which this chapter is written should perhaps be emphasized. The fundamental observation on which the many conjectures made here are based is that lipids in membranes do not, as a general rule, assume a bilayer organization upon hydration. In our view this leads to the strong possibility that those lipids preferring nonlamellar organization play functional roles which are not necessarily related to maintenance of bilayer structure. We have pointed out that many factors known to regulate membrane-mediated phenomena (divalent cations, pH, membrane protein, anesthetics, etc.) can strongly affect the macromolecular structures assumed under conditions which are not unduly removed from the physiological

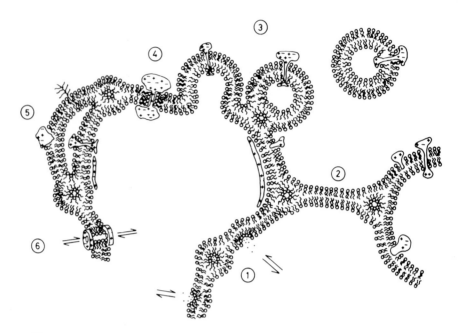

Fig. 31. A metamorphic mosaic model of biological membranes illustrating various structures and processes suggested by the ability of lipids to assume nonbilayer configurations. In part 1 transbilayer transport of polar molecules (e.g., divalent cations) is facilitated by intermediary formation of inverted micelles, whereas part 2 indicates membrane continuity between membrane bound compartments. In part 3 a process of budding off of a membrane bound vesicle is illustrated, as discussed elsewhere. The protein in part 4 is shown to assume a transmembrane configuration without the requirement for an apolar sequence of amino acids. The protein penetrates the membrane through a (short) cylinder of phospholipid. In part 5 compartmentalization is depicted within a continuous membrane system, whereas part 6 indicates possibilities of transmembrane transport where hexagonal (H_{II}) phase lipids form an aqueous pore through the membrane. This lipid configuration is stabilized in an orientation perpendicular to the plane of the surrounding bilayer by doughnut-shaped proteins with hydrophilic and hydrophobic sides, which could also serve as selectivity filters. Reproduced with permission from Cullis et al. [57].

situation. In addition we show that for a function such as fusion, which logically requires some nonlamellar intermediate, there are strong correlations between the availability of nonlamellar organizations and the expedition of fusion. Although the picture that emerges is by no means complete, the lamellar–nonlamellar characteristics of lipids lead to recognition of a new basic shape property of lipids, leading in turn to a different understanding of reasons for lipid diversity. Although none of the functional roles of lipids have been unambiguously identified in terms of their molecular shape, it clearly provides a rich hypothesis on which future experimentation may be based. A synopsis of these possibilities is given in Fig. 31.

References

1. Cullis, P. R., and Grathwohl, Ch. (1977). *Biochim. Biophys. Acta* **471**, 213–226.
2. Cullis, P. R., and de Kruijff, B. (1979). *Biochim. Biophys. Acta* **559**, 399–420.
3. Warren, G. B., Houslay, M. D., Metcalfe, J. C., and Birdsall, N. J. M. (1975). *Nature (London)* **255**, 684–687.
4. Luzzatti, V., Gulik-Kryzwicki, T., and Tardieu, A. (1968). *Nature (London)* **218**, 1031–1034.
5. Deamer, D. W., Leonard, R., Tardieu, A., and Branton, D. (1970). *Biochim. Biophys. Acta* **219**, 47–60.
6. Verkleij, A. J., and Ververgaert, P. H. J. Th. (1975). *Ann. Rev. Phys. Chem.* **26**, 101–121.
7. Verkleij, A. J., and de Gier, J. (1981). *In* "Liposomes: From Physical Structure to Therapeutic Applications" (E. Knight, ed.), Chapter 4, pp. 83–102. Elsevier and North Holland Publ., Amsterdam.
8. Cullis, P. R., Verkleij, A. J., and Ververgaert, P. H. J. Th. (1978). *Biochim. Biophys. Acta* **513**, 11–20.
9. Chapman, D., Williams, R. M., and Ladbrooke, B. D. (1967). *Chem. Phys. Lipids* **1**, 445–475.
10. Shipley, G. G., Avecilla, L. S., and Small, D. M. (1974). *J. Lipid Res.* **15**, 124–140 (1974).
11. Wieslander, A., Ulmius, J. Lindblom, G. and Fontell, K. (1978). *Biochim. Biophys. Acta* **554**, 340–357.
12. Shipley, G. G. (1973). *In* "Biological Membranes" (D. Chapman and D. F. H. Wallach, eds.), Vol. 2, pp. 1–89. Academic Press, New York.
13. Reiss-Husson, F. (1967). *J. Mol. Biol.* **25**, 363–373.
14. Rand, R. P., Tinker, D. O., and Fast, P. G. (1971). *Chem. Phys. Lipids* **6**, 333–342.
15. Minnikin, D. E., Abdolrahimzadeh, H., and Baddiley, J. (1971). *Biochem. J.* **124**, 447–448.
16. Cullis, P. R., and de Kruijff, B. (1976). *Biochim. Biophys. Acta* **436**, 523–540.
17. Demel, R. A., and de Kruijff, B. (1976). *Biochim. Biophys. Acta* **457**, 109–132.
18. Cullis, P. R., and de Kruijff, B. (1978). *Biochim. Biophys. Acta* **507**, 207–218.
19. Cullis, P. R., van Dijck, P. W. M., de Kruijff, B., and de Gier, J. (1978). *Biochim. Biophys. Acta* **513**, 21–30.
20. Verkleij, A. J., Mombers, C., Leunissen-Bijvelt, J., and Ververgaert, P. H. J. Th. (1979). *Nature (London)* **279**, 162–163.
21. de Kruijff, B. *et al.* (1979). *Biochim. Biophys. Acta* **555**, 200–209.
22. Verkleij, A. J., and de Kruijff, B. (1981). *Nature (London)* **290**, 427–428.
23. Miller, R. G. (1980). *Nature (London)* **287**, 166–167.
24. Hui, S. W., and Stewart, T. P. (1981). *Nature (London)* **290**, 427–428.
25. Verkleij, A. J., van Echteld, C. J. A., Gerritsen, W. J., Cullis, P. R., and de Kruijff, B. (1980). *Biochim. Biophys. Acta* **600**, 620–624.
26. Rand, R. P., and Sengupta, S. (1972). *Biochim. Biophys. Acta* **255**, 484–492.
27. Verkleij, A. J., de Maagd, R., Leunissen-Bijvelt, J., and de Kruijff, B. (1982). *Biochim. Biophys. Acta* **684**, 255–262.
28. Farren, S. B., Hope, M. J., and Cullis, P. R. (1982). *Biochem. Biophys. Res. Commun.* (submitted).

29. Hope, M. J., and Cullis, P. R. (1980). Biochem. Biophys. Res. Commun. 92, 846–852.
30. Papahadjopoulos, D., Jacobsen, K., Poste, G., and Shepherd, D. (1975). Biochim. Biophys. Acta 394, 483–491.
31. de Kruijff, B., and Cullis, P. R. (1980). Biochim. Biophys. Acta 602, 477–490.
32. Tilcock, C. P. S., and Cullis, P. R. (1981). Biochim. Biophys. Acta 641, 189–201.
33. Farren, S. B., and Cullis, P. R. (1980). Biochem. Biophys. Res. Commun. 97, 182–191.
34. Nayar, R., Schmid, S., Hope, M. J., and Cullis, P. R. (1982). Biochim. Biophys. Acta 688, 169–176.
35. Bally, M. B., Tilcock, C. P. S., Hope, M. J., and Cullis, P. R. (1982). Can. J. Biochem. (submitted).
36. Zwaal, R. F. A., Comfurius, P., and van Deenen, L. L. M. (1977). Nature (London) 268, 358–360.
37. Hope, M. J., and Cullis, P. R. (1979). FEBS Lett. 107, 323–326.
38. White, J. G. (1974). Am. J. Pathol. 77, 507–518.
39. Burnell, E., van Alphen, L., Verkleij, A. J., and de Kruijff, B. (1980). Biochim. Biophys. Acta 597, 492–501.
40. de Grip, W. J., Drenthe, E. H. S., van Echteld, C. J. A., de Kruijff, B. and Verkleij, A. J. (1979). Biochim. Biophys. Acta 558, 330–337.
41. de Kruijff, B., van den Besselaar, A. M. H. P., Cullis, P. R., van den Bosch, H., and van Deenen, L. L. M. (1978). Biochim. Biophys. Acta 514, 1–8.
42. Stier, A., Finch, S. A. E., and Bösterling, B. (1978). FEBS Lett. 91, 109–112.
43. Tarashi, T., van Echteld, C. J. A., de Kruijff, B., and Verkleij, A. J. (1982). Biochim. Biophys. Acta 685, 153–161.
44. van Echteld, C. J. A., van Stigt, R., Verkleij, A. J., Leunissen-Bijvelt, J., and de Gier, J. (1981). Biochim. Biophys. Acta 648, 287–291.
45. Fry, M. and Green, D. E. (1980). Biochem. Biophys. Res. Commun. 93, 1238–1246.
46. Goormaghtigh, E., Chatelain, P., Caspers, J., and Ruysschaert, J. M. (1980). Biochem. Pharmacol. 29, 3003–3010.
47. Goormaghtigh, E., van den Branden, M., Ruysschaert, J. M., and de Kruijff, B. (1981). Biochim. Biophys. Acta. In press.
48. Bachmann, E., Weber, E., and Zbinden, G. (1975). Agents et Actions 55, 383–393.
49. de Kruijff, B., and Cullis, P. R. (1980). Biochim. Biophys. Acta 601, 235–240.
50. Cullis, P. R., and Hope, M. J. (1978). Nature (London) 271, 672–675.
51. Hope, M. J., and Cullis, P. R. (1981). Biochim. Biophys. Acta 640, 82–90.
52. Poste, G., and Allison, A. C. (1973). Biochim. Biophys. Acta 300, 421–465.
53. Verkleij, A. J., Mombers, C., Gerritsen, W. J. Leunissen-Bijvelt, J., and Cullis, P. R. (1979). Biochim. Biophys. Acta 555, 358–362.
54. Hope, M. J., Walker, D., and Cullis, P. R. (1982). Biochem. Biophys. Res. Commun. (submitted).
55. Hope, M. J., Nayar, R., and Cullis, P. R. (1982). Biochem. Biophys. Res. Commun. (submitted).
56. Winkler, H., and Smith, A. D. (1975). In "Handbook of Physiology," Sect. 7 Endocrinology Vol. 6, Ch. 23, pp. 321.
57. Cullis, P. R., de Kruijff, B., Hope, M. J., Nayar, R., and Schimd, S. (1980). Can. J. Biochem. 58, 1091–1100.
58. Nayar, R., Hope, M. J., and Cullis, P. R. (1982). Biochemistry (in press).
59. Rothman, J. E., and Leonard, J. (1977). Science 195, 743–753.
60. Noordam, F., van Echteld, C. J. A., de Kruijff, B., and de Gier, J. (1981). Biochim. Biophys. Acta 646, 483–487.

61. Gerritsen, W. J., de Kruijff, B., Verkleij, A. J., de Gier, J., and van Deenen, L. L. M. (1980). *Biochim. Biophys. Acta* **598**, 554–560.
62. van den Besselaar, A. M. H. P., de Kruijff, B., van den Bosch, H., and van Deenen, L. L. M. (1978). *Biochim. Biophys. Acta* **570**, 242–255.
63. Zilversmit, D. B., and Hughes, M. E. (1977). *Biochim. Biophys. Acta* **469**, 99–110.
64. Serhan, C., Anderson, P., Goodman, E., Durham, P., and Weissman, G. (1981). *J. Biol. Chem.* **256**, 2736–2741.
65. Tyson, C. H., Zande, H. V., and Green, D. E. (1976). *J. Biol. Chem.* **251**, 1526–1332.
66. Salmon, D. M., and Honeyman, T. W. (1980). *Nature (London)* **284**, 344–345.
67. Putney, J. W., Weiss, S. J., van der Waals, C. M., and Haddaj, R. A. (1980). *Nature (London)* **284**, 345–347.
68. Mollenhauer, H. H., Morre, D. J., and Vanderwoude, W. J. (1975). *Mikroskopie* **31**, 257–272.
69. Morre, D. J., Kartenbeck, J., and Franke, W. W. (1979). *Biochim. Biophys. Acta* **559**, 71–152.
70. Israelachvili, J. N., Mitchell, D. J., and Ninham, B. W. (1976). *J. Chem. Soc. Faraday Trans. II* **72**, 1525–1568.
71. Madden, T. D., and Cullis, P. R. (1981). *Biochim. Biophys. Acta* **684**, 149–153.
72. Rand, R. P., Pangburn, W. A., Purdon, A. D., and Tinker, D. O. (1975). *Can. J. Biochem.* **53**, 189–195.
73. van Echteld, C. J. A., de Kruijff, B., Mandersloot, J. G., and de Gier, J. (1981). *Biochim. Biophys. Acta* **649**, 211–220.
74. Jain, M. K., van Echteld, C. J. A., Ramirez, F., de Gier, J., de Haas, G. H. and van Deenen, L. L. M. (1980). *Nature (London)* **284**, 486–487.
75. Hornby, A. P., and Cullis, P. R. (1981). *Biochim. Biophys. Acta* **647**, 285–292.
76. van Zoelen, E. J. J., de Kruijff, B., and van Deenen, L. L. M. (1978). *Biochim. Biophys. Acta* **508**, 97–108.
77. de Kruijff, B., van Zoelen, E. J. J., and van Deenen, L. L. M. (1978). *Biochim. Biophys. Acta* **509**, 537–542.
78. Gerritsen, W. J., van Zoelen, E. J. J., Verkleij, A. J., de Kruijff, B., and van Deenen, L. L. M. (1979). *Biochim. Biophys. Acta* **551**, 248–259.
79. van der Steen, A. T. M., de Jong, W. A. C., de Kruijff, B., and van Deenen, L. L. M. (1981). *Biochim. Biophys. Acta* **647**, 63–72.
80. Wieslander, A., Christiansson, A., Rilfors, L., and Lindblom, G. (1980). *Biochemistry* **19**, 3650–3656.
81. Silvius, J. R., Mak, N., and McElhaney, R. N. (1980). *Biochim. Biophys. Acta* **597**, 199–215.
82. Cronan, J. E., and Gelmann, E. P. (1975). *Bact. Rev.* **39**, 232–256.
83. Seeman, P. (1972). *Pharmacol. Rev.* **24**, 583–655.
84. Israelachvili, J. N. (1977). *Biochim. Biophys. Acta* **469**, 221–225.
85. Cullis, P. R., and de Kruijff, B. (1978). *Biochim. Biophys. Acta* **513**, 31–42.
86. de Kruijff, B., Rietveld, A., and Cullis, P. R. (1980). *Biochim. Biophys. Acta* **600**, 343–357.
87. Farren, S. B., and Cullis, P. R. (1982). *Biochim. Biophys. Acta* (submitted).
88. Comfurius, P., and Zwaal, R. F. A. (1977). *Biochim. Biophys. Acta* **488**, 36–42.
89. Cullis, P. R., and Hope, M. J. (1980). *Biochim. Biophys. Acta* **597**, 533–542.
90. Tilcock, C. P. S., and Cullis, P. R. (1982). *Biochim. Biophys. Acta* (submitted).
91. Cullis, P. R., de Kruijff, B., Hope, M. J., Nayar, R., Rietveld, A., and Verkleij, A. J. (1980). *Biochim. Biophys. Acta* **600**, 625–635.
92. Kachar, B. and Reese, T. S. (1982). *Nature* (London) **296**, 464–467.

Chapter 3

Diversity in the Observed Structure of Cellular Membranes

Fritiof S. Sjöstrand

Introduction. 84
The Approach and the Methods. 84
    Requirements. 84
    Theoretical Basis. 86
    Methods. 89
    Testing the Methods. 92
The Crista Membrane in Mitochondria. 93
    Observations and the First Step in Interpretation. 93
    The Second Step in Interpretation. 107
    The Third Step in Interpretation. 108
    A Fourth and a Fifth Step in Interpretation 110
    Intracristal Spaces and the Outer Compartment. 115
Surface Membranes in Mitochondria. 116
    The Inner Surface Membrane. 116
    The Outer Surface Membrane. 119
Mitochondrial Membranes: Conclusions 121
Outer Segment Disks in Photoreceptor Cells. 122
    Polarization Optical Analysis. 122
    X-Ray Diffraction Analysis 123
    Low Denaturation Embedding and Freeze-Fracturing. 124
    Function. 133
The Plasma Membrane of the Outer Segment 134
    Structure. 134
    Function. 135
Outer Segment of Photoreceptor Cells: Conclusions 138
References. 140

83

Introduction

From a technical point of view, the present situation allows the structure of certain types of membranes to be analyzed at the 25–30 Å level by direct imaging in the electron microscope. This requires, however, that the membranes consist of a single layer of protein molecules arranged in a crystalline order. It is then possible to improve the image quality by image processing procedures such as optical filtering, which leads to an improvement of the signal-to-noise ratio. In one case where the analysis also included the electron diffraction pattern produced by the membrane it was possible to extract information at the 7 Å level. This involved the analysis of the purple membrane in *Halobacterium halobium* (Unwin and Henderson, 1975). A membrane of this kind can only consist of a few species of protein molecules, hence the potential for complex function is limited. In the case of the purple membrane, only a single protein is involved, bacteriorhodopsin. Membranes with a complex function consist of too many different types of molecules to assume a structure similar to that of a single layer crystal. They must therefore be analyzed by applying a different methodological approach.

In this chapter some efforts to solve these technical problems will be described. The results will be reviewed and it will be shown that it is possible to obtain information which casts doubt on the now generally accepted universal concept of membrane structure.

The Approach and the Methods

REQUIREMENTS

When trying to develop a suitable methodology for analysis of the molecular structure of membranes, it is practical to define the requirements that must be satisfied by the methodology. The first requirement is that the method should introduce limited changes in the conformation of protein molecules. The extent of conformation changes that can be accepted depends upon the resolution at which the analysis can be pursued with respect to electron optical imaging. The first goal will be to retain the globular shape of globular protein molecules. This requirement can be satisfied even if the molecules undergo conformation changes leading to inactivation of enzymes.

A second requirement is that there should be a minimal extraction of lipids. According to a third requirement, the membranes should be analyzed *in situ* because membranes with a complex structure are likely to be too labile to be isolated without undergoing considerable structural modifications. This is illustrated by the extensive modification of the crista membrane in mito-chondria when isolated mitochondria are broken up to allow isolation of submitochondrial particles (Sjöstrand *et al.*, 1964). A fourth requirement stipulates that the interior of the membrane should be made available for analysis. An analysis of the surface topography of such membranes does not reveal sufficient information to show the structure of the membrane, in contrast to the situation when membranes consisting of a single layer of protein molecules in crystalline order are analyzed.

The methods that satisfy these requirements are freeze-fracturing and thin sectioning of embedded material. Freeze-fracturing has the advantage that, when properly executed, it does not involve any denaturation of proteins before fracturing. During fracturing proteins are exposed to plastic deforma-tion, which can lead to changes in the shape of molecules and complexes of globular protein molecules. Thus there is a certain distortion involved which varies in magnitude with the arrangement of the molecules. The effects of plastic deformation can, however, be recognized, and in spite of this distor-tion the structure is fairly well preserved at the 40–50Å level, which repre-sents the limit of resolution of the freeze-fracture technique when applied to nonperiodic structures. This limit is determined by the size of the metal grains formed when platinum is deposited onto the exposed surface.

Freeze-sectioning offers the advantage of eliminating dehydration and embedding. However, the material is instead exposed to enormous surface forces which can lead to denaturation of proteins. Frequently the sections are also collected on a medium that denatures proteins. Extensive fixation and slow freezing without cryoprotection also lead to protein denaturation. In fact, most published pictures of freeze-sectioned material reveal extensive denaturation of proteins. The resolution is limited when applying this tech-nique due to the limitations with respect to the minimum thickness of the sections and to the limits of resolution of negatively stained sections.

The conclusion is that it is highly justifiable to develop a method for embedding tissues in a plastic for thin sectioning. There is no obvious limit to the attainable resolution when analyzing such sections because an elec-tron optical resolution of 8–10 Å has been achieved when analyzing ex-tremely thin sections (Sjöstrand, 1967). It can therefore be expected that sectioned material could be analyzed at a rather high specimen resolution, and that this resolution limit would be determined by how well the prepara-tory procedures preserve the structure.

THEORETICAL BASIS

When developing a method for embedding tissues for analysis at a molecular level, we start by considering certain theoretical aspects. First, the transfer of globular proteins to a plastic involves enormous risks for protein denaturation. This becomes clear when we realize that the native globular conformation is imposed on the peptide chains by the aqueous medium and that water is a unique medium. The problem therefore involves finding the conditions that will minimize the conformation changes expected when protein molecules are transferred to a nonaqueous environment.

First consider the factors that determine the globular conformation. It has been shown that the introduction of nonpolar compounds into water leads to an unfavorable free energy change due to a loss in entropy. This effect has been explained as nonpolar groups tending to introduce structural order in water. In the case of lipid molecules the hydrocarbon tails of the fatty acids expose nonpolar groups whereas the head group is polar. When the concentration exceeds a certain value, the critical micellar concentration, the lipid molecules aggregate into micelles in which the hydrocarbon tails are buried in the interior whereas the polar head groups face the water and shield the hydrocarbon tails from contact with water. In this way the entropy effect is reduced.

In protein molecules a rather high percentage of the amino acids are nonpolar or consist of sequences of nonpolar groups. According to Kauzmann (1959), in an aqueous environment the peptide chain folds up in such a way that these groups become buried in the interior of the molecule, which assumes a globular shape. The packing of the peptide chain is so tight that water molecules cannot penetrate the globular protein molecule. In both these cases the exposure of nonpolar groups to contact with water molecules is minimized by a sequestering of these groups in the interior of the micelle and of the globular protein, respectively. The correctness of this deduction by Kauzmann has been confirmed by X-ray crystallographic analysis of the conformation of globular proteins. These effects of water have been referred to as the hydrophobic effect and have been discussed extensively by Tanford (1973).

When the proteins are transferred to an organic solvent, or to a plastic, the situation changes from a thermodynamic point of view. The exposure of nonpolar groups no longer leads to a similar reduction of entropy. In fact, the entropy will increase by randomizing the conformation of the protein molecules. In the extreme case, the peptide chain therefore assumes a random coil conformation. The conformation changes vary in extent, however, depending upon a variety of factors. They can lead to partial unfolding of the peptide chain or to a globular conformation that is different from the native conformation. It is, however, common that the peptide chain becomes less tightly packed due to an expansion of the molecule. The denaturation is a complex phenomenon and the effects of different denaturing conditions differ. In addition there are considerable differences in the sensitivity and in the reaction of various types of proteins to the same denaturing conditions (see monograph by Joly, 1965).

The conventional electron microscopic technique involves a complex combination of different denaturing conditions and it is not possible to predict to what extent the denaturation modifies the conformation of globular protein molecules in complex cellular structures. It can, however, be established by direct observation that the conformation changes must be extensive because there are no traces of globular protein molecules in membranes even when the protein content is 80% of the dry weight of the membrane. Only extensive modification of protein conformation can explain the enormous differences in the structural information obtained from freeze-fractured materials as compared to material that has been embedded according to conventional techniques. That the denaturation has led to an extension modification of the structure of protein-rich membranes is also shown by the experiments involving intentional denaturation of tissue proteins by means of heat or low pH (Sjöstrand and Barajas, 1968). The appearance of the membranes was similar to that after conventional embedding of aldehyde-fixed material.

The denaturation of the proteins is combined with the extraction of lipids and with the appearance of a particular pattern associated with membranes in general, the unit membrane pattern. This pattern can be produced by lipid bilayers as well as by proteins. It therefore does not allow any conclusions regarding the structure of the membrane if this structure is not known in advance, as in the case of the myelin sheath. This is shown by the triple-layered appearance of mitochondrial membranes after extraction of more than 90% of the 25% lipids in mitochondria (Fleischer *et al.*, 1965). Our first goal will be to reduce conformation changes to such an extent that the globular shape of protein molecules is retained. An obvious approach is to stabilize the conformation as a first step in the procedure. Extensive stabilization can be achieved by proper inter- and intramolecular cross-linking of the proteins. The unfolding of the peptide chain is due to thermal vibration of the chain. Cross-linking adjacent peptide chains reduces the amplitude of the thermal vibration. The denser the arrangement of protein molecules the more efficiently the intermolecular cross-linking will inhibit an unfolding of the peptide chains. Cross-linking is therefore particularly efficient in the case of membranes that contain a high concentration of closely packed proteins.

The stabilizing effect of cross-linking has been used widely as a means of stabilizing protein crystals for X-ray crystallographic analysis. Quiocho and

Richards (1964, 1966) showed that crystals of carboxypeptidase A became mechanically stable after cross-linking with glutaraldehyde, and that they retained enzymatic activity. Furthermore this activity was retained without any reduction even after storage of the cross-linked crystals for several months at room temperature, showing that the stability of the enzyme had improved. Crystallographically there were no indications of any conformation changes introduced by the cross-linking.

It has also been shown that certain functions involving complex multi-enzyme systems are retained after glutaraldehyde cross-linking. Photosystems I and II in chloroplasts are active after glutaraldehyde cross-linking (Hallier and Park, 1969a,b). The same applies to the respiratory chain in mitochondria (Utsumi and Packer, 1967). However the extent of cross-linking affected the function. Quiocho and Richards (1964, 1966) showed that the enzymatic activity of carboxypeptidase A was reduced with increased cross-linking, and Lenard and Singer (1968) demonstrated by means of circular dichroism measurements that proteins can undergo conformation changes when exposed to glutaraldehyde under conditions similar to those applied in conventional fixation of tissues. In this case the cross-linking is extensive due to the high concentration of glutaraldehyde and the long fixation time. These are only a few examples that show that brief cross-linking with glutaraldehyde is a feasible method of achieving a certain stabilization of protein conformation.

The second consideration involves an elimination of exposure of the proteins to a denaturing organic solvent for dehydration. If dehydration by means of an organic solvent is applied, the weakest denaturing solvent should be chosen. The weakest denaturing solvents are ethylene glycol and glycerol. Through the extensive analysis of the effect of ethylene glycol on protein conformation (Tanford *et al.*, 1955, 1962), it has been shown that ethylene glycol is a unique organic solvent for globular proteins. Conformation changes could not be observed until the concentration of ethylene glycol had been raised to considerably higher concentrations than those at which other solvents denature proteins. Certain globular proteins thus could tolerate an exposure to 90% ethylene glycol.

A more or less complete unfolding of the peptide chains in a denaturing medium requires a certain amount of time. According to a third consideration, therefore, the time the proteins are exposed to denaturing conditions should be as short as possible.

The unfolding can be slowed down by lowering the temperature. In this respect, much experience has been gained, first from preparative biochemical work, and more recently from low temperature enzyme kinetic studies. Acetone, which denatures proteins at room temperature, is useful as a protein solvent at −15 to −20°C. The enzyme kinetic studies which have been pursued most systematically by Douzou and coworkers (for a review see Douzou, 1977) require a transfer of enzymes to organic solvents like methanol or ethanol to make it possible to pursue the analysis at temperatures as low as $-100°C$. At this temperature enzymes can tolerate exposure to 90% ethanol without losing enzymatic activity. The substrate–enzyme interactions are then slowed down or quenched to make intermediate stages in this interaction accessible for analysis.

These studies have shown that low temperature can slow down protein denaturation even when the medium consists of ethanol or methanol at concentrations that efficiently denature proteins at room temperature. However the low temperature does not offer an absolute protection against denaturation. It slows down denaturation to such an extent that experiments extending over a certain time can be conducted. The experience from storage of frozen biological material at a low temperature has shown that under such conditions denaturation can be inhibited for long periods of time.

Inactivation of isolated enzymes by cold occurs in the case where the enzyme consists of several subunits aggregated through hydrophobic interaction. Lowering the temperature weakens this interaction. However such inactivation does not necessarily occur when the enzyme is incorporated in a membrane. The F_1 ATPase in mitochondria is cold sensitive only when isolated (i.e., not when in the crista membrane) which explains why mitochondria can be isolated with retained function in ice-cold media. The same is likely to apply to other cold-sensitive enzymes. The cross-linking can be expected to reduce the risk of dissociation for the few enzyme complexes which are known to dissociate when isolated in a cold medium.

On this basis three different methods were tried in our laboratory for the embedding of tissues for a structural analysis at a molecular level.

METHODS

The first method shares with conventional embedding techniques the use of an organic solvent for dehydration. However the weakest denaturing solvent is used, ethylene glycol, and the exposure time is as short as possible (Sjöstrand and Barajas, 1968; Sjöstrand, 1980).

Step 1. Stabilization of the structure by brief cross-linking with glutaraldehyde. A 1% glutaraldehyde solution in Tyrode's solution is used and the cross-linking time is 3–15 min. Whenever possible the glutaraldehyde solution is perfused through the tissue.

Step 2. In order to dehydrate the tissue as quickly and as uniformly as possible, the tissue is homogenized very gently in an all-glass Potter-Elfvehjem homogenizer. In this way single cells and small groups of cells are obtained.

Step 3. The homogenized tissue is dehydrated in 90 or 100% ethylene glycol at 0°C for 2–5 min.

Step 4. The material is transferred to Vestopal (20% Vestopal 120 and 80% Vestopal 310).

In order to pursue the embedding this quickly, the homogenized material is pelleted after homogenization and after dehydration using a Beckman Microfuge. The centrifugation times are: after homogenization, 30 sec; after dehydration, 1–2 min.

Ethylene glycol and Vestopal mix poorly and it is therefore important to remove as much ethylene glycol as possible by blotting with filter paper before the transfer to Vestopal. The high viscosity of Vestopal also contributes to a slow inflitration of the material. To speed up the infiltration a special centrifuge head was designed (Sjöstrand and Halma, 1978) which allows the material to be centrifuged back and forth in a large volume of Vestopal for 24 to 48 hr. After infiltration, Vestopal is cross-linked at cold room temperature or at −15°C using a weak UV lamp as an energy source.

Vestopal was chosen as embedding medium because it is suitable for sectioning of extremely thin sections with less distortion than many other embedding media. It also appeared to be a weak lipid solvent and therefore fairly polar. Ethylene glycol is a poor lipid solvent but still extracts lipids efficiently enough to introduce risks of removal or perturbation of lipids. Because of the risk of lipid extraction this technique has been used in our laboratory for the analysis of membranes with a low lipid content, like the crista membrane in mitochondria. However the lipid-rich outer mitochondrial membrane and the myelin sheath are preserved after embedding with this method.

The second method is more theoretically satisfying than the first method. It makes extensive use of the slowing down of protein denaturation at low temperatures (Sjöstrand and Barajas, 1968; Sjöstrand and Kretzer, 1975).

Step 1. The cross-linked homogenized material or fresh homogenized material is frozen rapidly by spray freezing in propane chilled to −180°C by liquid nitrogen, according to Bachmann and Schmidt (1971). No cryoprotection is required in this case.

Step 2. The frozen material is dried by vacuum distillation at −80 to −90°C. This low temperature is chosen to prevent crystallization or recrystallization of water in the tissue.

Step 3. The dried tissue is infiltrated with a plastic at −80°C under high vacuum. Lowicryl HM20 is used and is a better embedding medium than hydroxypropylmethacrylate, which was used originally.

Step 4. The temperature is raised to −50°C and the plastic is polymerized by means of weak UV irradiation.

The temperature at which the tissue is infiltrated is of crucial importance. It must be high enough so that the viscosity of the plastic is sufficiently low to allow proper infiltration and low enough to slow down protein denaturation. Both Lowicryl HM20 and HPMA denature proteins at room temperature but seem to be satisfactory when used at −50 to −80°C.

The third method involves low temperature embedding without freezing. It involves a stepwise lowering of the temperature as the freezing point of the dehydrating medium is lowered. The following scheme can illustrate the procedure, which is still being explored. Kellenberger and co-workers have applied low temperature embedding but their procedure is different.

Step 1. The cross-linked, homogenized material is transferred to 30% ethylene glycol isosmolar to Tyrode's solution. The temperature is lowered to −10°C.

Step 2. The material is transferred to 50% ethylene glycol and the temperature is lowered to −35°C. These concentrations of ethylene glycol have been shown to be inert to globular proteins at room temperature according to the studies by Tanford and co-workers (Tanford *et al.*, 1964, 1966).

Step 3. The material is transferred to 80% ethylene glycol, and the temperature is lowered to −42°C.

Step 4. The material is transferred to 100% methanol and the temperature is lowered to −80°C.

Step 5. Transfer to 100% Lowicryl HM20 in which 0.6% benzoin methyl ether has been dissolved.

Step 6. Polymerization of the plastic at −50°C using a weak UV source.

The time of each step is 10 min. when changing the media the material is pelleted using a Beckman Microfuge kept at the temperature of each step. The centrifugation time is 30 sec, which is short enough to prevent any warming of the material. The pellets are resuspended by stirring with a piece of thin piano wire inserted in the chuck of a small hand drill.

Testing the Methods

The First Test

If the new methods do not lead to as extensive denaturation as the conventional methods, the appearance of membranes should differ from their appearance when the material has been prepared according to conventional methods. However a difference in the appearance does not prove that the new methods do not perturb the structure sufficiently to lead to a different artifactual presentation of the membrane structure.

The Second Test

All three methods should lead to similar results because they are all based on conditions that should reduce protein denaturation.

The Third Test

The structure should appear reasonable when considering the known chemical composition of the membranes. For instance, there should be some indication of the presence of 75–80% globular proteins in the crista membrane of mitochondria.

The Fourth Test

The methods should make it possible to reveal differences in the structure of membranes with different functions, if such differences exist.

The Fifth Test

Since freeze-fracturing is a method that allows the analysis of the structure at the 40–50 Å level with minimal distortion, the observations made on material prepared according to the new techniques can be compared to the same type of material prepared by freeze-fracturing. Both methods should give comparable results.

The Sixth Test

The freeze-sectioning technique also allows a comparison of at least certain features of membranes, and observations made when applying this technique should agree with those made on material prepared according to the new methods.

All these tests were satisfied by the new embedding techniques. It is therefore concluded that these methods make it possible to preserve the globular proteins well enough that the structure is retained with less perturbation than with conventional methods. The combination of these methods and freeze-fracturing makes it possible to analyze the molecular structure of membranes at the 40–50 Å level. The new methods will be referred to as low denaturation-embedding techniques.

The Crista Membrane in Mitochondria

OBSERVATIONS AND THE FIRST STEP IN INTERPRETATION

Low Denaturation-Embedded Material

The low denaturation-embedding techniques were first applied in a study of the structure of mitochondria (Sjöstrand and Barajas, 1968; Sjöstrand, 1977, 1980). In this material the membranes appeared lightly stained in contrast to the more intensely stained matrix (Fig. 1–3). In conventional material the intensity of the staining reflects the mass density distribution. It therefore would be expected that the cristae, with their higher mass density as compared to the matrix, would bind the stain more effectively than the matrix. This anomalous staining can be explained by referring to the above discussion of the conformation of globular protein molecules. The concentration of such molecules in the crista membrane is high, about 80%, and they are to a considerable extent interacting hydrophobically. The interior of these molecules is predominantly nonpolar and not accessible to stain ions in the native state of conformation. Furthermore there are no binding sites for stain in the nonpolar interior. Certain charged groups are not accessible to binding stain. This is shown by the increase in the number of titratable groups following denaturation. The globular protein molecules therefore should appear as lightly stained particles with the staining confined to the periphery of the particles. In the case of aggregates of hydrophobically interacting molecules, nonpolar regions would be expected to extend through groups of molecules and the unstained region would involve several molecules.

To test whether the staining was anomalous, unstained sections were analyzed in the dark-field mode of illumination in the electron microscope.

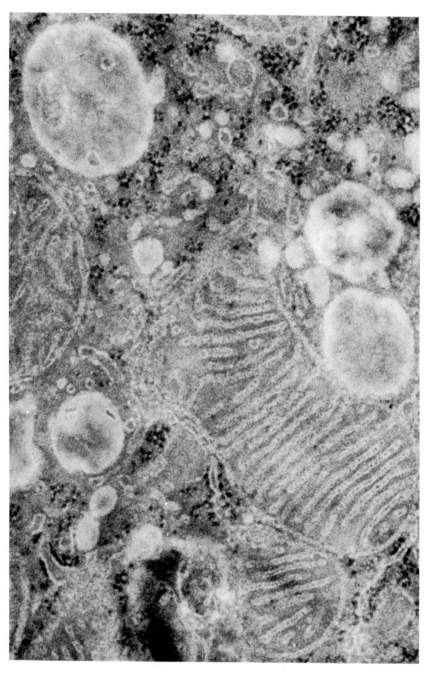

Fig. 1. Survey picture of apical cell region in proximal convoluted tubule cell in the rat kidney. Embedding according to method 1 with dehydration in 100% ethylene glycol for 2 min. The picture reveals a rather complex structure of this cell region with mitochondria and lysosomes. Free ribosomes appear to consist of a central mass from which processes extend. Magnification: 90,000×.

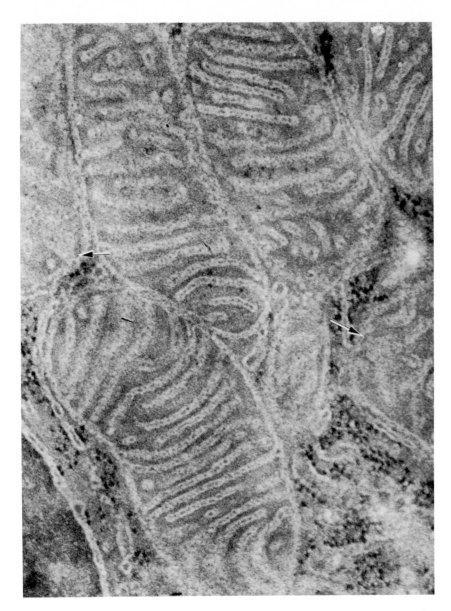

Fig. 2. Mitochondria in proximal convoluted tubule cell in rat kidney. Embedding according to method 1. The cristae are seen in different orientations, perpendicular, obliquely, and close to parallel to the plane of the section, and appear lighter than the matrix. When oriented perpendicular to the plane of the section, more intensely stained areas in the center of the cristae are lined up in a fairly regular way. These opaque areas are due to the superposition of considerably smaller stained spots as is shown in cristae which have an oblique orientation. The appearance of the cristae in profile view shows that the affinity for the stain is particularly low at the matrix surface of the crista membrane, which agrees with the location of the lipids interacting hydrophobically with proteins at that surface. Some stalklike connections extend from cristae viewed face-on to the inner surface membrane (arrows). Magnification: 107,000×.

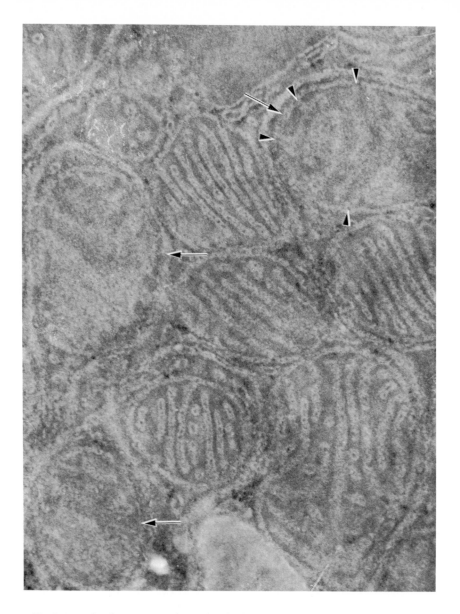

Fig. 3. Mitochondria in proximal convoluted tubule cell in rat kidney. Embedding according to method 1. The cristae appear at various orientations relative to the plane of the section. In two mitochondria (arrows), the cristae are seen in face-on views and a particulate structure is then revealed with the "particles" being lightly stained and delimited by somewhat more intensely stained areas. Since the staining is anomalous and the lightly stained areas therefore have a high mass density and do not represent voids, it is justified to consider them to be real particles delimited by the staining confined to their periphery. Arrowheads point to stalklike connections between cristae and the inner surface membrane. Magnification: 90,000×.

In darkfield, elastically scattered electrons are collected for imaging and, since elastic scattering is proportional to mass density, the pictures reveal the relative mass-density distribution in the specimen. The dark-field analysis (Fig. 4) showed that the mass density of the cristae was considerably higher than that of the matrix (Sjöstrand *et al.*, 1978). The staining is therefore anomalous and the explanation presented above is reasonable.

One striking piece of information which could be extracted from the electron micrographs of low denaturation-embedded isolated mitochondria involved the thickness of the mitochondrial membranes (Fig. 5). The crista membrane measured 120–130 Å in thickness whereas the two membranes at the surface of the mitochondria were considerably thinner, with the inner of the two membranes measuring 60–70 Å in thickness and the outer membrane 40–50 Å (Sjöstrand, 1977). Such differences in the thickness show that both surface membranes are different compared to the membrane of the cristae. We therefore must distinguish between the crista membrane and the inner and the outer surface membranes.

In face-on views of the crista membrane a particulate structure was observed, consisting of lightly stained "particles" outlined by the faint staining (Fig. 3). Knowing that the staining of the membranes is anomalous, these "particles" must contribute to the high mass density of the crista membrane and must be real particles and not voids. It can be assumed that the light staining of these particles is due to the compact packing of nonpolar amino acid side chains in the interior of globular protein molecules and of complexes of such molecules, as discussed above. This was, in fact, the predicted appearance of the protein molecules if the protein had not been denatured. The observation of a particulate structure satisfied one of the requirements mentioned above, that the observed structure should agree with what is known about the chemical composition of the membrane. The 75–80% globular protein in the membrane should give the membrane a particulate structure.

Freeze-Sectioning

These observations were subjected to a test by the application of two other methods, freeze-sectioning and freeze-fracturing. The freeze-sectioning technique was applied under conditions where protein denaturation by surface forces, or by the medium used for collecting the sections, would be minimal. As in the low denaturation-embedded material, the membranes of the cristae were closely apposed and the thickness of the individual crista membrane was 120 Å (Fig. 6), verifying the observation made on low denaturation-embedded material (Sjöstrand and Bernhard, 1976). The sections

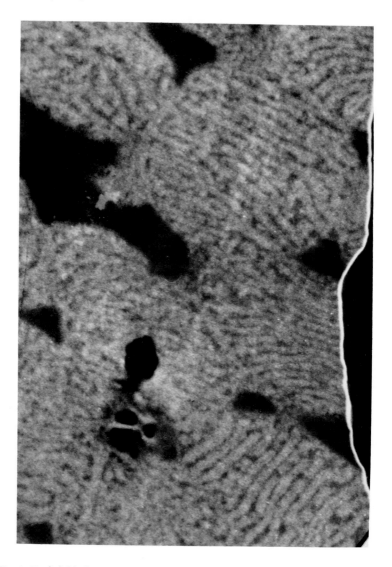

Fig. 4. Dark-field electron micrograph of unstained section through pelleted isolated heart muscle mitochondria embedded according to method 1. The section was mounted on a film pierced by holes and the edge of the photographed hole is seen at the right edge of the picture with a strong Fresnel fringe. The cristae appear bright, showing that their mass density is higher than that of the matrix. The thickness of the cristae varies due to different extent of "compression" imposed during sectioning. The mitochondrion in the lower right corner shows the proper thickness of the cristae because the cristae are oriented parallel to the direction of sectioning. The white streak across the picture is a knife mark indicating this direction. Magnification: 80,000×. From Sjöstrand *et al.*, 1978.

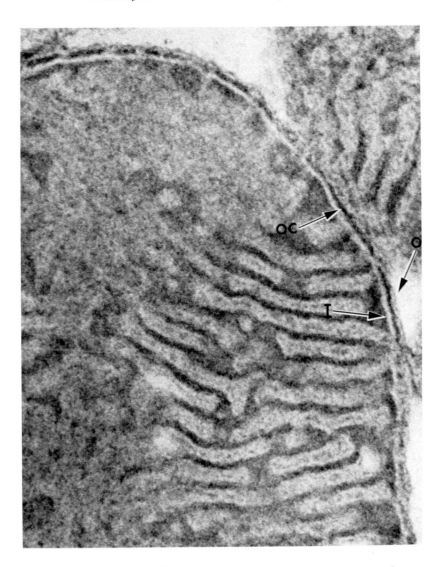

Fig. 5. Mitochondrion isolated from rat heart muscle tissue. The cristae are oriented more or less parallel to the plane of the section. Due to the isolation procedure the two membranes at the surface of the mitochondrion have become separated. This way their thickness can be measured individually. The outer surface membrane (O) is considerably thinner than the inner surface membrane (I). Both surface membranes are thinner than the half width of the cristae which corresponds to the thickness of the crista membrane. OC = outer compartment extending between the two surface membranes. Magnification: 210,000×. From Sjöstrand, 1977.

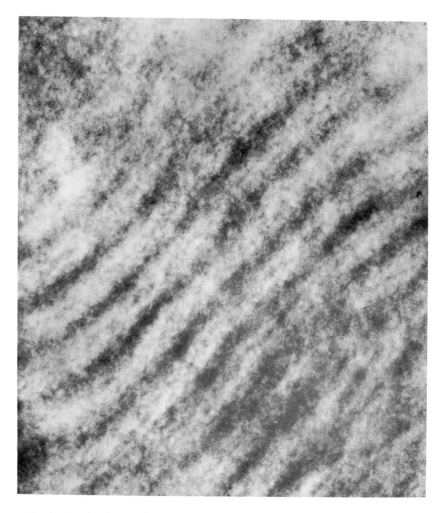

Fig. 6. Mitochondrion in frozen section of rat heart muscle tissue fixed 5 min in formalin vapor and collected on sucrose droplet according to Tokuyasu (1973), negative staining with 2% silicotungstate. The stain is predominantly located in the matrix, some faint staining of the cristae reveals a particulate structure, no intracristal space. Magnification: 275,000×. From Sjöstrand and Bernhard, 1976.

were analyzed after negative staining, which is required to reduce the destructive effects of surface forces during the drying of the sections. It was characteristic that the negative stain had not penetrated the cristae, although penetration would be expected if there were an intracristal space present because the stain had free access to any such space at the cut edge of the cristae. The stain furthermore did not infiltrate the crista membrane which shows that the molecules in the membrane are closely packed. Any modification of the technique that favored protein denaturation led to cristae with an intracristal space and to a thinner crista membrane (Fig. 7).

Freeze-Fracturing

Mitochondria had been studied earlier in freeze-fractured material but no really representative pictures of the cristae had been published. It was difficult to obtain good fractures exposing the cristae but it was easy to obtain fractures exposing the inner surface membrane. This membrane was considered identical to the crista membrane, and so it was assumed to represent the phosphorylating membrane. It was now with great suspense that the freeze-fracturing technique was applied. Fortunately, the conditions were found which made it possible to obtain good fracture faces at the cristae (Sjöstrand and Cassell, 1978a). There is a problem involved in the interpretation of pictures of freeze-fractured material. It is impossible to interpret the pictures correctly if the location of the fracture plane is not known. When the fracture plane is oriented parallel to a membrane, it must be determined whether it is located at one of the surfaces or in the interior of the membrane. Many times this is difficult to do. According to an international agreement the fracture plane is always located in the center of the membranes (Branton *et al.*, 1975). This agreement appeared to be an unsatisfactory way to solve the most crucial problem involved in the application of the freeze-fracturing technique. It is clear that if the accepted dogma is wrong the consequence will be that all interpretations of the observed structure which are based on the dogma will be erratic. It therefore seemed to be rather risky to rely on the dogma. When the experimental evidence which was considered to solidly support the dogma was analyzed, it became clear that some of this evidence, instead of proving the correctness of the dogma, proved that the dogma was wrong (Sjöstrand, 1979). It was furthermore obvious that an interpretation of the structure which is based on the dogma can never lead to a result disqualifying the dogma. It therefore eliminates all possibilities to subject the accepted interpretation to a test. The dogma does not explain a very important feature of freeze-fractured material. It leaves the lack of structural complementarity of complementary fracture faces unexplained. One would expect that the inability to explain such an obvious and important piece of information should cast some doubt on the correctness of the dogma (see below). Realizing the importance of locating the fracture faces correctly, an approach was adopted whereby the analysis involved fracture faces the location of which could be determined in an unambiguous way.

The considerable thickness of the cristae as judged from the observations made on low denaturation-embedded material should make it possible to

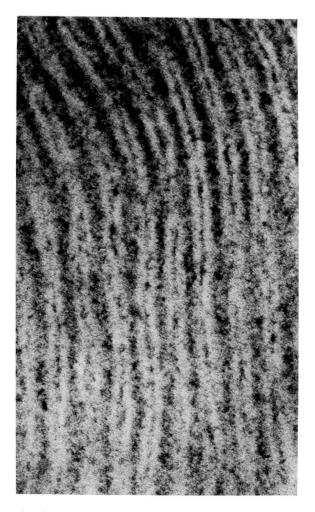

Fig. 7. Mitochondrion in frozen section of rat heart muscle tissue. The tissue was fixed in formaldehyde vapor for 5 min, dehydrated in ethanol and rehydrated before freeze-sectioning. Reduced thickness of crista membrane and an intracristal space. Magnification: 3000,000×. From Sjöstrand and Bernhard, 1976.

obtain informative cross and oblique fractures through cristae. The ambiguity with respect to location of the fracture planes applies to planes oriented parallel to the membrane surface but not to cross and oblique fractures. The freeze-fractured material showed that the cristae were of a similar thickness to that determined on low denaturation-embedded material and the prediction turned out to be correct. It was possible to obtain oblique fractures across the cristae and even fractures passing through the cristae at a slanting angle.

As an example, Fig. 8 and 9 show cristae that have been fractured in such a way that the fracture enters the cristae at a slanting angle. This is shown by the fact that the appearance of the fracture face changes abruptly from a fairly smooth appearance to a particulate appearance without jumping from one plane to another. If it had jumped, a step would have been indicated by a sharp shadow along the line of transition. The fracture has progressed into the interior of practically the entire crista in Fig. 8. The fracture faces always revealed a particulate structure when they exposed the interior of the cristae. In addition to particulate fracture faces, two rather smooth faces were observed, one of which could be identified as exposing the matrix. The other face was determined to be located at the matrix surface of the crista membrane because the information obtained regarding the inner structure of the cristae made it unlikely that any smooth fracture face could be located in the interior of the crista membrane or at the surface facing the center of the cristae (Fig. 9).

The fracture could also pass through the mitochondria in steps revealing alternately rather smooth and particulate faces (Fig. 10). Since the smooth face had been found to represent the matrix surface of the cristae and the interior of the entire crista had been shown to be particulate, it was possible to explain the regular stepwise fracturing as due to a jumping of the fracture plane from the matrix surface to the middle of the cristae. The particulate face then revealed the surface of the crista membrane that faced the center of the crista.

For the freeze-fracturing technique to give meaningful information, there is one requirement which must be fulfilled. The fracturing must expose the fractured material in such a way that basic structural properties of the material are revealed. If this is not the case, the method is meaningless. Fortunately in practice it has been shown that the method satisfies this requirement. The structural properties that can be revealed are properties affecting the path of the fracture through the material. This path is likely to proceed where the interatomic bonds are weakest. If the material consists of globular protein molecules in an aggregated form, the interatomic bonds are stronger within the molecules than between the molecules. The interior of the molecules is characterized by a dense concentration of covalent bonds whereas the bonding between the molecules involves charge interaction, nonpolar interaction, and hydrogen bonding. With a similar density of material, the latter bonds should break more easily than covalent bonds when exposed to the same force. Globular protein molecules should therefore appear as particles on the fracture face provided their diameter exceeds the resolution limit for the freeze-fracturing technique, 40–50 Å. If, on the other hand, the

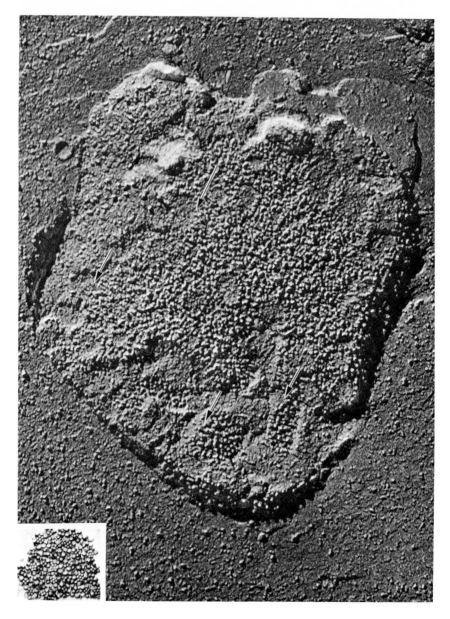

Fig. 8. Freeze-fractured rat heart muscle mitochondrion. The fracture plane has entered a crista at a slanting angle. Arrows point to the abrupt transition from a fairly smooth face to a densely particulate face without any step indicating an abrupt change in the level at which the fracture has progressed. The insert shows a photograph of the model for the crista membrane that was proposed in 1968 and presented pictorially in 1970 by Sjöstrand and Barajas. Magnification: 104,000×. From Sjöstrand and Cassell, 1978a.

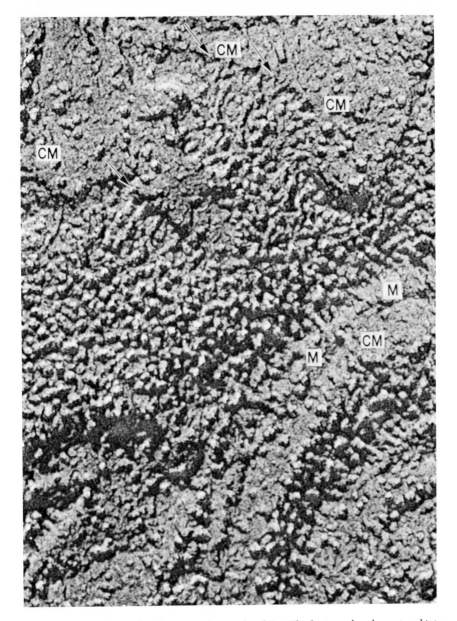

Fig. 9. Freeze-fractured rat heart muscle mitochondrion. The fracture plane has entered into the interior of the crista at a slanting angle from above. Arrows indicate the transition from the relatively smooth matrix face (CM) of the crista and the densely particulate face exposing the structure of the interior of the crista. Fracture through the matrix is indicated by M. Magnification: 246,000×. From Sjöstrand and Cassell, 1978a.

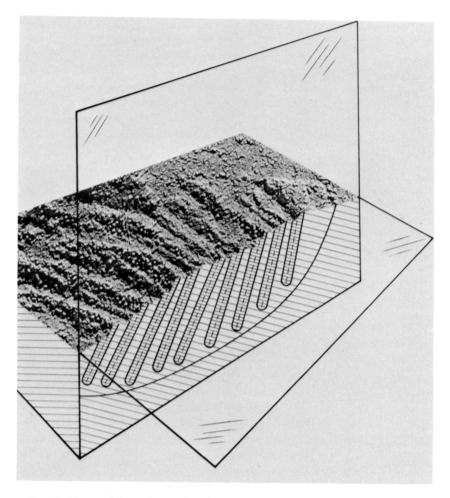

Fig. 10. Picture of freeze-fractured rat heart muscle mitochondrion with a plane oriented perpendicular to the fracture plane drawn to illustrate the relationship between the stepwise arrangement of the fracture and the orientation of the cristae. From Sjöstrand, 1979.

material consists of molecules which are too small to be observed with this technique, the fracture face should be smooth, provided that there are no large aggregates of molecules bonded more strongly than the average bonding strength in the material. Lipids would therefore give rise to smooth fracture faces.

As a consequence a material consisting of 80% globular protein molecules should appear as a particulate material when exposed by fracturing. Conversely, we can conclude that if we observe a particulate fracture face when fracturing through such a material, the globular protein molecules must be responsible for the particulate structure, and the fracture reveals the molecular structure of the material at a resolution of 40–50 Å with a certain distortion due to plastic deformation.

On the other hand, a material consisting partially of molecules that are too small to be observed at a resolution of 40–50 Å should give rise to a partially smooth fracture face, provided that these molecules form large enough patches and are not uniformly distributed among the large molecules. Conversely, a relatively smooth fracture face can be interpreted to reveal accumulations of small molecules. In the cristae there are 20% lipids, and it is justifiable to conclude that the observed, relatively smooth, fracture face associated with the matrix surface of the cristae is due to the presence of accumulations of lipid molecules at this surface.

THE SECOND STEP IN INTERPRETATION

A discussion of the meaning of the recorded pictures like the one presented above constitutes the first step in the interpretation of the observations. The second step involves a translation of the observations into a concrete concept describing the molecular structure of the crista membrane. This structure is most easily expressed in the form of a molecular model. We then consider the various observations one at a time and try to deduce their significance.

1. The first structural feature of the crista membrane to consider is its thickness, 120–130 Å. Since the average diameter of protein molecules or of subunits of protein molecules is considerably less than this dimension, it follows that protein molecules and subunits of protein molecules must form a three-dimensional structure. This agrees with the three-dimensional subunit structure of isolated cytochrome oxidase (Fuller *et al.*, 1979), cytochrome reductase (Hovmöller *et al.*, 1981), and ATP synthase (Soper *et al.*, 1979).

2. The close packing of the observed particulate structure shows that the protein molecules are closely aggregated in the membrane.

3. The relatively smooth matrix surface of the crista membrane makes it justifiable to locate lipids at the matrix surface and to assume that they are in a bilayer arrangement because they are in contact with the aqueous medium in the matrix. The thickness of such bilayers in biological material has been determined to be about 50 Å (see, for instance, Fettiplace *et al.*, 1971) due to

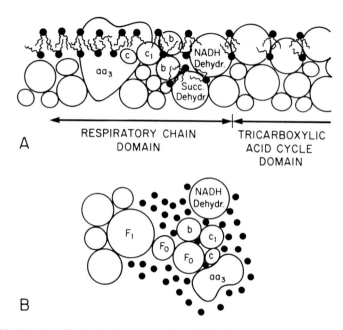

Fig. 11. Drawings illustrating the proposed model for the molecular structure of the crista membrane. **A:** a cross section through the membrane which passes through a respiratory chain and a tricarboxylic acid cycle domain. Patches of lipid bilayer are associated predominantly with the respiratory chain and to a lesser extent with the tricarboxylic acid cycle domain. Some lipid molecules are assumed to be associated with certain proteins outside the patches of lipid bilayer to contribute to the establishment of nonpolar diffusion paths in the interior of the membrane allowing diffusion of ubiquinone. Succinate dehydrogenase can equally well be assumed to be associated with the lipid bilayer structure like NADH dehydrogenase. **B:** face-on view of the respiratory chain domain illustrating the proposed relationship between the respiratory chain and the ATP synthase complex. Black dots indicate lipid molecules. From Sjöstrand, 1982.

the liquid state of the lipids. This means that the thickness of the bilayers is only a little more than one third the thickness of the membrane.

Fig. 11 illustrates the deduced membrane model.

THE THIRD STEP IN INTERPRETATION

From the observed structure illustrated in the membrane model, we now want to deduce some basic properties of the membrane. The three-dimensional packing of protein molecules and the absence of an aqueous space in the center of the cristae means that there is not a sufficiently large contact area between the membrane and an aqueous medium to make it possible for all polar surfaces of the protein molecules to have access to an aqueous medium. As a consequence polar surfaces as well as nonpolar surfaces must be buried in the interior of the cristae. Since it is likely that polar surfaces face each other, and the same applies to nonpolar surfaces, polar and nonpolar regions or domains will be mixed in the interior of the membrane.

According to a second deduction, the stability of the membrane must be determined primarily through protein–protein interaction. A large part of the membrane structure therefore can be compared to that of a protein aggregate. In this case the protein molecules expose sufficiently large nonpolar surfaces to make covering up of these surfaces by aggregation a thermodynamically favorable arrangement. To the stability of such an aggregate contribute the interaction of nonpolar groups through London's dispersion forces and intermolecular hydrogen bonding. The aggregates are characterized by a particular ordered arrangement of the subunits which shows that there are features that allow the subunits to recognize each other. Nonrandomness is therefore a characteristic feature of such aggregates. The same may very well apply to the crista membrane, which then would consist of domains within which the molecules are arranged according to particular patterns.

The third conclusion is based on the close packing of large molecules in the membrane. This must mean that the movements of the molecules are restricted with respect to amplitude. As a consequence the viscosity of the membrane must be high. This, in turn, could favor the formation of domains within which molecules form ordered aggregates even when the bonding is weak. Molecular interactions within such aggregates would be possible through the kind of fluidity proposed by Sjöstrand and Barajas (1968), according to which sequential interactions are possible through rotational and oscillatory movements of the molecules. The conflicting results reported with respect to the motility of cytochrome oxidase are discussed in a recent review (Sjöstrand, 1982). A fourth conclusion is based on the location of lipids at the matrix surface. These lipids could form a nonpolar barrier at this surface by a nonpolar interaction between bilayer regions and proteins located at the matrix surface.

The properties of the crista membrane discussed so far are all based directly on the observed structural features of the membrane and on known principles for molecular interactions. The stabilization of the membrane through nonpolar protein–protein interaction is a well known feature reflected in the low water-solubility of a large part of the membrane proteins. The ability of protein molecules within the membrane to aggregate to form well-defined complexes is illustrated by cytochrome oxidase. In this case the three most hydrophobic proteins are synthesized in the mitochondria and are coded for by the mitochondrial DNA while four components are synthesized in the cytoplasm and are coded for by nuclear DNA. Still these seven components can aggregate in the crista membrane in the presence of other protein molecules to form a complex with a highly ordered structure. The same applies to the ATP synthase where, in the F_1 factor, components synthesized in the mitochondria aggregate with subunits synthesized in the cytoplasm. The cytochrome reductase bc_1 complex of the respiratory chain has also been isolated as a complex in such a pure form that its dimensions and part of its shape could be determined (Hovmöller *et al.*, 1981).

It is highly likely that these various complexes are present as such in the membrane and are not products of the preparatory procedure. Nothing excludes larger aggregates from being present, such as the respiratory chain combined with the ATP synthase. The larger the complexes are, the more difficult it must be to isolate them intact in a pure form with present techniques. The interactions with other complexes in the membrane through bonds of a strength similar to those contributing to the stability within the complex will reduce the selectivity in bond strength required for isolation of the hypothetical large complexes in a pure form. As a consequence only pieces that are particularly strongly bonded through nonpolar and charge interaction have so far been isolated.

The close packing of the protein molecules in the crista membrane could lead to an establishment of long-range order in the molecular arrangement. A very faint indication of such order was reported by Sjöstrand (1980a). This possibility is presently being explored. The structural lability of the crista membrane reflects that the molecules are partially associated through weak bonding. This increases the difficulties in revealing any possible long range order in the membrane structure.

A Fourth and a Fifth Step in Interpretation

The Respiratory Chain

The next step in the interpretation of the observed structure involves trying to evaluate the effects of the structure on molecular interactions. The membrane is, in this case, considered to offer a particular environment for electron and proton transport and for enzyme catalysis. These aspects have been discussed in a recent review (Sjöstrand, 1982).

The fifth step in the interpretation leads us even further in our speculations. It means that we try to deduce the contribution of the structure to specific membrane functions, such as oxidative phosphorylation. We then arrive at the following concept. The respiratory chain components are forming one multimolecular aggregate with the cytochrome reductase bc_1 complex associated with the cytochrome oxidase–cytochrome c complex. This association favors successive molecular interactions responsible for electron transport and proton translocation by the close topographic arrangement of interacting centers and through rotation and thermal vibration of the molecules within the complexes (Sjöstrand and Barajas, 1968, 1970; Sjöstrand, 1982).

Cytochrome oxidase has been shown to have the shape of a somewhat distorted Y with a total length of the complex of 110 Å (Fuller *et al.*, 1979). When incorporated with lipids in a single layer crystal, the two arms are embedded in the lipid bilayer to the extent that only small areas at the arms are exposed at the surface of the bilayer. These areas are located at the matrix surface. In contrast the opposite end of the complex extends 40–60 Å out from the bilayer. The asymmetric association of cytochrome oxidase with the bilayer agrees with the distribution of nonpolar binding sites exposed at the surface. This association of cytochrome oxidase with the lipid bilayer makes it easy to accomodate the complex in the membrane model discussed here because, in this model, lipid bilayer regions are located at the matrix surface and the thickness of the membrane makes it possible to accomodate the part that extends far out from the bilayer (Fig. 11).

The monomeric cytochrome reductase consists of at least eight different subunits (Weiss and Kolb, 1979) including two cytochrome b (MW $\simeq$ 30,000), one cytochrome c_1 (MW $\simeq$ 31,000), the iron–sulphur subunit (MW $\simeq$ 25,000) and five additional subunits with molecular weights $\simeq$ 50,000, 45,000, 14,000, 12,000 and 8,000. The complex is partially stabilized by charge interactions as shown by its cleavage when the ionic strength of the medium is increased. This way a subunit complex consisting of two cytochrome b, one cytochrome c_1 and three small peptides with the molecular weights 14,000, 12,000 and 8,000 can be isolated. Dimers of both the entire cytochrome reductase complex and the cytochrome bc_1 complex have been crystallized with lipids to form monolayer crystals. The analysis of electron micrographs and electron diffraction patterns of these crystals showed that the size of the entire cytochrome reductase complex and that of the cytochrome bc_1 subunit complex were roughly the same in a face-on projection. In a direction perpendicular to the single layer crystal, the cytochrome reductase measured about 150 Å whereas the cytochrome bc_1 subunit complex measured about 70 Å. The monomer of the cytochrome bc_1 subunit complex measured 70 × 50 Å in a face-on view. Its dimensions will therefore be 70 × 50 × 70 Å.

It is assumed that the cytochrome bc_1 subunit complex is associated with the lipid bilayer at the matrix surface and that it extends 70 Å in a direction perpendicular to the crista membrane. The entire cytochrome reductase complex would then extend across the entire membrane in the case where the complex has a similar conformation in the crista membrane as in the artificial lipid crystal membrane. That this is not necessarily the case is indicated by the fact that the complex cannot be cleaved when exposed to a medium of high ionic strength when in the crista membrane or in an artificial phospholipid bilayer, whereas it is cleaved when dispersed in Triton X-100. It is possible that, in the membrane, interaction with phospholipid molecules in the lipid bilayer leads to an exposure of nonpolar groups and that the nonpolar interaction which then is added to charge interaction is strong enough to prevent cleavage in a medium of high ionic strength. In our hypothetical model the cytochrome reductase complex is positioned next to cytochrome oxidase (Fig. 11). We see that the observed thickness of the crista membrane can accomodate cytochrome oxidase and cytochrome reductase.

ATP Synthase

The ATP synthase has been isolated as a tripartite complex with the F_1 ATPase headpiece connected to a base piece by a stalk. The diameter of the F_1 is 90 Å and that of the base piece about 60 Å (Soper *et al.*, 1979). The total length of the complex has been determined to be 150 Å in yeast ATP synthase (Todd and Douglas, 1981). The conformation of this complex when incorporated in the membrane is unknown. The entire complex must be embedded in the membrane because no particles with the dimensions of the F_1 headpiece have been observed in the crista membrane when in its native state. It was shown by Sjöstrand *et al.* (1964) that they appeared in connection with the rupturing of isolated mitochondria preferentially in a medium of low osmolality. The cristae then were transformed into tubular structures showing extensive modifications of the membrane structure. These tubules had earlier been interpreted to be intact cristae viewed in profile.

With such extensive modifications of the membrane structure the meaning of the appearance of stalked particles ("elementary particles") seemed rather obscure. Were they particles existing as such in the membrane and released during the transformation, or were they artificial aggregates? In fact, it remained at that time to be proven that the particles were present as such in the membrane and had become visible by popping out from the membrane surface and that they were not an artificial aggregate formed during the transformation of the membrane into tubules. This was a conservative and critical way to evaluate the observation based on an acknowledgement of the importance of ruling out the possibility that electron microscopic pictures present the structure in a distorted way as artifacts. Not until Racker and co-workers demonstrated that the particles could be isolated and given a function was their real nature demonstrated. Still, the characteristic shape and size of these particles has only been observed when they are released from the membrane. It is therefore not known whether the subunits of the ATP synthase are aggregated in the same compact way when the complex is incorporated in the membrane. If we assume that F_1 ATPase is incorporated with the rest of the ATP synthase complex as a tripartite particle similar in appearance to the isolated ATP synthase, it is likely that the base piece and the stalk are associated with a lipid bilayer region at the matrix surface of the crista membrane. In order to incorporate the F_1 complex in the membrane, it is then necessary to orient the long axis of the ATP synthase parallel to the plane of the membrane. Thus the F_1 complex could be partially located outside the bilayer region and in contact with other protein molecules at the matrix surface (Figure 11B). The possibility that the respiratory chain and ATP synthase are associated to form aggregates within the membrane has not been ruled out.

The Soluble Proteins

In liver mitochondria 67% of the mitochondrial proteins are easily brought into solution (Schnaitmann and Greenawalt, 1968) whereas the rest require detergents for extraction. The former proteins have been assumed to be located in the matrix without any real justification. This would mean that the concentration of proteins in the matrix would be so high that it is questionable whether they can be in true solution as pointed out by Srere (1980). The structural analysis using low denaturation-embedding or freeze-fracturing revealed few particles present in the matrix. If the soluble proteins were located in the matrix, the fracture face exposing the matrix should be almost as particulate as that exposing the crista membrane and it would be practically impossible to distinguish between matrix and crista. Since there was no indication of the presence of any high concentration of globular protein molecules in the matrix in low denaturation-embedded material, Sjöstrand and Barajas (1968) proposed that the soluble proteins were located in the crista membrane but loosely bound to the membrane. This interpretation was the forerunner to the "peripheral" proteins of Singer and Nicolson (1972).

In our hypothetical membrane model the tricarboxylic acid cycle enzymes are located together in the crista membrane in tricarboxylic acid cycle domains. A particular organization of the enzymes would allow direct substrate transfer between the enzymes of the cycle.

Oxidative Phosphorylation

Next to these domains there would be cytochrome chain domains, and the NADH and succinate hydrogenases would be located at the boundary between the domains. Since the molar ratio of NADH dehydrogenase and cytochrome chains is about 1:7 electron transfer from each dehydrogenase would involve several respiratory chains. This makes it unlikely that there is a direct electron transfer between dehydrogenases and the cytochrome chain, and the important role of ubiquinone becomes clear. It is assumed that ubiquinone can diffuse between dehydrogenases and the cytochrome chains along nonpolar paths, one of which would be located in the hydrocarbon layer of the lipid bilayer regions.

With an organization of the membrane structure according to this proposal, there would be no need for any long-range proton translocation to establish a proton gradient. The translocation would involve a distance of about 20 Å across the hydrocarbon layer of the lipid bilayer regions and translocation within the membrane over distances of tenths of Ångströms. The proton gradient could be an intramembrane gradient as proposed by Williams (1961, 1978) and the structure of the membrane would allow the maintaining of high charge density locally.

When mitochondria are isolated their structure is modified, with the appearance of an outer compartment which communicates with the suspension medium. An aqueous space then extends into the cristae as an intracristal space and the surface of the crista membrane that faces this space becomes highly hydrated. In this manner, protons can diffuse into the outer compartment and into the medium with pH changes as one consequence. The transmembrane proton gradient that is created this way is likely to be less efficient for driving the phosphorylation of ADP than the localized intramembrane gradients assumed to represent the situation in native mitochondria.

The transmembrane proton gradient postulated by Mitchell (1961, 1967, 1977) would require proton translocations over long distances even if we only consider the translocation of protons, ADP, and P_i within the ATP synthase complex, where the total distance of translocation would be 150 Å. It would be a proton translocation within a protein complex, which means that exactly the same requirements must be satisfied as in the case of translocation within the membrane. The difficulties in conceiving of intramembrane proton translocation therefore also apply to a transmembrane proton gradient. There is nothing in Mitchell's chemiosmotic theory that requires a transmembrane proton gradient, and referring to the F_0 component of ATP synthase as a "proton well" by Mitchell does not furnish any explanation for proton translocation within the ATP synthase complex.

INTRACRISTAL SPACES AND THE OUTER COMPARTMENT

In the low denaturation-embedded material, the two membranes of each crista were always closely apposed and there was no indication of the existence of an intracristal space. The two surface membranes were also closely apposed, which means that there was no indication of the presence of an outer compartment. The same observations were made on freeze-sectioned and freeze-fractured material. In fact, no intracristal space can be observed after freeze-drying and conventional embedding (Sjöstrand and Baker, 1958), after conventional embedding of material fixed in aldehydes without postfixation in OsO_4, and of material fixed in potassium permanganate. The only occasion where intracristal spaces occur in mitochondria fixed *in situ* is after osmium fixation, whether preceded by glutaraldehyde fixation or not.

The situation is, however, different when analyzing isolated mitochondria. In this case the two surface membranes are separated by an interspace which makes it possible to measure the thickness of the individual membranes. If the isolation of liver mitochondria has been carried out in a pure sucrose medium, there are intracristal spaces present in all cristae. These spaces close when substrate is made available and remain closed during oxidative phosphorylation (Sjöstrand and Candipan, unpublished observations). The latter observations show that there is a mechanism capable of transporting water from the intracristal spaces to the matrix and this mechanism must be located in the crista membrane. This mechanism prevents the opening up of an intracristal space. The implication of this observation with respect to Hackenbrock's (1966, 1968) claim that the crista membrane undergoes conformation changes when the state of metabolism changes has been discussed in a recent review (Sjöstrand, 1982).

The observations justify the conclusion that an outer compartment involving a space separating the two surface membranes and intracristal spaces is due to a modification of the native structure of mitochondria caused by the isolation procedure. The space in the cristae and that separating the two surface membranes communicate through the stalklike connections extending from the cristae to the inner surface membrane, which were first shown by Andersson-Cedergren (1959) and later confirmed by Daems and Wisse (1966) in three-dimensional reconstructions of the mitochondria. These connections can be seen in low denaturation-embedded material when the cristae are oriented more or less parallel to the plane of the section (Fig. 2 and 3).

Surface Membranes in Mitochondria

The Inner Surface Membrane

The inner surface membrane was shown to be about half as thick as the crista membrane in low denaturation-embedded material (Sjöstrand, 1977). This clearly shows that the two membranes must be structurally different. It was also observed that there was a particulate structure associated with the surface membranes. Since the images of both membranes were superimposed in the electron micrographs, it could not be determined whether this structure referred to both surface membranes. The analysis of the freeze-fractured mitochondria revealed a particulate structure at the outer surface of the inner surface membrane whereas the matrix surface was somewhat smoother (Fig. 12 and 13). The particles were not quite as densely arranged as in the crista membrane and the particle size distribution was very different from that in the crista membrane. It showed a single maximum at 110 Å and a fairly narrow distribution of the values around this maximum (Sjöstrand and Cassell, 1978b). The freeze-fracturing also confirmed the difference in thickness of the two surface membranes. The thinness of the inner surface membrane excluded that fracture faces with an oblique orientation would appear. The fracture was either a cross-fracture or it followed either surface of the membrane, sometimes combined with a cross-fracture. The size of the particles made it justifiable to assume that the membrane consists of a single layer of particles. This would exclude a location of the fracture plane in the center of the membrane. The interpretation of the molecular structure of the inner surface membrane is illustrated in Fig. 14. Elevated areas were dispersed in a rather regular fashion on the matrix surface of the inner surface membrane (Fig. 13). These areas corresponded in distribution and frequency to the stalklike connections between the cristae and the inner surface membrane. They can therefore be identified as those connections which had been broken when the cristae were removed during fracturing.

The discovery that the inner surface membrane is different from the crista membrane has obvious implications with respect to mitochondrial function. It means that the exchange between the matrix and the cytosol is controlled by membranes other than the crista membrane, in contrast to the generally accepted concept. It furthermore means that the carriers involved in this

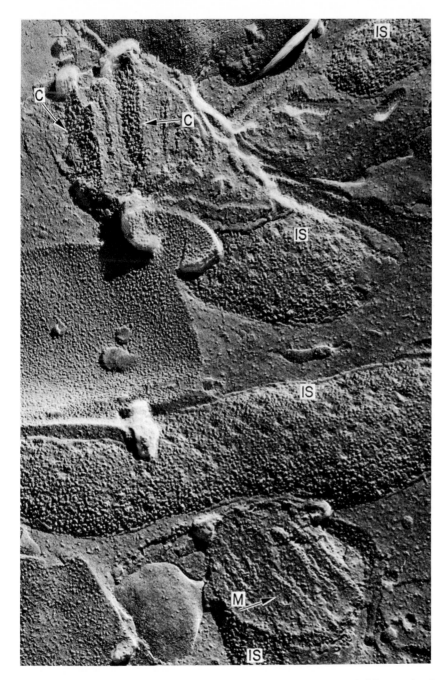

Fig. 12. Freeze-fractured rat kidney mitochondria. The fracture has revealed the peripheral surface of the inner surface membrane (IS) of three mitochondria and the interior of the cristae (C) in one mitochondrion. There is a considerable difference in the density of the arrangement of particles in the inner surface membrane and in the cristae. In still another mitochondrion the fracture exposes the matrix (M). Magnification: 74,000×.

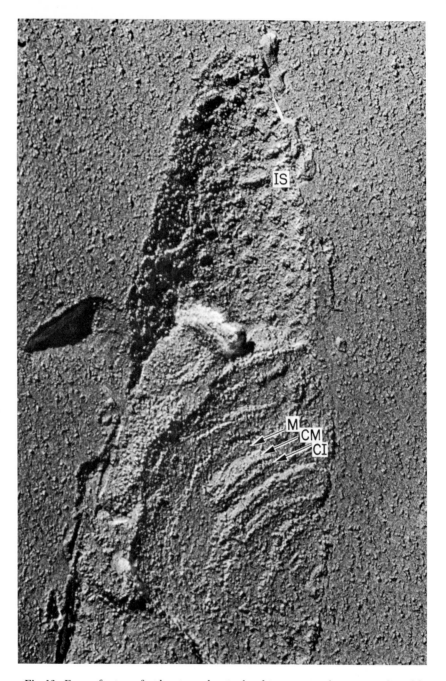

Fig. 13. Freeze-fracture of rat heart muscle mitochondrion exposing the matrix surface of the inner surface membrane (IS) with rather regularly arranged elevations which are the broken stalklike connections between the cristae and the inner surface membrane. In the lower half of the picture, the fracture has passed through the interior of the mitochondrion exposing the

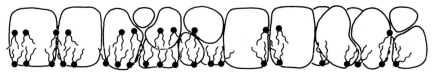

Fig. 14. Drawing illustrating the proposed model for the inner surface membrane of mitochondria. The particles should be separated partially to illustrate that the packing of particles is not a close packing.

exchange are likely to be located predominantly in the inner surface membrane, which is more particulate than the outer surface membrane. It is proposed that the ADP–ATP translocase of Klingenberg and coworkers (Klingenberg *et al.*, 1974; Klingenberg, 1979) is located in the inner surface membrane. The fact that ADP–ATP translocation and other carrier functions can be demonstrated only to a very small extent in submitochondrial particles is then easily explained by these particles consisting predominantly of crista membrane vesicles. Inhomogeneity among submitochondrial particles has been demonstrated, for instance, by Huang *et al.* (1973). This can also be explained by the fractions containing mixtures of vesicles derived from the crista membranes and from the inner surface membrane (see Sjöstrand, 1982).

THE OUTER SURFACE MEMBRANE

Both in low denaturation-embedded and in freeze-fractured material the outer surface membrane appears as a structurally much simpler membrane than the other two mitochondrial membranes. In freeze-fractured material both its surfaces were to a great extent smooth with large particles raised over the smooth surface (Fig. 15). These particles became rearranged in specimens which had been kept at 0°C and could then form a netlike pattern (Sjöstrand and Cassell, 1978b). This shows that this membrane has a certain fluidity which allows translational movements of particles. The thickness of this membrane was determined to be 40–50 Å on low denaturation-embedded material. That the membrane is thin was also obvious when analyzing freeze-fractured material. The steps from the outer surface of the membrane to the outer surface of the inner surface membrane thus practically always cast short shadows.

The dimensions and the smoothness of the fracture faces associated with the outer surface membrane make it justifiable to conclude that a large part

---

matrix (M) and several cristae with a fairly smooth matrix surface (CM) of one crista membrane and a particulate intracristal surface of the second crista membrane (CI). Magnification: 100,000×.

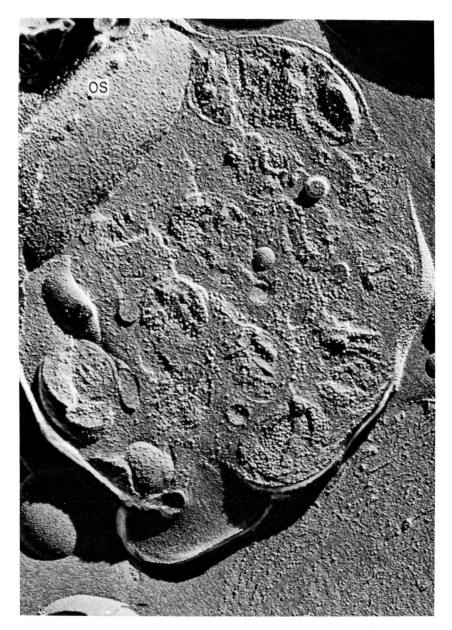

Fig. 15. Freeze-fracture across inner segment of photoreceptor cell in the guinea pig retina showing fractures through several mitochondria and in one case a fracture along the outer surface of one mitochondrion (OS). The particulate interior of many cristae is revealed. Magnification: 73,000×.

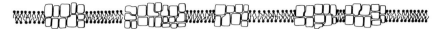

Fig. 16. Drawing illustrating the proposed model for the structure of the outer surface membrane in mitochondria. The large patches seen on the two surfaces of this membrane are thought to consist of large aggregates of protein molecules. From Sjöstrand, 1980b.

of this membrane consists of lipids in a bilayer arrangement. This is consistent with the high lipid content of this membrane—45% (Parsons *et al.*, 1966). The size of the particles makes it reasonable to assume that they consist of large aggregates of protein molecules. Fig. 16 illustrates this interpretation of the structural information.

Mitochondrial Membranes: Conclusions

The mitochondria offer exceptionally favorable conditions for making a comparison between the structure of different membranes because three different membranes can be analyzed side by side and can therefore be compared in the same picture. This eliminates the possibility that preparatory procedures and the recording method can have provoked spurious differences. Furthermore the differences are so extensive that simple methods are sufficient to reveal the differences, such as measurements of membrane thickness and of particle size distributions. Already these three membranes demonstrate such a diversity with respect to structure that it is impossible to make them suit any universal structural pattern. The observations show that the generally accepted universal membrane model of Singer and Nicholson (1972) is not applicable to all mitochondrial membranes. It is applicable to the outer surface membrane if the model is modified to involve large complexes of protein molecules instead of individual protein molecules dispersed in a lipid bilayer. These complexes might well consist of organized protein aggregates wherein the conditions for molecular interaction are similar to those in the crista membrane. To what extent the inner surface membrane conforms with the Singer–Nicolson model is difficult to judge. The packing of the particles appears to be too dense to accomodate a continuous lipid bilayer extending between the particles. It seems likely that the bilayer is discontinuous and forms patches of bilayers interposed between large aggregates of particles. This could account for a certain fluidity of this membrane.

The crista membrane does not in any respect conform with the Singer–Nicolson model and the dense packing of protein molecules and of complexes of protein molecules excludes this membrane from having the fluidity that characterizes this model. Instead the fluidity is likely to be of the kind suggested originally by Sjöstrand and Barajas (1968). According to the Singer–Nicolson (1972) model there is no long range order in membranes, and molecular interactions are due to favorable random collisions between molecules. Furthermore, in the Singer–Nicholson model all polar groups are considered to be in contact with water and all molecular interactions take place in an aqueous environment. Even though the Singer–Nicholson model allows great variety in the arrangements of peripheral proteins, there is no possibility of making the crista membrane conform with that model.

Outer Segment Disks in Photoreceptor Cells

POLARIZATION OPTICAL ANALYSIS

The outer segment of photoreceptor cells is functionally of particular interest because it is associated with the transduction of absorbed light to a signal that changes the permeability of the plasma membrane and thereby affects the state of polarization of the photoreceptor cell membrane. In the dark the plasma membrane is "leaky" for Na^+. This leakiness is reduced when the photoreceptor cell is exposed to light. As a consequence the cell hyperpolarizes. The efficiency by which light can affect the permeability of the plasma membrane is extremely high. A single absorbed photon has been estimated to be sufficient to affect the state of membrane polarization in dark-adapted rod cells.

It was shown that the energy transduction is associated with a membrane structure by the demonstration that the entire outer segment consists of a pile of double membrane disks (Sjöstrand, 1948, 1949, 1953). Polarization optical analysis had revealed earlier that the outer segments are birefringent. The most extensive analysis of this has been pursued by Schmidt (1928, 1935a,b,c, 1937). The birefringence had a positive sign before extraction of lipids and the sign changed to negative after extraction. This information made it likely that the lipid molecules were responsible for the positive birefringence and that they were oriented parallel to the long axis of the outer segment. The negative birefringence observed after lipid extraction, which also involved denaturation of proteins, showed the presence of an anisodiametric structure predominantly oriented perpendicular to the long axis of the outer segment. Schmidt later demonstrated (1935c, 1937) that the negative birefringence was form birefringence, which indicated that it was due to a layered arrangement of the denatured protein. Schmidt (1935c, 1937) also showed dichroism in the dark-adapted outer segments and the disappearance of dichroism after the bleaching of rhodopsin. This showed that the rhodopsin molecules had a preferred orientation.

Schmidt concluded that the outer segment consisted of alternating lipid and protein layers. However the polarization optical method did not allow a determination of the thickness of these layers. It was furthermore not possible to eliminate to what extent protein denaturation had contributed to the negative birefringence observed after extraction of the lipids. The conclusions that can be drawn on the basis of a polarization optical analysis are limited and the concept presented by Schmidt in his model was one of several possible interpretations of the observations. It was therefore not surprising that the electron microscopic analysis revealed a rather different structure. Instead of the thick layers of lipids and proteins proposed by Schmidt, the electron microscopic analysis revealed the presence of a complex membrane structure. The unit structure consisted of two membranes which extended across the entire cross section of the outer segment in the form of a disk with a special structural specialization at the edge of the disk, the edge structure (Sjöstrand, 1948, 1949, 1953). A stack of such disks filled the entire outer segment. Furthermore the disks were separated by a thin cytoplasmic space. The center-to-center separation of the disks was found to be about 300 Å. The dimensions of the disks showed that each disk membrane could only contain a single lipid bilayer. A layer of protein was proposed to be located between the two bilayers (Sjöstrand, 1960).

X-Ray Diffraction Analysis

X-ray diffraction analysis of the outer segments is hampered by the limited information contained in the diffraction patterns. It appears, however, that the analysis has clearly revealed the presence of extensive areas of lipid bilayers with two bilayers belonging to each disk, as had been concluded on the basis of a combination of the observations made in the electron microscopic and in the polarization optical analysis (Sjöstrand, 1960).

Considerable effort has been devoted to localizing rhodopsin relative to the lipid bilayers. Various X-ray crystallographers have interpreted the diffraction patterns very differently. The rhodopsin molecules have been assumed to be embedded eccentrically in the bilayer (Gras and Worthington, 1969; Worthington, 1973, 1974), located symmetrically relative to the bilayer (Blaurock and Wilkins, 1969, 1972; Blaurock, 1972; Vanderkooi and Sundaralingham, 1970), or at the cytoplasmic surface of the bilayer (Corless,

1972; Yeager, 1975, neutron diffraction). The only position that has not been proposed on the basis of X-ray diffraction analysis is that at the surface of the bilayer facing the center of the disk. These many alternatives reflect the lack of order in the arrangement of the rhodopsin molecules. They therefore only contribute to a minor modification in the diffraction pattern produced by the lipid bilayers.

Low Denaturation Embedding and Freeze-Fracturing

Observations

Since the outer segment membrane is rich in lipids, the low denaturation-embedding technique referred to earlier as method number 1 is not suitable. Therefore the number 2 method was used, which involves rapid freezing, freeze-drying and low temperature embedding. This method made it possible to determine that the thickness of the disk membrane is about 100 Å. This piece of information turned out to be of crucial importance for the interpretation of the observations made on freeze-fractured outer segments.

Several researchers have published pictures of freeze-fractured outer segments which revealed one smooth and one particulate fracture face associated with the disks. They have, however, either abstained from an interpretation of the observations or they have tried to apply the dogma that the fracture face is located in the center of the disk membrane, which leads automatically to a classification of the particles as intramembrane particles. It has been shown that the smooth and the particulate fracture faces are complementary faces. A recent review by Röhlich (1981) reveals the inability to explain the lack of structural complementarity of these faces. He refers to the fact that this does not only apply to the photoreceptor membranes and "is still an unsolved problem in freeze-fracture morphology."

When the fracture passes obliquely across the outer segment, smooth and rough fracture planes alternate in a regular fashion as the fracture passes stepwise through the outer segment (Fig. 17). If shadows are cast at the steps, the heights of the step can be calculated because we know that the center-to-center distance between disks is 300 Å in a well-preserved outer segment. This distance is divided into two steps and the relative heights of these steps can be determined from the lengths of the shadows. This does not require a knowledge of the shadowing angle. From the relative heights of the shadows the absolute heights of the steps can be calculated because the sum of the heights of the two steps is equal to 300 Å. It was found that the ratios of the lengths of the shadows (Fig. 18 and 19) could be either 1:2 or 1:5 (Sjöstrand and Kreman, 1978; Sjöstrand, 1979). The ratio 1:2 had been

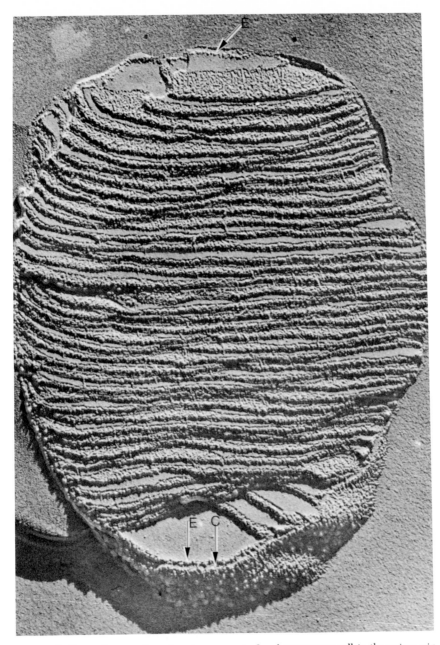

Fig. 17. Freeze-fracture through outer segment of a photoreceptor cell in the guinea pig retina. The fracture has passed stepwise through the regularly arranged outer segment disks and reveals one smooth and one particulate face associated with each disk. The edge structure (E) is exposed in several places. The outer surface of the plasma membrane is exposed in the lower part of the picture and shows a particulate structure. The fracture has cut across the plasma membrane at C, which makes it possible to measure its thickness. Magnification: 74,000×.

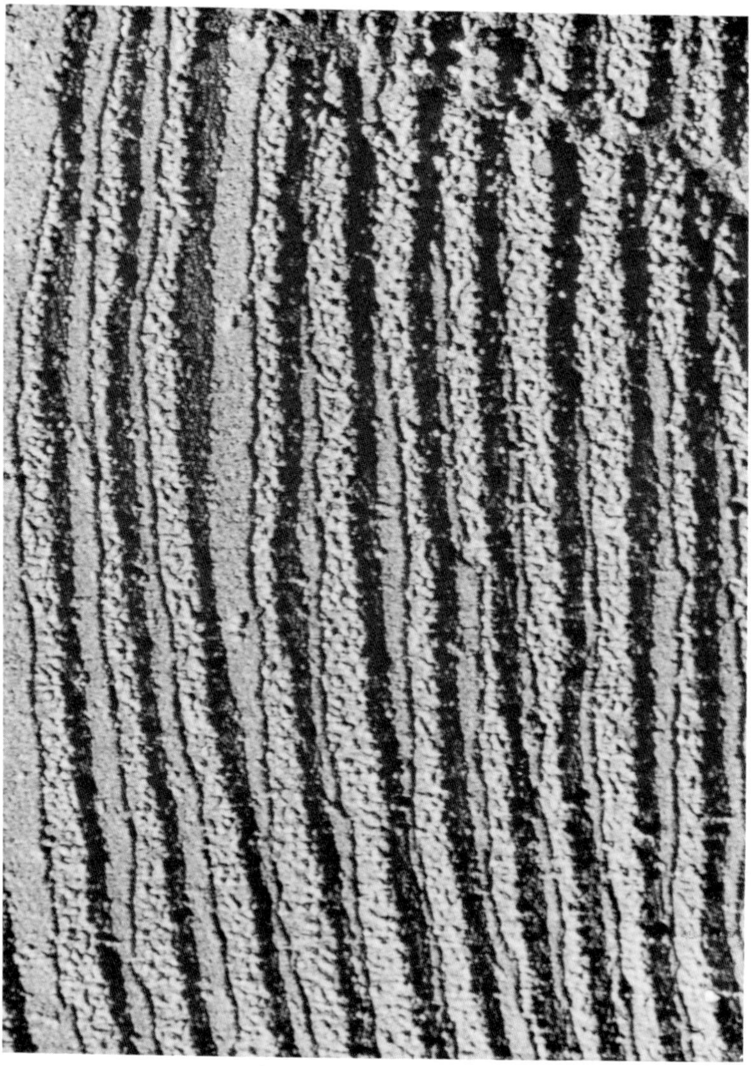

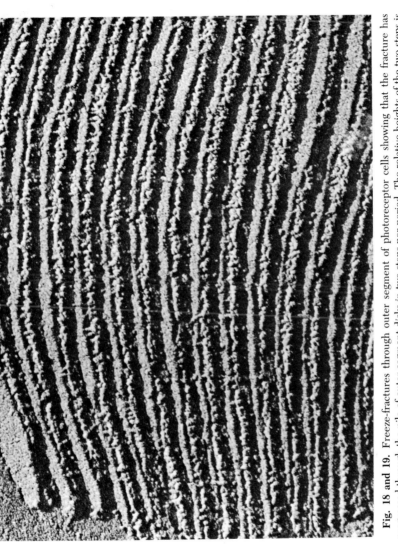

Fig. 18 and 19. Freeze-fractures through outer segment of photoreceptor cells showing that the fracture has progressed through the pile of outer segment disks in two steps per period. The relative heights of the two steps is revealed by the lengths of the shadows cast at the steps. The lower step is associated with the disks whereas the higher step cuts across part of the disk and the entire cytoplasmic space interposed between the disks. The sum of the heights of the two steps is equal to the period 300 Å, which includes one disk (200 Å) and one cytoplasmic space (100 Å). Since the dimension of the period is known, the absolute height of the steps can be calculated from the relative heights which are 1:5 in Figure 18 (top) and 1:2 in Figure 19 (bottom). Magnification: 150,000×.

observed earlier by Corless *et al.* (1976) and had led these researchers to conclude that the fracture planes were located in the center of the disk membrane. The absolute heights which correspond to these ratios are 100 and 200 Å for the first ratio, and 50 and 250 Å for the second ratio.

The smooth faces were found to be associated with the disks because fractures through the cytoplasm which also revealed smooth faces could easily be distinguished from the smooth disk faces. As a consequence each disk was represented by two fracture faces, one smooth and one particulate. The fact that the fracture could jump either 50 Å or 100 Å down from the smooth face, and in both cases revealed a particulate face, makes it rather easy to interpret the structure. It means that at both these levels, 50 Å and 100 Å below the smooth face, the fracture faces expose an identical particulate structure. This shows that a particulate material is located at a level that extends from 50 Å to more than 100 Å below the smooth fracture face.

The edge structure of the disks appears clearly in the freeze-fractured material, and it could be established that the particles in this structure differed from those in the particulate membrane faces with respect to their dimensions (Fig. 17).

Interpretation

Since the disk structure is centrosymmetric and the thickness of the disk is known to be about 200 Å, the location of the particulate fracture face 100 Å below the smooth fracture face must be in the middle of a zone consisting of particulate material. The fact that particulate fracture faces can be located either 50 Å or 100 Å below the smooth fracture face can furthermore be interpreted to show that the particulate material is arranged in two layers, about 50 Å thick, which are in mutual contact. The only possible location for these particulate layers will then be in the center of the disk because a location at the cytoplasmic surface would mean that they would be separated either by a cytoplasmic space with a width of 100 Å or by smooth material with approximately the same thickness. As a consequence the material exposing a smooth fracture face must be located at the cytoplasmic surfaces of the disk and must be about 50 Å thick. The smooth fracture face must then be the cytoplasmic surface of the disk, which agrees with the observation that this face always faces the cytoplasm and is directly associated with the fracture face that exposes the cytoplasm. The disk membrane is thus a layered structure consisting of two different materials separated into two layers with about the same thickness, 50 Å.

There are approximately equal parts of lipids and proteins in the outer segments, and in rod cells 85% of the protein is rhodopsin with a molecular diameter of 40–50 Å (Heller, 1968). Thus they are large enough to be ob-

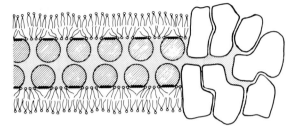

Fig. 20. Drawing illustrating the deduced structure of the outer segment disks with one lipid bilayer at each side of the disk and two layers of photopigment molecules in an aqueous environment in the center. The interaction of rhodopsin with the lipid bilayer occurs through the retinal (thick black line) interacting with the hydrocarbon layer of the bilayer through openings between the head groups of the lipid bilayer. This interaction leads to some perturbation of the lipid bilayer structure which is maximal in the dark-adapted state when the orientation of retinal interferes most extensively with the hydrocarbon layer. To the right the edge structure is shown consisting of large protein complexes. Modified from Sjöstrand, 1979.

served when exposed by fracturing. The two layers can therefore be accounted for by lipids and proteins being located in separate layers in the disk membrane. Fig. 20 illustrates the deduced structure of the disk.

The interpretation has in a straightforward way been based on observations and available information regarding the chemical composition of the outer segment. No other assumption has been introduced than the one on which the usefulness of the freeze-fracturing method is based: that fracture faces reveal structural properties of the material that has been exposed by fracturing. This means that a material that exposes a smooth face must be different from a material that exposes a particulate face.

Etching was not applied in this study because it has been established that it leads to the deposition of a layer of contamination onto the membrane surface that is exposed by etching (Sjöstrand, 1979). It has been shown by others (Corless *et al.*, 1976) that neither the smooth nor the particulate faces are etchable. Our interpretation is supported by the relationships of the smooth and particulate faces to the edge structure. An edge structure could only be observed on smooth fracture faces as an aggregation of particles somewhat raised above the plane of the face (Fig. 17). When particulate faces reached to the edge of the disk, no edge structure was observed and there was a high step separating the particulate face from the cytoplasmic face. The height of this jump reflects the fact that the edge is thicker than the rest of the disk.

We then arrive at the simplest and most straightforward interpretation of the observations according to which each disk membrane consists of two layers, one lipid and one protein layer, each with a thickness of about 50 Å.

This accounts for the observed thickness of the disk membrane. The lipid layer is located at the cytoplasmic surface of the disk and due to its contact with an aqueous medium it is assumed to consist of a single lipid bilayer. The assumption that the lipids are present in the form of a bilayer is supported by the polarization optical and X-ray diffraction data. The lipid bilayer is assumed to be in a liquid state. The protein layer consists predominantly of rhodopsin in rod cells and the concentration is likely to be considerably higher than 85% of the proteins because some of the proteins other than rhodopsin are concentrated in the edge structure. The layered structure of the disk membrane explains that complementary fracture faces can appear very different, smooth and particulate, respectively. It is a consequence of the fact that the two complementary faces expose materials with greatly different composition.

The rhodopsin molecules are known to interact hydrophobically with the lipids and to be oriented. Furthermore the retinal group is oriented in a plane roughly parallel to the plane of the disk membrane. It is therefore assumed that the rhodopsin molecules interact hydrophobically with the hydrocarbon layer of the lipid bilayer through openings between the polar head groups of the lipid molecules without being immersed in the hydrocarbon layer. In a liquid lipid bilayer with a thickness of 50 Å there are conditions fulfilled for the headgroups being separated by large enough distances to allow such an interaction. It is furthermore assumed that the retinal group is involved in the hydrophobic interaction and that this interaction is responsible for the orientation of the rhodopsin molecules. This interaction of rhodopsin with the hydrocarbon layer and a packing density of about 0.6 explains the large motility of the rhodopsin molecules both with respect to rotational and translational movements. The latter motility would be determined by the liquid state of the lipid bilayer which will lead to constant lateral changes in the position of the site of rhodopsin–lipid interaction, the rhodopsin molecules moving with the lipid molecules.

Verification of Interpretation

The analysis has led to locating the rhodopsin in a way that had not been proposed on the basis of X-ray crystallographic analysis. It therefore appeared important to try to verify the interpretation of the pictures of freeze-fractured outer segments. This was done by the development of a technique to isolate outer segment disks intact (Sjöstrand and Durstenfeld, unpublished work). Membranes which had earlier been isolated from outer segments had never been intact disks but were vesicular membrane fragments. The freeze-fracture experiments showed that the disks easily disintegrate into vesicles which can have a particulate surface facing either outward or inward. Such material is therefore not suitable to determine on which side of the membrane rhodopsin is located. To isolate intact disks it is necessary to first stabilize the disk structure by cross-linking with glutaraldehyde. With the proper homogenization technique, stacks consisting of a few disks were obtained which were analyzed after negative staining or after freeze-drying.

It was shown that even very extensive cross-linking did not appreciably change the appearance of the disks in freeze-fractured outer segments. This agrees with the observation by Brown (1972) who showed that it requires extensive cross-linking with glutaraldehyde to immobilize the rhodopsin molecules as demonstrated by photodichroism in the outer segments. They were thus cross-linked in 5% glutaraldehyde for 16 hr at 25°C. No photodichroism could be observed with less extensive cross-linking.

The isolated disks exposed a smooth cytoplasmic surface, which confirms that the interpretation of the location of the fracture planes is correct. Röhlich (1981) has published a picture of an outer segment fixed according to conventional methods with the exception that the tissue had been treated with tannic acid after double fixation with glutaraldehyde and osmium tetroxide. The picture showed each disk to consist of two layers located at the two cytoplasmic surfaces of the disk. Each of these layers appeared triple layered with a more faintly stained middle layer sandwiched between two more intensely stained layers. Between these two triple-layered components there was an ~100 Å-wide middle layer which was intensely stained. This is exactly the pattern that would be expected to be observed when a disk with the structure like that proposed here is viewed in a crosssection in conventionally fixed outer segments where extraction of lipids and proteins have been minimized. The triple-layered structure of the layers located at the cytoplasmic surfaces of the disk corresponds to the appearance of crosssections through lipid bilayers. The appearance of the opaque material in the middle of the disk corresponds to what can be expected from a layer of denatured protein.

The particle size distribution in the disk membrane was rather wide, from 40 Å to 90 Å. It did not reflect the predominance of a particle with a particular dimension or of aggregates of such a particle. The size distribution therefore did not correspond to what would be expected from a layer consisting predominantly of rhodopsin molecules. The packing of the particles was not as dense as that in the crista membrane. This agrees with the estimated packing density according to which there is sufficient space to surround each rhodopsin molecule by a 5 Å-wide water layer if uniformly distributed (Sjöstrand and Kreman, 1978). The discrepancy between the observed size distribution of the particles and the expected one can be explained by plastic deformation of partially aggregated particles.

In order to show that the particulate structure really was due to rhodopsin molecules and aggregates of rhodopsin molecules, experiments were carried out in which early stages in the extraction of rhodopsin were analyzed using cetyltrimethylammonium bromide as a solvent (Sjöstrand *et al.*, 1979). This led to a loss of particles. Instead of alternating particulate and smooth fracture faces, sequences of smooth fracture faces were observed (Fig. 21). After partial extraction of rhodopsin, the particles were separated by large enough distances that individual particles attached to a smooth surface could be measured with respect to their diameters. It then was shown that the particle size distribution exhibited two maxima, one close to 50 Å and the other at

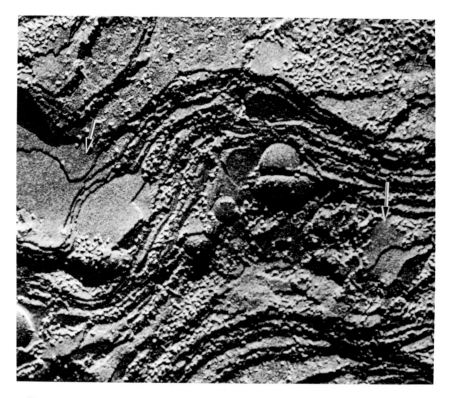

Fig. 21. Freeze-fracture through outer segment of photoreceptor cell in the guinea pig retina after partial extraction of rhodopsin. The particles on the particulate faces are considerably fewer than in normal outer segments and are completely absent on large parts of the particulate faces. Arrows point to an area wherein a sequence of membranes all membrane surfaces are smooth in contrast to the alternating smooth and particulate surfaces observed in outer segments that have not been extracted. Notice that the particles are partially separated by large enough spaces to make it possible to measure the diameter of individual particles positioned on a smooth surface, a condition required for reliable measurements. Magnification: 115,000×.

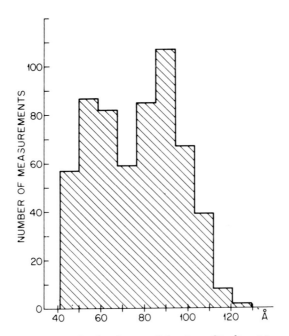

Fig. 22. Diagram showing the distribution of the sizes of isodiametric particles in outer segment disks after partial extraction of rhodopsin. In contrast to the particle size distribution in nonextracted retinas, the size distribution in the extracted retinas shows two maxima which agree with the presence of single rhodopsin molecules and tetrameres of rhodopsin molecules assuming that the diameter of the molecules is 40–50 Å. From Sjöstrand *et al.*, 1979a.

90 Å. This is the distribution expected from the rhodopsin molecules and tetramers of rhodopsin molecules (Fig. 22). The fact that rhodopsin could be removed to an appreciable extent without breaking down the lipid part of the membrane agrees with the concept that the membrane is a layered structure.

FUNCTION

In rod cells the outer segment disks are not connected to the plasma membrane. The effect of light on the state of polarization of the rod cell must therefore involve a transmission of a signal through the cytoplasm from the site of absorption of light by rhodopsin molecules in the disk membrane to the plasma membrane. It has been proposed that calcium may function as an internal transmitter with light releasing Ca^{2+} from the disks by making the membrane leaky for Ca^{2+} (Hagins, 1972).

To try to deduce a mechanism for the transmission of a signal with the limited knowledge available must necessarily lead to a highly speculative proposal. The fact that a single photon is sufficient to affect the state of polarization of the rod cell shows that the transmission is very efficient and is likely to involve an amplification mechanism. Our speculation is based entirely on an interpretation of the observed structure of the outer segment disks. These disks consist of two different components, the disk membrane and the edge structure. The disk membrane is the site for the primary photochemical reactions as is shown by the location of rhodopsin in this membrane. To find a function for the edge structure we can point to the location of this structure very close to the plasma membrane and to the fact that it consists of molecules that are probably not rhodopsin as judged from the large size of the particles in the edge structure. We have two different structures and two different functions to account for: energy transduction and signal transmission. Structurally it is reasonable to associate the edge structure with the latter function. The short distance separating the edge structure from the plasma membrane means that this structure is in a favorable position topographically for the transmission of a signal across the cytoplasm. It was therefore proposed that the edge structure is the site at which the transmitter, which can be Ca^{2+}, is released (Sjöstrand and Kreman, 1978). This requires, however, that a signal be transmitted to the edge structure from the rhodopsin molecules that have absorbed light. According to Lewis and co-workers' analysis by means of resonance Raman spectroscopy, a proton is released during the early photochemical reaction of rhodopsin (Lewis *et al.*, 1973; Lewis and Spoonhower, 1974). The disk structure encloses the rhodopsin molecules between two charge insulating lipid bilayers. It therefore could function as a disk-shaped conductor and the release of protons could lead to a conduction of a charge to the edge structure. To achieve an amplification the edge structure could respond with a cascade type of release of Ca^{2+}. The merit of this speculation is that it focuses the interest on the chemical nature of the edge structure.

The Plasma Membrane of the Outer Segment

STRUCTURE

In freeze-fractured outer segments the plasma membrane exposed one smooth and one particulate fracture face (Fig. 23). These faces represented an extreme case of lack of structural complementarity (Sjöstrand and Kreman, 1978). Scattered large particles were distributed over the smooth face. They extended high above the smooth surface. The particles on the particulate face were to a certain extent separated by narrow interparticle spaces which showed that they were not closely packed. Particles were missing completely within patches of varying size. The particulate face could be considerably distorted by plastic deformation. The thickness of the plasma membrane was determined to be about 100 Å on cross fractures exposing elevated edges of the membrane (Fig. 24). The membrane was considerably thinner at the smooth patches. The particulate face always faced the extracellular space whereas the smooth face was associated with fracture faces exposing the cytoplasm. These observations together with the complete lack of structural complementarity and the measured thickness of the membrane make it justified to locate the two fracture faces at the peripheral and the cytoplasmic surfaces of the membrane with the particulate face being the peripheral surface.

The particle size distribution in the particulate face differed from that of the disk membrane. The measurements were made on both types of membranes in the same electron micrographs to eliminate, as far as possible, differences introduced by varying conditions for plastic deformation which vary with the temperature of the tissue during cleavage. The observed difference shows that the two membranes are different and makes it justified to conclude that the difference involves the membrane proteins. Since the disk membrane is formed from folds that originate at the plasma membrane (Sjöstrand, 1959; Nilsson, 1964), it appears clear that these folds are not invaginations of the plasma membrane. Instead they consist of a special membrane which is assembled in the plasma membrane in the form of folds.

An interpretation of the observations with respect to the molecular structure of the plasma membrane can be seen in Fig. 25. This model is similar to that proposed for the disk membrane, with respect to the layered structure, with one lipid bilayer accounting for the smooth cytoplasmic surface of the membrane and one predominantly protein layer accounting for the particulate peripheral surface of the membrane. The measured thickness of the membrane accomodates both layers. Large complexes of protein molecules account for the large particles observed on the smooth face and are assumed to penetrate the bilayer. The possibility that other protein complexes penetrate the bilayer is also indicated.

FUNCTION

A main function of the plasma membrane is to form a barrier for ions and to control the ionic composition of the cytoplasm by active ion transport. The presence of a lipid bilayer that is predominantly free from penetrating pro-

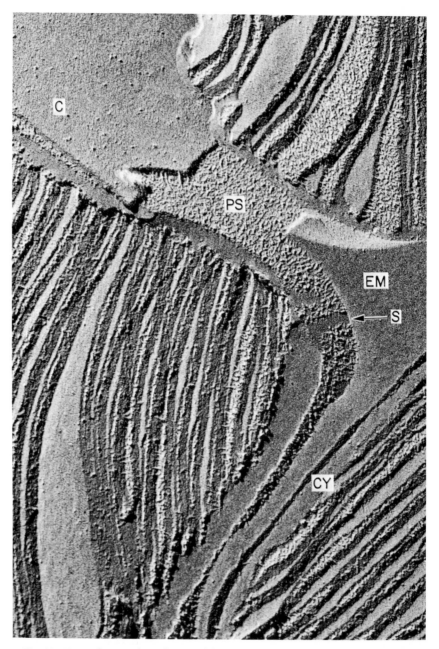

Fig. 23. Freeze-fracture through parts of three outer segments in photoreceptor cells in the guinea pig retina revealing the structure of the plasma membrane. The particulate peripheral surface (PS) shows some smooth patches (S). This surface faces the extracellular medium (EM). In the upper left corner and the lower right corner, the cytoplasmic surface of the plasma membrane (C) is exposed and in the latter location it is clearly shown that it faces the cytoplasm (CY). Magnification: 98,000×. From Sjöstrand and Kreman, 1979.

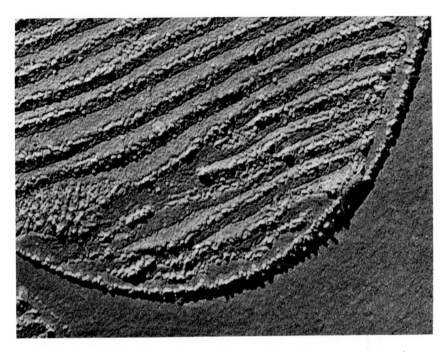

Fig. 24. Freeze-fracture of outer segment of photoreceptor cell in guinea pig retina, showing a cross-fracture through the plasma membrane which makes it possible to measure the thickness of the membrane. Magnification: 130,000×. From Sjöstrand and Kreman, 1979.

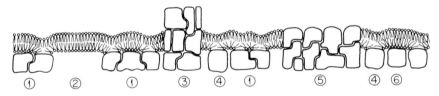

Fig. 25. Drawing illustrating the deduced structure of the plasma membrane of the outer segment of photoreceptor cells. The various numbers refer to different possible relationships of protein molecules and the lipid bilayer: 1. Aggregates of protein molecules which partially interact hydrophobically with the bilayer. 2. Lipid bilayer without association with protein molecules. 3. Large multimolecular protein complex penetrating the lipid bilayer. 4. Protein molecules interacting individually and hydrophobically with the bilayer. 5. Complex of protein molecules extending across entire membrane. 6. Protein molecule bound to the membrane by charge interaction with polar heads of lipid molecules. From Sjöstrand and Kreman, 1979.

tein molecules means that the bilayer structure is extensively used as a barrier for charged particles. The incorporation of proteins in artificial bilayers is associated with a considerable reduction of the ohmic resistance (Mueller *et al.*, 1962, 1964). This shows that such incorporation can have a deleterious effect on the barrier function. The large particles on the smooth face are assumed to be protein complexes involved in active ion transport.

Other functions of the plasma membrane are communication with other cells, offering of receptor sites for hormones, and interaction with neighboring cells. In the case of the outer segment, this interaction involves the pigment epithelium cells. The location of the proteins predominantly in the peripheral surface of the membrane appears as an adaptation to such functions, which all involve participation of proteins. Special proteins can act as recognition sites or antigenic sites and others as receptor sites. The latter would be associated with local transmembrane signal paths.

Outer Segment of Photoreceptor Cells: Conclusions

Both the outer segment disk membrane and the plasma membrane of the outer segment were found to be layered structures with one predominantly lipid layer and one predominantly protein layer. The lipids in these membranes can in this way form a lipid bilayer that is only broken up to a limited extent by the membrane proteins. This structure is reminiscent of the Danielli–Davson model for the plasma membrane. This model must, however, be modified extensively to satisfy the observed structural features of the disk membrane and the outer segment plasma membrane. The lipid bilayer is not an uninterrupted layer as assumed by Danielli and Davson. Instead, complexes of protein molecules penetrate the bilayer. Furthermore, there is no evidence for two layers of unfolded peptide chains sandwiching the lipid bilayer. Instead, the proteins retain a globular conformation when associated with the bilayer. They are in addition arranged asymmetrically with respect to the bilayer.

From a structural point of view, conditions are fulfilled for considerable motility of the protein molecules because the particles in the particulate fracture faces are not closely packed, in contrast to the situation in the crista membrane. The observed diffusion of rhodopsin molecules in the outer segment can therefore be explained. A similar motility of the protein molecules is also likely to apply to the plasma membrane. The particle-free patches in the plasma membrane can be artifactual and a consequence of a phase change in the lipid bilayer in connection with the immersion of the tissue in a cold fixative. This could explain the great variation in the presence of such areas, which can be missing completely from even large areas exposed by fracturing. Until an artifactual formation of these patches has been ruled out, they should not be considered seriously as a special structural feature of the plasma membrane. If the pictures of the freeze-fractured membranes had been interpreted in the conventional way, it would have been impossible to deduce a structure of the membranes that involved two layers. All particles would then automatically have been interpreted to be intramembrane particles and the deduced membrane model would have been a repetition of the theme now monotonously repeated and illustrated in published papers showing how membranes have been cleaved into two halves with intramembrane particles attached to the exposed surfaces. The 100 Å thickness of the edge of the membrane would in this case represent half the thickness of the membrane which therefore would be about 200 Å thick, a thickness which is highly unrealistic. The lack of complementarity would be impossible to explain. Such a way to interpret the information would thus leave certain basic aspects of the observations unexplained.

The analysis of the structure of the disk membrane and of the plasma membrane has added still another structural pattern to those deduced for the mitochondrial membranes. Neither of these membranes conform with the Singer–Nicolson (1972) membrane model and these additional examples make it even more justified to conclude that no universal membrane model is applicable but represents an unrealistic oversimplification.

With respect to membrane fluidity, the observations support the concept that, at least in certain types of membranes, protein complexes and protein molecules can diffuse within the membrane. It is, however, unlikely that such fluidity applies to all membranes. In membranes with a complex metabolic function like the crista membrane, the fluidity is likely to be restricted to the kind of molecular motility proposed by Sjöstrand and Barajas (1968). It is also likely that the same restricted motility applies to the molecules within the large molecular complexes in the outer surface membrane of mitochondria and in the plasma membrane. This restricted motility can be of crucial importance to the function by allowing a maintenance of a particular type of molecular organization within these complexes. The conditions for molecular interactions within these complexes might in this way be similar to those characterizing the crista membrane in mitochondria by offering a similar environment and similar facilitation of molecular interactions. The molecular organization of the crista membrane could, in principle, represent a universal model for metabolically active membranes and for enzymatically active domains in membranes like the domains involved in active transport.

References

Andersson-Cedergren, E. (1959). *J. Ultrastruct. Res. Suppl. 1*.

Bachmann, L., and Schmidt, W. W. (1971). *Proc. Nat. Acad. Sci. USA* **68**, 2149.

Blaurock, A. E. (1972). *Chem. Phys. Lipids* **8**, 285–291.

Blaurock, A. E., and Wilkins, M. H. F. (1969). *Nature (London)* **233**, 906–909.

Blaurock, A. E., and Wilkins, M. H. F. (1972). *Nature (London)* **236**, 313–314.

Branton, D., Bullivant, S., Gilula, N. B., Karnovsky, M. J., Moor, H., Mühlethaler, K., Northcote, D. H., Packer, L., Satir, B., Speth, U., Staehelin, L. A., Steere, R. L., and Weinstein. R. S. (1975). *Science* **190**, 54–56.

Brown, P. K. (1972). *Nature (London)* **236**, 35–38.

Corless, J. M. (1972). *Nature (London)* **237**, 229–231.

Corless, J. M., Cobbs, W. H. III, Costello, M. J., and Robertson, J. D. (1976). *Exp. Eye Res.* **23**, 295–324.

Daems, W. TH., and Wisse, E. (1966). *J. Ultrastruct. Res.* **16**, 123.

Douzou, P. (1977). *Adv. Enzymol.* **45**, 157.

Fettiplace, R., Andrews, D. M., and Haydon, D. A. (1971). *J. Membrane Biol.* **5**, 277.

Fleischer, S., Fleischer, B., and Stoeckenius, W. (1965). *Fed. Proc.* **24**, 296.

Fuller, S. D., Capaldi, R. A., and Henderson, R. (1979). *J. Mol. Biol.* **134**, 305–327.

Gras, W. J., and Worthington, C. R. (1969). *Proc. Nat. Acad. Sci. USA* **63**, 233–238.

Hackenbrock, C. R. (1966). *J. Cell Biol.* **30**, 269.

Hackenbrock, C. R. (1968). *J. Cell Biol.* **37**, 345.

Hagins, W. A. (1972). *Ann. Rev. Biophys. Bioeng.* **1**, 131.

Hallier, U. W., and Park, R. B. (1969a). *Plant Physiol.* **44**, 535–539.

Hallier, U. W., and Park, R. B. (1969b). *Plant Physiol.* **44**, 544–546.

Heller, J. (1968). *Biochemistry* **7**, 2906–2913.

Hovmöller, S., Leonard, K., and Weiss, H. (1981). *FEBS Lett.* **123**, 118–122.

Huang, C. H., Keyhani, E., and Lee, C. P. (1973). *Biochim. Biophys. Acta* **305**, 455.

Joly, M. (1965). "A Physico-chemical Approach to the Denaturation of Proteins." Academic Press, New York.

Kauzmann, W. (1959). *Adv. Protein Chem.* **14**, 1–63.

Klingenberg, M. (1979). *Trends Biochem.* **4**, 249.

Klingenberg, J., Riccio, P., Aquila, H., Schmiedt, B., Grebe, K., and Topitsch, P. (1974). *In* "Membrane Proteins in Transport and Phosphorylation" (G. F. Azzone, M. E. Klingenberg, E. Quagliariello, and N. Siliprandi, eds.), p. 229. North-Holland Publ., Amsterdam.

Lenard, J., and Singer, S. J. (1968). *J. Cell Biol.* **37**, 117–121.

Lewis, A., and Spoonhower, J. (1974). *In* "Spectroscopy in Biology and Chemistry" (S. Chen and S. Yip, eds.), Chapter 11. Academic Press, New York.

Lewis, A., Fager, R., and Abrahamson, E. W. (1973). *J. Raman Spectrosc.* **1**, 465.

Mitchell, P. (1961). *Nature (London)* **19**, 144.

Mitchell, P. (1967). *Fed. Proc.* **26**, 1370.

Mitchell, P. (1977). *FEBS Lett.* **78**, 1.

Mueller, P., Rudin, D. O., Tien, H. T., and Wescott, W. C. (1962). *Nature (London)* **194**, 979–980.

Mueller, P., Rudin, D. O., Tien, H. T., and Wescott, W. C. (1964). *Recent Prog. Surf. Sci.* **1**, 379–393.

Nilsson, S. E. G. (1964). *J. Ultrastruct. Res.* **11**, 581.

Parsons, D. F., Williams, G. R., and Chance, B. (1966). *Ann. N.Y. Acad. Sci.* **137**, 643–666.

Quiocho, F. A., and Richards, F. M. (1964). *Proc. Nat. Acad. Sci. USA* **52**, 833–839.

Quiocho, F. A., and Richards, F. M. (1966). *Biochemistry* **5**, 4062–4079.

Röhlich, P. (1981). *Acta Histochem. Suppl.* **23**, 123–136.

Schmidt, W. J. (1928). *Arch. Exp. Zellforsch.* **6**, 350–366.

Schmidt, W. J. (1935a). *Ber. Oberhess. Ges. Natur Heilk. Giessen Naturwiss. Abt.* **16**, 170–174.

Schmidt, W. J. (1935b). *Zool. Anz.* **109**, 245–251.

Schmidt, W. J. (1935c). *Z. Zellforsch. Mikrosk. Anat.* **22**, 485–522.

Schmidt, W. J. (1937). "Die Doppelbrechung von Karyoplasma, Zytoplasma und Metaplasma." Gebrüder Bornträger, Berlin.

Schnaitman, C., and Greenawalt, J. W. (1968). *J. Cell Biol.* **38**, 158.

Singer, S. J., and Nicolson, G. L. (1972). *Science* **175**, 720.

Sjöstrand, F. S. (1948). *J. Appl. Phys.* **19**, 1188.

Sjöstrand, F. S. (1949). *J. Cell. Comp. Physiol.* **33**, 383–403.

Sjöstrand, F. S. (1953). *J. Cell. Comp. Physiol.* **42**, 15.

Sjöstrand, F. S. (1959). *Rev. Mod. Phys.* **31**, 301; *In* "Biophysical Science - A study Program" (J. L. Oncley, F. O. Schmitt, R. C. Williams, M. D. Rosenberg, and R. H. Bolt, eds.). Wiley, New York.

Sjöstrand, F. S. (1960). *Radiation Res. Suppl.* **2**, 349–386.

Sjöstrand, F. S. (1967). "Electron Microscopy of Cells and Tissues," Vol. 1. Academic Press, New York.

Sjöstrand, F. S. (1977). *J. Ultrastruct. Res.* **59**, 292–319.

Sjöstrand, F. S. (1979). *J. Ultrastruct. Res.* **69**, 378–420.

Sjöstrand, F. S. (1980a). *J. Ultrastruct. Res.* **72**, 174–188.

Sjöstrand, F. S. (1980b). *Biol. Cell.* **39**, 217–220.

Sjöstrand, F. S. (1982). *In* "Subcellular Biochemistry," (D. B. Roodyn, ed.), Vol. 9. (in press).

Sjöstrand, F. S., and Baker, F. S. (1958). *J. Ultrastruct. Res.* **1**, 239–246.

Sjöstrand, F. S., and Barajas, L. (1968). *J. Ultrastruct. Res.* **25**, 121–155.

Sjöstrand, F. S., and Barajas, L. (1970). *J. Ultrastruct. Res.* **32**, 293–306.

Sjöstrand, F. S., and Bernhard, W. (1976). *J. Ultrastruct. Res.* **56**, 233–246.

Sjöstrand, F. S., and Cassell, R. Z. (1978a). *J. Ultrastruct. Res.* **63**, 111–137.

Sjöstrand, F. S., and Cassell, R. Z. (1978b). *J. Ultrastruct. Res.* **63**, 138–154.

Sjöstrand, F. S., and Halma, H. (1978). *J. Ultrastruct. Res.* **64**, 216–269.

Sjöstrand, F. S., and Kreman, M. (1978). *J. Ultrastruct. Res.* **65**, 195–226.

Sjöstrand, F. S., and Kreman, M. (1979). *J. Ultrastruct. Res.* **66**, 254–275.

Sjöstrand, F. S., and Kretzer, F. (1975). *J. Ultrastruct. Res.* **53**, 1–28.

Sjöstrand, F. S., Andersson-Cedergren, E., and Karlsson, U. (1964). *Nature (London)* **202**, 1075–1078.

Sjöstrand, F. S., Dubochet, J., Wurtz, M., and Kellenberger, E. (1978). *J. Ultrastruct. Res.* **65**, 23–29.

Sjöstrand, F. S., Kreman, M., and Crescitelli, F. (1979a). *J. Ultrastruct. Res.* **69**, 53–67.

Soper, J. W., Decker, G. W., and Pedersen, P. L. (1979b). *J. Biol. Chem.* **254**, 11170–11176.

Srere, P. A. (1980). *Trends Biochem. Sci.* **5**, 120.

Tanford, C. (1973). "The Hydrophobic Effect: Formation of Micells and Biological Membranes." Wiley, New York.

Tanford, C., Hauenstein, J. D., and Rands, D. G. (1955a). *J. Am. Chem. Soc.* **77**, 6409.

Tanford, C., Buckley, C. E. III, De, P.K., and Lively, E. P. (1962). *J. Biol. Chem.* **237**, 1168.

Tanford, C., Swanson, S. A., and Shore, W. S. (1955b). *J. Am. Chem. Soc.* **77**, 6414.

Tanford, C., Marler, E., Jury, E. *et al.* (1964). *J. Biol. Chem.* **239**, 4034–4040.

Tanford, C., Kawahara, K., and Lapanje, S. (1966). *J. Biol. Chem.* **241**, 1921–1923.

Todd, R. D., and Douglas, M. G. (1981). *J. Biol. Chem.* **256**, 6984–6989.

142   Fritiof S. Sjöstrand

Tokuyasu, K. T. (1973). *J. Cell Biol.* **57**, 551.

Unwin, P. N., and Henderson, R. (1975). *J. Mol. Biol.* **94**(3), 425–440.

Utsumi, K., and Packer, L. (1967). *Arch. Biochem.* **120**, 404–412.

Vanderkooi, G., and Sundaralingham, M. (1970). *Proc. Nat. Acad. Sci. USA* **67**, 233–238.

Weiss, H., and Kolb, H. J. (1979). *Eur. J. Biochem.* **99**, 139–149.

Williams, R. J. P. (1961). *J. Theoret. Biol.* **1**, 1.

Williams, R. J. P. (1978). *In* "Current Topics in Bioenergetics" (D. R. Sanadi, ed.), Vol. 3, p. 79. Academic Press, New York.

Worthington, C. R. (1973). *Exp. Eye Res.* **17**, 487–501.

Worthington, C. R. (1974). *Annu. Rev. Biophys. Bioeng.* **3**, 53–80.

Yeager, M. J. (1975). *In Brookhaven Symp. Biol.* (B. P. Schoenborn, ed.), Vol. 27, p. III-3.

Chapter *4*

Correlation of Membrane Models with Transmission Electron Microscopic Images

Ronald B. Luftig and Paul N. McMillan

Introduction: The Unit Membrane Model and the Unit
   Membrane Image.. 143
Problems of Adequate Fixation for Erythrocyte Ghosts................. 146
   The Unit Membrane versus the Dense Band-Image................. 147
   Analysis of Artifacts Caused by Classical OsO_4
      Fixation: A Biochemical and Immunological Approach 153
   Problems with Glutaraldehyde Fixation........................... 158
   Preservation of Membrane Structure by Other Fixatives............. 161
Fixation in Other Membrane Systems.............................. 163
New Techniques.. 165
References... 168

Introduction: The Unit Membrane Model and the Unit Membrane Image

The thin skin or membrane that encompasses the outer surface of a wide variety of cells from different organisms serves many functions, e.g., it provides selective permeability channels, adhesion sites for various substrata, or receptor sites for signaling macromolecules (MacLennan *et al.*, 1971; Spatz and Strittmatter, 1973; Hynes, 1976; Oppenheim and Rosenstreich, 1976; Bergman and Haimovitch, 1977; Ishii and Nakae, 1980). The membrane also acts as a structural barrier, separating the cytoplasmic contents of the cell from its outer milieu (Steck, 1974; Yu and Branton, 1976). Most, if not all, of these membrane functions are carried out by proteins although, in some cases, we cannot rule out the functional involvement of lipid components, as in the methylation of phospholipids that occurs after mitogen stimulation (Hirata *et al.*, 1980). How the membrane proteins carry out such diverse functions and where they are localized at the cell surface has been a puzzle to cytologists and cell biologists for over fifty years. Only now, as specific membrane systems (e.g., human erythrocytes, gram-negative bacteria, rat CNS myelin, bovine rod outer segments and slime molds) are being dissected into their component protein parts is it possible to probe these questions at the molecular level. Before we consider the question of protein localization as well as structure and function in these specific membrane systems, we will provide a historical perspective of what constitutes an accurate general model of membrane structure.

The idea that all membranes have a similar backbone or bilayer composed of phospholipids was originally proposed by Danielli and Davson (1935); this concept has held up through the onslaught of many modern biophysical techniques over the past forty-five years. It was derived from experimental observations of Gorter and Grendel (1925) as well as consideration of the constraints imposed on the constituent phospholipids to remain in a bilayer configuration, namely, polar head groups facing out to the aqueous phase and hydrophobic tails buried within the bilayer. This burying of the hydrophobic tails of phospholipids itself provides for a force based on repulsion whereby the assembly of the cell membrane backbone can occur. Quantitation, in thermodynamic terms, of the various stages of membrane assembly using this "hydrophobic effect" has been examined in detail by Tanford (1973, 1978). Briefly, the alkyl chains of amphiphilic molecules (polar head group plus one hydrocarbon moiety) or phospholipids (which contain two hydrocarbon chains per head group) are postulated to be "squeezed out of the aqueous medium" and aggregate in the middle of the bilayer. Gradually vesicles are formed as the concentration of phospholipid molecules increases and, finally, proteins are bound to the membranes by tight hydrophobic anchors (integral proteins) or are loosely associated by anionic or electrostatic interaction with polar head groups at the bilayer surface (peripheral proteins). The classification of membrane proteins as integral or peripheral was proposed by Singer and Nicolson (1972) in their "fluid mosaic model" and it has gained wide acceptance over the years. The fluidity of the membrane bilayer, and thereby the rates at which certain integral proteins move laterally within the bilayer is determined by the amount and type of phospholipid in the bilayer as well as the amount of cholesterol present. Cholesterol tends to decrease the fluidity and thereby the mobility of proteins associated with the bilayer. For example, as shown by Warren *et al.* (1975), when phospholipids in the lipid bilayer surrounding a calcium transport protein are replaced by cholesterol, there is an inactivation of membrane ATPase activity. The phospholipid annulus surrounding the protein would normally exclude the cholesterol present in the membrane so that the proteins are free to segregate laterally. Additional cholesterol enrichment studies showed similar alterations, namely, the biconcave shape of human erythrocytes, which would be altered in hypotonic saline (0.42% NaCl), is maintained when 10 μ*M* cholesterol sulfate is added (Bleau *et al.*, 1975). The addition of cholesterol also alters the surface labeling of spectrin, actin, and band 3 (Borochov *et al.*, 1979). However, this latter result needs to be interpreted with some caution since it has been shown that enriching erythrocyte ghosts with 65–100% cholesterol leads to no difference in the accessibility of exposed regions of band 3 to proteases (Kirby and Green, 1980). Other techniques that have been developed to examine how membrane lipids interact with integral proteins will be presented later.

The bilayer concept of membrane structure discussed above (Danielli and Davson, 1935) proved to be consistent with the trilamellar image of membrane structure which arose from X-ray diffraction analysis (Schmitt *et al.*, 1935; Bear *et al.*, 1941; Finean and Burge, 1962) and electron microscopy (Robertson, 1957) of the myelin sheath of peripheral nerves. The myelin sheath appears as a repeating unit structure of about 60–80 Å by both techniques. Other studies correlating X-ray diffraction and electron microscopy of retinal rod outer segments (Blaurock and Wilkins, 1969; Gras and Worthington, 1969; Corless, 1972; Robertson, 1972) supported this repeating unit membrane structure. Further, the observation in the electron microscope of a trilamellar image for a variety of membrane systems led Robertson (1959) to propose the general term "unit membrane image" for the structure of all membranes. This concept proved to be useful for describing the underlying phospholipid bilayer of all membranes; however as scientists became more interested in determining how the different proteins, which play diverse functional roles, were localized in membranes, a better representation of membrane structure was sought. In the unit membrane or trilamellar image, the representation of proteins was solely at the outer and inner surfaces of the phospholipid bilayer. It is clear from the fluid mosaic membrane model as well as freeze-fracture, nuclear magnetic resonance, and immunological studies, however, that most membrane systems contain integral proteins which protrude partly or completely through the bilayer. Some examples of this are found in the membranes of erythrocyte ghosts (Bretscher, 1973), rod outer segments (Röhlich, 1976), and the sarcoplasmic reticulum (Saito *et al.*, 1978). In freeze-fracture electron micrographs, these embedded proteins appear as intramembrane particles. This has been seen with the vertebrate photoreceptor membranes (Mason *et al.*, 1974), erythrocyte ghosts (Pinto da Silva and Nicholson, 1974; Yu and Branton, 1976), *Acholeplasma laidlawii* (Tourtellote and Zupnik, 1973), and even myelin (Pinto da Silva and Miller, 1975). It should be further noted that the biochemical composition of most of these membranes is roughly 50% protein and 50% lipid. An oddity in this regard is the camel erythrocyte membrane where the protein-to-lipid ratio is 3:1 (Eitan *et al.*, 1976). This membrane is particularly rich in integral proteins and intramembranous particles which are more closely organized than in human erythrocytes. Myelin is also an exception in that it contains only 20% protein. However in all of these membranes integral as well as surface proteins are key structural components. Then why, we ask, has not some transbilayer structure been visualized for these systems by thin-section electron microscopy? Moreover why do all membranes exhibit a unit membrane image? One certainly would expect that membranes with different protein compositions, performing different functions, should exhibit different images in the electron microscope. An answer to this is that the earlier use of X-ray diffraction analysis, which was apparently appropriate for determining the periodicity of repeated unit structures such as phospholipid bilayers or myelin sheaths, was in most instances not useful for analyzing the location of protein molecules that are oriented within the plane of the membrane. A preliminary study suggests, however, that with appropriate manipulation, e.g., removing nonintegral proteins from erythrocyte ghosts (Lesslauer, 1980), some useful information may be obtained by this technique.

In summary, we contend that although the original unit membrane model (Danielli and Davson, 1935) and its more recent version, the fluid mosaic model (Singer and Nicholson, 1972), provide for an accurate representation vis á vis the underlying lipid bilayer structure of membranes, the unit membrane image, which ascribes a trilamellar image to all membranes (Robertson, 1959), needs to be reinvestigated.

Problems of Adequate Fixation for Erythrocyte Ghosts

The human erythrocyte membrane is probably the most extensively studied biological membrane. This is not only because erythrocyte membranes can be prepared in large quantities in homogeneous form by simple hypotonic lysis procedures (Dodge *et al.*, 1963), but also because they represent a readily accessible cell for studies of the molecular basis of human disease states (Sauberman *et al.*, 1979) and for studying how minor changes in proteins are related to genetic polymorphisms (Harrel and Morrison, 1979).

In reexamining the methods by which human erythrocyte ghosts are fixed and processed for thin-section electron microscopy, we have come to the conclusion that the trilamellar image represents, for the most part, an artifact due to the removal and/or degradation of proteins by treatment with 0.1 to 1% osmium tetroxide (McMillan and Luftig, 1973, 1975). Surprisingly even after membrane proteins have been cross-linked with 5% glutaraldehyde, up to 70% of the proteins can still be solubilized by postfixation with 1% OsO_4 (McMillan and Luftig, 1973). The evidence supporting these contentions, and a discussion of alternative fixation protocols, will be provided below.

THE UNIT MEMBRANE VERSUS THE DENSE-BAND IMAGE

We first showed (McMillan and Luftig, 1973, 1975) that when 5% glutaraldehyde alone was used to fix erythrocyte ghosts, an entirely different image from the classic trilamellar image was observed, namely, an electron-dense band image with a membrane width of about 160 Å was seen (Fig. 1C). The classic trilamellar image of about 80 Å was only seen if the ghosts were fixed in 1% OsO_4, with or without prior fixation in 5% glutaraldehyde (Fig. 1A and B). As a matter of technical interest, it should be pointed out that these initial studies were quite difficult to perform since the extensively washed erythrocyte ghosts did not form a cohesive pellet, and they were also difficult to visualize in the EPON block as it was being sectioned. We overcame these problems by mixing the glutaraldehyde-fixed membranes with an equal volume of 1% Bacto-agar to form a cohesive pellet, then staining with Wright's stain (a histological stain for erythrocytes; Wright, 1902) after the sample hardened. The denseband image we found with glutaraldehyde fixation alone (Fig. 1C) appears to be a valid representation of the erythrocyte membrane since it is comparable to the Triton X-100 insoluble fibrillar matrix seen by Yu *et al.* (1973). Further, when contrasted with the less dense membrane images of Fig. 1A and B, it appears to us that treatment with 1% OsO_4 has caused the leaching of material from the erythrocyte membrane. This contention has been supported by several lines of evidence: (*a*) there is a direct correlation between fixation with increasing OsO_4 concentrations and the increased appearance of the trilamellar image (Table I); (*b*) the amount of protein found in washes after fixation and dehydration of the ghosts prior to embedding is eightfold greater after 1% OsO_4 treatment than

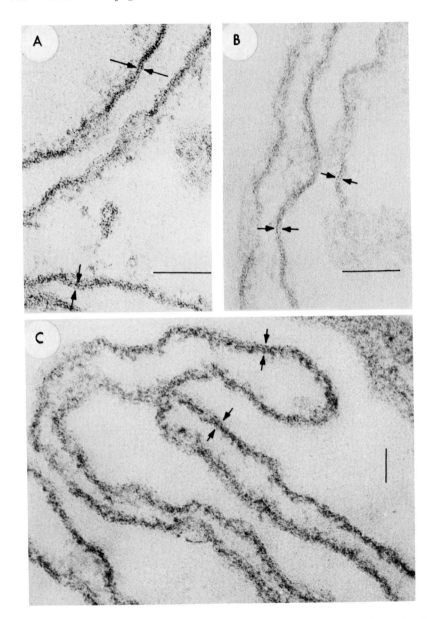

Fig. 1. Human erythrocyte ghost membranes fixed in (**A**) 1% OsO₄; (**B**) 5% glutaraldehyde followed by 1% OsO₄; and (**C**) 5% glutaraldehyde alone. Arrows designate membrane widths. (**A**) and (**B**) are shown at a magnification (174,000×) twice that of (**C**) (87,000×) to better illustrate the trilamellar appearance of the membrane. The bar represents 1 μm in all cases. Adapted from McMillan and Luftig (1973), courtesy of Proceedings of the National Academy of Sciences.

TABLE I

Quantitation of the Percentage Electron-Dense and Trilamellar Image Obtained
after Postfixation of Erythrocyte Ghosts at Several Concentrations of OsO$_4$[a]

Fixative (w/v)	Morphology of ghost image (%)[b]		
	Trilamellar	Dense-band	Unmeasurable[c]
1.0% OsO$_4$	31.0	8.1	60.9
0.1% OsO$_4$	42.0	9.8	48.2
0.05% OsO$_4$	46.5	26.0	27.5
0.025% OsO$_4$	7.8	44.1	48.1
5% glutaraldehyde	4.2	45.2	50.6

[a] Adapted from McMillan and Luftig (1975), courtesy of the Journal of Ultrastructural Research.

[b] At least 20 separate ghosts were measured for each point. Our determination of trilamellar and dense-band regions are typically characterized by the examples seen in Fig. 1A and Fig. 1C, respectively.

[c] On the average, about 50% of the total region for a single ghost was unmeasurable. This probably reflects partial fragmentation of erythrocyte ghosts or the cutting of a region of the ghost in a tangential section.

after 5% glutaraldehyde-only fixation; and (c) exposure to increasing concentrations of OsO$_4$ decreases the stability of membrane proteins. This latter point was determined by using an assay where the amount of protein solubilized from ghosts after exposure to a 5 mM EDTA solution was measured. We found by this assay that after fixation of ghosts with 1% OsO$_4$ for 2 hr, 5mM EDTA solubilized over 90% of the membrane proteins. In fact even lower OsO$_4$ concentrations (e.g., 0.1%) still led to extensive solubilization of membrane proteins (e.g., 50%). Only when concentrations of OsO$_4$ were used in the range of 0.006% was the extraction minimal. The data for this experiment are shown in Table II. The molecular basis for this phenomenon, i.e., the release of protein after OsO$_4$ fixation, appears due in part to the breaking of covalent bonds by OsO$_4$ (Maupin-Szamier and Pollard, 1978), although cross-linking of phospholipids associated with proteins in the bilayer may play a secondary role. In summary, we have shown thus far that a direct correlation exists between the relative solubility and release of membrane proteins and the appearance of the trilamellar image.

In addition to the above experiments utilizing thin-section electron microscopy, still other correlations exist between erythrocyte ghost images obtained after OsO$_4$ fixation and protein release. For example, as seen in Figs. 2 and 3, there is a 1:1 relationship between the exposure of membranes to increasing concentrations of OsO$_4$ followed by 5 mM EDTA solubiliza-

TABLE II

Solubilization of Erythrocyte Ghost Proteins
by 5 mM EDTA Treatment
after Fixation with OsO_4[a,b]

OsO_4 (w/v) used (%)	Protein solubilized (%)
1.0	78.9
0.1	58.9
0.05	40.2
0.012	14.1
0.006	2.6

[a] Exposure to 5 mM EDTA (pH 7.5) was for 2 hr at 20°C after ghosts were fixed with OsO_4. Protein extraction was measured by the Lowry et al. (1951) assay. Over 90% of the starting material could be accounted for as a sum of the supernatant and pellet protein remaining after solubilization. An average of 12.0% protein was solubilized when 5% glutaraldehyde fixation alone was employed instead of OsO_4. This is considered background and was subtracted from each sample point.

[b] Adapted from McMillan and Luftig (1975), courtesy of the Journal of Ultrastructural Research.

tion, and the disappearance of intramembrane particles as assayed by freeze-fracture electron microscopy. These intramembrane particles correlate in some as yet undefined way with the state of integral proteins in the membranes (Hong and Hubbell, 1972; Parish, 1975; Pinto da Silva and Nicholson, 1974). With erythrocyte ghosts it is believed that they represent an oligomeric form of band 3, the major transmembrane protein which is looped through the membrane more than once and has its amino terminus exposed to the cytoplasm (Steck, 1978). Yu and Branton (1976) showed that such particles could be observed when band 3 protein was reconstituted with lipid vesicles *in vitro*, and Weinstein et al. (1978) showed that such particles could be removed by selective enzymatic digestion of band 3 protein as assayed by using band 3 protein specific antisera. Thus it can be said that the use of OsO_4 also leads to the removal of integral membrane proteins.

At this point it may be argued, though, that even if the trilamellar image is an artifact of fixation due to the removal of proteins, the electron-dense band

$OsO_4(\%)$ PF   EF

0

0,1

0,025

0,006

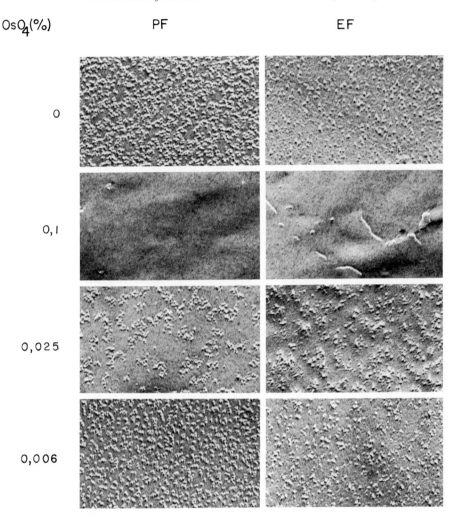

Fig. 2. Freeze-fracture appearance of human erythrocyte ghosts after exposure to OsO_4 at various concentrations followed by 5 mM EDTA solubilization. PF and EF signify protoplasmic and external fracture faces, respectively. Note that 0.1% OsO_4 and higher concentrations lead to complete solubilization of all intramembranous particles (unpublished observations). Magnification is 63,000×. Reproduced from Luftig *et al.* (1977), courtesy of Life Sciences.

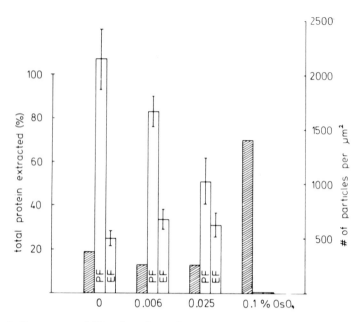

Fig. 3. Quantitation of EF and PF freeze-fracture particles seen after 5 mM EDTA solubilization of OsO_4-fixed human erythroctye ghosts. Shaded bars represent percentage of protein
solubilized. Reproduced from Luftig *et al.* (1977), courtesy of Life Sciences.

observed in Fig. 1C may, itself, be an artifact. The dense-band image could
be thought of as arising as a result of the collapse of membrane proteins. This
putative collapse could occur because phospholipids are extensively removed during the processing of glutaraldehyde-fixed ghosts for thin-section
electron microscopy, i.e., the ghosts are dehydrated through organic solvents and, with glutaraldehyde-only fixation, we expect that there would be
a substantial loss of phospholipids (Korn and Weisman, 1966; McMillan and
Luftig, 1975). However it turns out that the dense-band image is not dependent on the percentage of lipid retained in the ghosts since: (*a*) use of a
relatively low OsO_4 concentration, e.g., 0.025%, which allows stabilization
of more than 80% of the phospholipids, results in images identical to those
found with 5% glutaraldehyde alone (McMillan and Luftig, 1975); and (*b*)
treatment of erythrocyte ghosts with Triton X-100, a detergent which re-
moves most of the lipid, leaves behind an insoluble fibrillar structure which
can be visualized as an interconnecting meshwork of protein-like material
similar to the dense-band image (Yu *et al.*, 1973).

Analysis of Artifacts Caused by Classical OsO$_4$ Fixation: A Biochemical and Immunological Approach

As indicated above, the trilamellar image, consisting of two electron-dense lines (about 20 Å each) separated by about a 30 Å clear area, had been taken for many years as a literal representation of the unit membrane. The clear area was considered the hydrophobic interior and the dense area represented polar head group–protein interactions. However, as we showed for the erythrocyte ghost, this relatively featureless image (Fig. 1A,B) which is observed for almost all membranes fixed by "classical" methods, e.g., utilizing 1% OsO$_4$ or 2–5% glutaraldehyde followed by 1% OsO$_4$, is an oversimplification caused by the removal of membrane proteins (McMillan and Luftig, 1973, 1975; Luftig *et al.*, 1977). This contention also supports earlier observations made by Sjöstrand and Barajas (1968) who examined mitochondrial membranes using similar glutaraldehyde-only fixation conditions and observed densely staining, presumably proteinaceous material appearing between the lines of the trilamellar image.

The evidence discussed thus far in support of our contention that the trilamellar image of erythrocyte ghosts is an artifact can be summarized as follows: increasing OsO$_4$ concentrations leads to a concomitant (*a*) increase in the trilamellar versus dense-band image; (*b*) increased solubilization of membrane proteins by 5 mM EDTA treatment; and (*c*) loss of intramembranous particles as visualized by freeze-fracture electron microscopy.

These studies lead us to ask two additional questions, namely, What specific proteins are removed from the ghosts? and How are they removed? With regard to the first question we have shown, in Table II, that 80% of the membrane protein can be removed after 1% OsO$_4$ fixation, and from the above discussion we have indicated that some of it is band 3 (nomenclature of Fairbanks *et al.*, 1971). We thus expect that among the remainder of proteins removed will be the peripherally associated spectrin complex (bands 1 and 2), which constitutes up to 40% of the membrane protein. This has been tested for with an immunological procedure, namely, the Ouchterlony (1949) double-immunodiffusion technique. An antiserum raised in rabbits against the distilled water extract of fresh, unfixed erythrocyte ghosts (generously provided to us by Dr. J. Reynolds, Duke University Medical Center), was reacted with proteins solubilized from OsO$_4$ treated ghosts. This extract included four major polypeptides with apparent molecular weights of 220,000, 200,000, 185,000, and 175,000, as analyzed by SDS–PAGE (Reynolds and Trayer, 1971). These polypeptides probably correspond to spectrin bands 1 and 2 as well as to the syndein bands 2.1 and 2.2 (Yu and Goodman,

1979) (see Fig. 6). Band 2.1 has been designated as ankyrin (Bennett and Stenbuck, 1980) because it is thought to anchor spectrin to the cytoplasmic portion of band 3. This has been confirmed in studies where the formation of noncovalent complexes between an exposed segment of band 2.1 and band 3 were followed by antibody competition analysis (Litman *et al.*, 1980). When we tested our antiserum against the extract used in raising it (control), four precipitin bands were observed, as expected. When the protein solubilized from 1% OsO_4-fixed ghosts by 5 mM EDTA treatment was tested against this antiserum, three precipitin bands were found (Fig. 4). Further, since these three bands were continuous with the three fastest migrating bands precipitated from the control antigen material, it appears that these antigens are the same. The most external of the bands may actually be two bands since in the control extract the two slowest bands migrate very closely together and then split at the antigen well region. Thus probably all four polypeptides seen in the extract are released after OsO_4 treatment. In conclusion we can say that both integral membrane proteins and peripheral proteins, namely, band 3 protein as well as spectrin and perhaps band 2.1, are solubilized after exposure to OsO_4. Fig. 4 also shows that relatively little material was solubilized when 5% glutaraldehyde-only fixation was employed.

With regard to the second question raised above, namely, How does OsO_4 fixation lead to protein removal from erythrocyte ghosts, we developed an alternative method to examine protein instability other than solubilization by subsequent 5 mM EDTA treatment. This approach was also designed to help us understand how 70% of the protein could still be solubilized from ghosts by 1% OsO_4 after they had been prefixed with 5% glutaraledhyde (McMillan and Luftig, 1973). It is particularly important to understand this latter mechanism because OsO_4 will likely continue to be utilized as a postfixation step after glutaraldehyde prefixation due to its lipid stabilization properties. The ability of OsO_4 to extensively cross-link unsaturated lipids was originally shown by Korn (1967) and is discussed in Hayat (1970). The formation of an osmate–diester cross-linked lipid network was determined by electron-spin reasonance because of the inhibition to free rotation of spin labels within the plane of the membrane bilayer (Jost and Griffith, 1973).

We ask, How could the stabilizing treatment just described possibly lead to the removal of proteins that have already been fixed by 5% glutaraldehyde? There appear to be at least three possibilities, each of which is not mutually exclusive of the others. First, OsO_4 could alter the conformation of nonexchanging phospholipids in the bilayer by cross-linking them to the bulk phospholipid. The fact that membrane phospholipids could be divided into two classes, one in the plane of the bilayer being free to migrate and the other more ordered and tightly bound to integral proteins, has been shown for several membrane systems (Packer *et al.*, 1974; Gulik-Krzywicki, 1975;

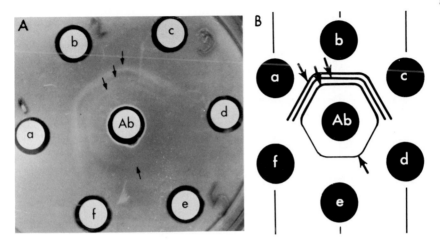

Fig. 4. Ouchterlony double-immunodiffusion of 5 m*M* EDTA-solubilized protein after 1% OsO$_4$ (wells (a)–(c)) or 5% glutaraldehyde (wells (d)–(f)) fixation. Arrows point to precipitin lines which are schematically represented in (**B**).

Laggner, 1975; Klausner *et al.*, 1979; Yeagle, 1980). We should be careful in generalizing this concept to all membranes unless a definition of the membrane system, protein concentration, time scale of measurement and limitation of the measurement technique used is provided (Chapman *et al.*, 1979). However almost all of the systems discussed in this chapter satisfy these criteria and thus, for them, the tightly bound class of phospholipid needs to be kept in a specific conformation in order for the function of the integral proteins to be expressed. If the tightly-bound phospholipid is altered by OsO$_4$ treatment, then we would speculate that this could release the integral proteins, e.g., band 3 protein of erythrocyte ghosts, from their protective shells and allow them to be extracted by a subsequent exposure to 5 m*M* EDTA. Such a solubilization by 5 m*M* EDTA also hints at the possibility that, in the erythrocyte ghosts, a release mechanism may be involved where Ca^{2+} or other internal divalent cation bridges are made accessible to external solvents.

A second, entirely different, explanation for how OsO$_4$ causes removal of proteins from membranes is based on the findings of Maupin-Szamier and Pollard (1978) who found that OsO$_4$ leads to the covalent breakage of actin filaments. Thus, in addition to the reactions mentioned above where it cross-links lipids, OsO$_4$ can potentially break down the fibrillar cytoskeleton of erythrocyte ghosts (composed of spectin–actin complexes) and perhaps also hydrophilic domains of integral membrane proteins. The total effect would be a cascade phenomenon where actin linked to spectrin anchored by band

2.1 to band 3 would be fragmented, resulting in the wholesale removal of proteins, even those previously cross-linked with glutaraldehyde, from membranes. Such a detrimental effect of OsO_4 on proteins is consistent with the findings by several laboratories, e.g., Lisak *et al.*, 1976 found that low concentrations of OsO_4 cleaved actin and ovalbumin into peptides and deaminated amino acids, and Deetz and Behrman (1980) found with lysozyme that cysteine and methionine residues were among the most reactive with OsO_4. Also, several years ago Hake (1965) had observed a similar oxidation of cysteine to cysteic acid and methionine to methionine sulfone in proteins and amino acids by OsO_4 treatment.

The third and final possibility for how OsO_4 can remove proteins previously fixed with glutaraldehyde relies on the general principle that glutaraldehyde is a bifunctional reagent which has the potential, by aldol condensation (Richards and Knowles, 1968), to form a polymeric, partially double-bonded structure with proteins or lipids. Glutaraldehyde or 1,5-pentanedialdehyde can cross-link proteins, by their exposed amino groups, to other proteins, or proteins to aminophospholipids. This putative cross-linked structure could then be cleaved by OsO_4, resulting in the removal of both protein and glutaraldehyde moieties. The extent of glutaraldehyde cross-linking depends on whether it is in its monomer form (Richards and Knowles, 1968; Hayat, 1970; Korn *et al.*, 1972) or in the form of polymers of variable length (Richards and Knowles, 1968; Morel *et al.*, 1971; Monsan *et al.*, 1975). In the monomer form, when hydrated, glutaraldehyde can be converted into a cyclical ring which bridges only two amino groups (Korn *et al.*, 1972). In the polymeric form, as stated above, an aldol condensation of several glutaraldehyde monomers can occur, leading to the formation of α, β-unsaturated regions, some of whose electrons are donated during cross-linking (Richards and Knowles, 1968). In the latter case a free $—(C{=}C)—$ bond can be formed which could subsequently be oxidized by OsO_4, leading to formation of an osmic diester (Korn, 1967; Criegee *et al.*, 1942) and thereby leaving the previously cross-linked proteins or amino-phospholipids in a less stable state and accessible to subsequent solubilization procedures. The following experiment performed to test this latter possibility shows that, in fact, [^{14}C]glutaraldehyde as well as protein moieties are released by OsO_4 postfixation.

The details of the labeling protocol are presented in Fig. 5. Briefly, erythrocyte ghosts adhered to a Formvar™ support film were fixed with a 60 mM solution of [1,5-^{14}C]glutaraldehyde (custom synthesized by New England Nuclear at 7.9 mCi/mmol) and subsequently exposed to either 1% OsO_4 or buffer for varying amounts of time; then the amount of label released was counted. As can be seen in Table III, in two separate experiments we found essentially the same result, namely, that after exposure to OsO_4,

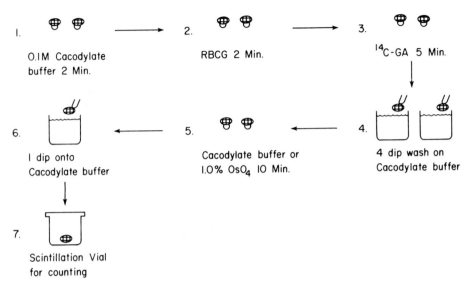

Fig. 5. Effect of OsO$_4$ postfixation on the retention of [^{14}C]glutaraldehyde in "fixed" human erythrocyte ghosts. Formvar ^{TM}-coated electron microscope grids were placed on top of buffer, erythrocyte ghosts, and [^{14}C]glutaraldehyde, respectively, in steps 1 through 3 (drop size was 25 μl). After removing most of the unbound label, the ghosts were exposed to 1% OsO$_4$ or buffer (control) prior to washing and counting.

about 70% of the tightly associated glutaraldehyde label was released as compared to the control. Although this experiment provides some support for the third explanation above, we still need to analyze the labeled material released and observe whether it is associated with protein or phospholipid before we can determine the relative degree of protein cross-linking. In the future we also need to analyze this supernatant material as well as the 5 mM EDTA-solubilized material obtained after OsO$_4$ treatment of erythrocyte ghosts by use of molecular sieve column chromatography, e.g., Sephadex G-75 or larger. Then we can determine what size proteins are released. Further, to show the generality of this reaction, we also need to use other labeled protein cross-linking reagents prior to OsO$_4$ treatment, e.g., sub-erimidate as well as bis-[^{35}S]-dithio-succinimidyl propionate (Lomant and Fairbanks, 1976). If it turns out that OsO$_4$ is breaking down glutaraldehyde and other cross-links, as postulated above, then we will try to develop methods to prevent the formation of potential α, β-unsaturated bonds by blocking the free, unreacted carbonyl groups after glutaraldehyde fixation. This could potentially be accomplished by the addition of several small molecular weight amino compounds (e.g., hexanediamine) to glutaraldehyde-fixed erythrocyte ghosts, then looking for the subsequent ability of 1% OsO$_4$

TABLE III

The Effect of OsO$_4$ Postfixation on the Retention of [^{14}C]Glutaraldehyde in "Fixed" Human Erythrocyte Ghosts

	Average cpm remaining	
Treatment[a]	Exp. 1[b]	Exp. 2[b]
1. + RBCG + [^{14}C]GA + 4 dip wash + 10 min buffer wash	821 ± 433	8562 ± 3000
2. + RBCG + [^{14}C]GA + 4 dip wash + 10 min OsO$_4$ fixation[c]	278 ± 114	2693 ± 1050
3. − RBCG + [^{14}C]GA + 4 dip wash + 10 min buffer wash	173 ± 70	707 ± 306

[a] The detailed steps for how [^{14}C]glutaraldehyde (GA)-fixed erythrocyte ghosts (RBCG) were dipped in OsO$_4$ and then washed is presented in Fig. 5.

[b] The procedures for Exp. 1 and 2 differed slightly in that all grids in Exp. 2 were treated with NCS solubilizer (Amersham) prior to the addition of scintillation fluid. This was done in order to digest all organic material from the grid and thereby provide an even suspension of labeled particles in the counting fluid. Omission of this step resulted in considerable quenching of counts.

[c] When the OsO$_4$ or cacodylate buffer drops from the 10 min incubations were transferred to filter papers and counted, the average count rate was 50,000 cpm in all cases.

postfixation to not induce the formation of a trilamellar image and/or the 5 mM EDTA solubilization of membrane proteins.

PROBLEMS WITH GLUTARALDEHYDE FIXATION

Thus far we have emphasized the fact that OsO$_4$ fixation, with or without prior glutaraldehyde fixation, leads to the solubilization and removal of most membrane proteins from erythrocyte ghosts. We have also argued that the electron-dense band image observed after glutaraldehyde-only fixation is itself not a major artifact due to the collapse of protein after removal of lipids or wide-scale denaturation of proteins. This is because similar fibrillar network images were seen by other techniques, e.g., the Triton X-100 cytoskeleton (Yu *et al.*, 1973). Also, by scanning electron microscopy, a network containing filaments 5–40 μm long was observed (Hainfeld and Steck, 1977) and a tangled fibrillar network was seen in thin sections when the mordant tannic acid was used along with glutaraldehyde during fixation (Tsukita *et al.*, 1980). However what we have not yet analyzed is to what degree this fibrillar image itself represents an artifact.

Thus, for example, when erythrocyte ghosts were treated with low concentrations (0.05%) of glutaraldehyde, the membrane appeared as a compact thickened band and a fibrillar network was not observed until a higher concentration, namely $\geq 0.1\%$, of glutaraldehyde was used (Luftig *et al.*, 1977). This implies that such high concentrations of glutaraldehyde can cause local denaturation of membrane proteins. Extrapolating from the experiments of Tilney and Detmers (1975) and Pinder *et al.* (1975), we would then suggest that there is a denaturation of spectrin by $\geq 0.1\%$ glutaraldehyde that can trigger formation of an extensive fibrillar network of actin. Also, reports that glutaraldehyde fixation can change the distribution of surface anionic sites in cell membranes of cultured BHK cells (Grinnell *et al.*, 1976), as well as a careful freeze-fracture analysis indicating that tight junction fibrils may be polymerization products caused by extensive glutaraldehyde cross-linking (Vandeurs and Luft, 1979), have led us to be concerned that, although glutaraldehyde-only fixation does stabilize membrane proteins, their morphological state can still be altered by this agent. We have thus examined the preservation of membrane structure by fixatives other than glutaraldehyde to give a broader perspective. This will be presented in the next section.

If we were to condense, from all of the above studies, a take-home lesson on how to fix membranes, it would be: (*a*) start with a relatively low concentration of glutaraldehyde (less than 0.1%), followed by OsO_4 at 0.025%; (*b*) if the material is not properly fixed, i.e., pellets are not cohesive, then try slightly higher concentrations of glutaraldehyde or other bifunctional protein cross-linkers (see below). The images obtained may not be conformationally accurate but at least almost all of the protein is retained and this is useful in itself. For example, we found that, when ghosts were prepared under conditions that caused removal of the enzyme glyceraldehyde 3-phosphate dehydrogenase (G3PD), i.e., ghosts were exposed to concentrations of 0.15 M or 0.5 M NaCl for 30–60 min, then gaps spaced around the perimeter of the dense-band image were observed for the first time (Fig. 6). If 1% OsO_4 postfixation was used these gaps were not seen; instead, a trilamellar image was visualized in both treated and untreated samples. The meaning of the gaps in the ghost membrane is not clear at this time; it may represent areas where localized concentrations of the deleted proteins were removed or weakened areas of the phospholipid bilayer. Further supporting studies are needed to see if such gaps will appear as well when G3PD is eluted from

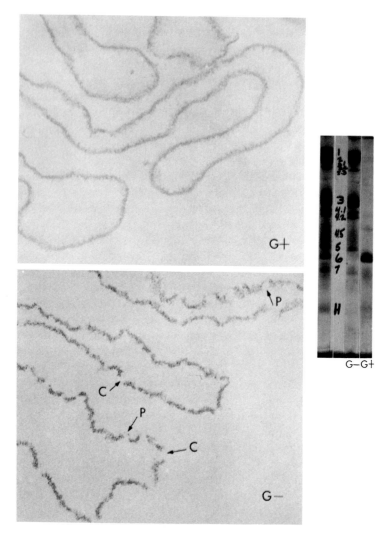

Fig. 6. Exposure of human erythrocyte ghosts to 0.5 *M* NaCl, under the conditions described in the text, leads to the removal of G3PD. Fixation of these treated ghosts by 5% glutaraldehyde alone permits the visualization of partial (P) or complete (C) gaps in the membrane whereas the untreated membrane (G+) shows the dense-band image. On the right is a set of three SDS–PAGE gels of erythrocyte ghosts prepared and labeled according to Fairbanks *et al.* (1971). The (G−) preparation shows the band pattern of ghosts seen after they have been exposed to 0.15 or 0.5 *M* NaCl; the (G+) preparation shows the pattern obtained from the supernatant fluids of the ghost suspension after salt exposure. Note the selective removal of G3PD (band 6). The gel on the far left is from an untreated preparation of ghosts and serves as a control. Reproduced from Luftig *et al.* (1977), courtesy of Life Sciences.

ghosts by other than salt treatment, e.g., 2 mM NADPH (Kant and Steck, 1973; Fossel and Solomon, 1979). If so, then fundamental information about the morphological state of G3PD in membranes will have been obtained.

PRESERVATION OF MEMBRANE STRUCTURE BY OTHER FIXATIVES

Another group of bifunctional cross-linking agents, other than glutaraldehyde, that offers promise as fixatives for localizing proteins in membranes includes the imidates. As reported originally by Hassell and Hand (1974), dimethyl suberimidate can adequately fix cells with little loss of protein or lipid. We noted that when it was used to fix erythrocyte ghosts at a concentration of about 0.1% it gave an image similar to that seen with low levels of glutaraldehyde, namely, a dense-band image. Furthermore, when we used dimethyl adipimidate, which is smaller than suberimidate by only a 2-carbon chain length and has been shown to effectively form covalent cross-links between dissimilar erythrocyte membrane proteins (Neihaus and Wold, 1970), a drastically different image was seen (Fig. 7) wherein the membrane appeared to have a patchy substructure. It thus appears that by using a variety of bifunctional cross-linking agents different membrane images can be observed. If, in the future, such images could be computerized and correlated with SDS–PAGE patterns of the cross-linked membrane proteins, it might be possible to provide a nearest-neighbor map of erythrocyte proteins. However we need to keep in mind that, before we analyze these cross-linked products on gels, we must ensure that they are of naturally occurring complexes rather than of artificial complexes due to random collisions between rapidly diffusing proteins. Thus experiments should also be performed with cleavable, photosensitive heterobifunctional reagents which can be flash-photolyzed in milliseconds (Kiehm and Ji, 1977). This will minimize possible artifacts and help in interpreting the cross-linking data. For erythrocyte ghosts it should be emphasized that essentially the same cross-linked products were found by the flash-photolysis technique as had been observed with reagents such as the imidates, *o*-phenanthroline–Cu chelate, or mild glutaraldehyde (Steck, 1972; Freedman, 1979). Thus, in both cases, band 3 dimers, band 6 tetramers, and spectrin dimers and tetramers were found (Kiehm and Ji, 1977), suggesting nearest-neighbor locations between these homo- and heterotypic groups of proteins.

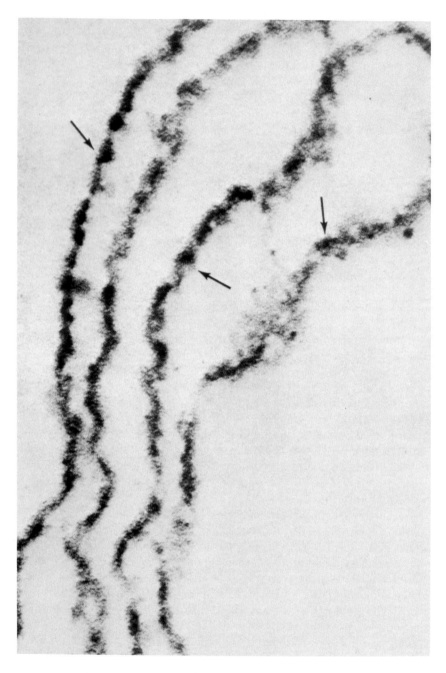

Fig. 7. Erythrocyte ghosts fixed in 0.1% dimethyl adipimidate. Note the irregularly spaced, dark-staining patches along the membrane (arrows). Magnification is 171,000×. Reproduced from McMillan and Luftig (1975), courtesy of the Journal of Ultrastructural Research.

Fixation in Other Membrane Systems

One of the clearest indications we had, from our earlier studies, that fixation of membranes with glutaraldehyde alone was meaningful, was that the images from different membrane systems appeared different (McMillan and Luftig, 1975). Thus for erythrocyte ghosts we saw a dense fibrillar image, whereas for rat CNS myelin we observed concentric layers of a less dense image (Fig. 8A). This latter image was expected because myelin has a low protein content. It was unexpected, however, that glutaraldehyde-only fixed myelin would give a different image than that obtained when OsO_4 was employed (compare Fig. 8A and 8B), i.e., there was essentially no highly dense periodic repeating line, and also the glutaraldehyde-alone fixed double membrane width was larger (160 Å versus 120 Å). As above we can account for the different images by suggesting that OsO_4 causes the removal of proteins from myelin as it did in the erythrocyte ghost system. Thus the dense lines seen with OsO_4 fixation may well represent a nonspecific deposition of osmium at regions where the myelin basic protein, involved in holding the myelin lamellae together (Smith and McDonald, 1979; Stollery *et al.*, 1980), has been removed.

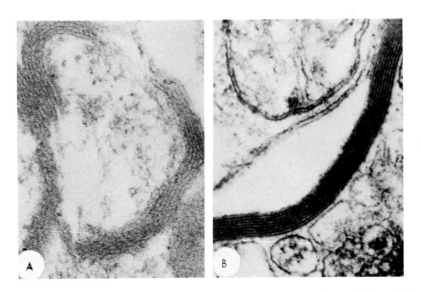

Fig. 8. A comparison of rat CNS myelin fixed in (**A**) 5% glutaraldehyde, and (**B**) 1% OsO_4. Magnification in both cases is about 73,600×. Adapted from McMillan and Luftig (1975), courtesy of the Journal of Ultrastructural Research.

For *Dictyostelium discoideum* and *Escherichia coli* membranes fixed with glutaraldehyde alone, we observed yet another feature, transverse projections which penetrated through the membrane bilayer. This was in contrast to the trilamellar image observed after OsO_4 fixation of these membranes. These projections may be related, in *E. coli*, to the porin sites on the outer membrane (Rosenbusch, 1974) (see arrows on Fig. 9A). Porin oligomers form channels in gram-negative bacteria such as *E. coli* and *S. typhimurium* that permit small solutes, such as sugars and amino acids, to penetrate through the outer membrane. For *E. coli* B, which is seen in Fig. 9, a single pore protein is produced and it accounts for as much as half of the total membrane protein. It has also been visualized by negative-stain and freeze-drying electron microscopy as a hexagonal lattice covering much of the cell surface (Steven *et al.*, 1977). The thin-section image seen with glutaralde-

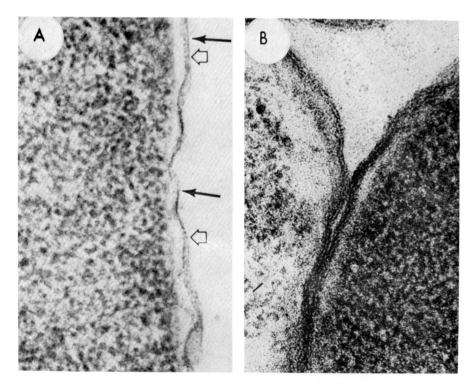

Fig. 9. *E. coli* fixed by (**A**) 5% glutaraldehyde, and (**B**) 1% OsO_4. Note that regions of the outer membrane (**A**, arrows) exhibit transmembranous projections which, in some cases, appear to completely traverse the membrane (arrow head). (**A**) is magnified 96,000×; (**B**) is 150,000×. Adapted from McMillan and Luftig (1975), courtesy of the Journal of Ultrastructural Research.

hyde-only fixation provides another view of this protein (Fig. 9A). This view may turn out to be useful in the future examination of different strains of *E. coli* and *S. typhimuium* that have different peptidoglycan-associated pore proteins (Lee *et al.*, 1979).

A similar increased visualization of membrane proteins over the trilamellar image has also been reported by Saito *et al.* (1978) for sarcoplasmic reticulum membrane vesicles when 2.5% glutaraledhyde supplemented with 1% tannic acid was used instead of 1% OsO_4 alone. These authors could now visualize a fibrillar structure on the outer surface of the vesicles. It should be noted, however, that in this study 1% OsO_4 was still utilized as a postfixation step. Perhaps the addition of tannic acid may stabilize these proteins to subsequent denaturation and removal by 1% OsO_4.

In conclusion, we want to reiterate our point that membranes from different systems have different morphologies and that new fixation techniques, which permit minimal denaturation and/or removal of these proteins, are needed to detect them.

New Techniques

Thus far we have focused on the precautions one needs to take with fixatives so as to accurately visualize membrane proteins in the electron microscope. These methods represent a good starting point in that approximately 80–90% of the proteins will be present; however the images seen, e.g., fibrillar dense-band for erythrocyte ghosts, do not alone give specific information as to the location of individual proteins. If we also choose to use imidates of different chain lengths to cross-link and map proteins, we need to be alert as well to problems with membrane protein denaturation and alterations in the intrinsic dynamic state of the membrane caused by these agents (Wang and Richards, 1974). To minimize all such problems, it is best to use a variety of approaches to localize proteins in membranes. Thus we should not limit ourselves to aldehydes and imidates but should also compare images obtained using several other classes of cross-linking agents as well, e.g., *cis*-diols (glycol) and photoactivable reagents. Then all of the images obtained could be correlated with two-dimensional SDS–PAGE profiles of cross-linked hetero- and homotypic protein complexes to provide a nearest-neighbor map of the membrane proteins.

The photoactivatable membrane-saturable cross-linking agents mentioned above will permit one to study associations between integral membrane proteins. These agents, such as [3H]adamantanediazirine (a lipophilic carbene precursor), are currently being used by several groups (Gupta *et al.*, 1979; Bayley and Knowles, 1980) in different membrane systems. After being intercalated into the hydrophobic interior of the membrane, they form a highly reactive photogenerated intermediate which can cross-link proteins to itself, as well as phospholipids to proteins. An interesting example of the specificity of such reagents is provided by Wu and Wisnieski (1979) who used a photoreactive glycolipid to label the filamentous phage M13 coat protein in synthetic bilayers. They found that only integral membrane peptides were labeled by the membrane-bound probe; it did not label externally added protein nor trypsin-cleavable protein sites.

If cross-linking agents such as those discussed above are used to fix membranes, and subsequently the membrane pellets are embedded in a nonplastic matrix, such as 30% bovine serum albumin, then we have the additional potential to apply specific antisera to the thin sections for localization of different membrane proteins. Further, if such antisera to different proteins were conjugated to correspondingly different sized markers (e.g., ferritin, sowbane mosaic virus or hemocyanin), then we can map membrane protein associations by yet another technique. Clearly there are technical difficulties inherent in this approach, e.g., specificity of antisera, distance of marker from antigen, cohesiveness of pellets after fixation with different cross-linking reagents; however the information we can obtain makes it worth considering this approach as well as the two-dimensional SDS–PAGE approach for mapping protein associations.

Another useful new approach to study membrane structure involves modification of the classical freeze-fracture and freeze-etching procedures. Since these techniques do not require a prefixation step, they can provide another perspective to localizing integral membrane proteins. For example, the recent modification where cytochemical labels are applied to platinum–carbon replicas (Pinto da Silva *et al.*, 1981) looks promising for detecting groups of integral proteins in the cross-fractured cytoplasm. In particular, this technique will be helpful because it allows one to determine whether surface residues of integral proteins have been translocated during freeze-fracture. Also, using this technique and selectively removing polypeptides by salt, low pH, enzyme, or detergent degradation, we can correlate changes in specific intramembranous particles with changes to specific proteins. Gerritsen *et al.* (1979) used this approach to show that, after stripping off extrinsic proteins by 0.01 M NaCl treatment, the intramembrane particles of erythrocyte ghosts could still be aggregated by incubation in 150 mM NaCl, 10 mM CaCl or a pH 5.5 buffer.

Another approach to studying the association between membrane proteins is to alter the cholesterol level in membranes and examine the effect on the proteins. Using this procedure Araki (1979) showed that cholesterol and proteins in the erythrocyte membranes can be partially segregated by exposure to low temperatures. In particular, microvesicles obtained from slow freezing of cells or ghosts were found to be enriched in both cholesterol and band 6. Perhaps the gaps seen in Fig. 6 with G3PD-depleted erythrocyte ghosts might represent such weak points in the membrane where G3PD becomes aggregated prior to release in microvesicles. Using ^{31}P-resonance shifts in a G3PD–glyceraldehyde-3-phosphate inside-out vesicle system, Fossel and Solomon (1979) have also shown, in support of this contention, that there is a functional linkage between transmembrane proteins, such as (Na^+/K^+)-ATPase and G3PD, at the cytoplasmic face.

As a final point, we note that there are several currently used biophysical techniques, e.g., flash-induced transient dichroism to measure rotational diffusion (Nigg *et al.*, 1980), ^{31}P-nuclear magnetic resonance (NMR) spectrosopy (Yeagle, 1980), and fluorescence photobleaching recovery (FPR) (Elson and Reidler, 1979; Wolf *et al.*, 1980), that represent still further valuable techniques with which we can provide information complementary to the thin-section electron microscopy studies described earlier. Nigg *et al.* (1980) showed that the rotational diffusion of band 3 protein in the presence of divalent antiglycophorin A antibodies was strongly reduced. With appropriate controls, it was concluded that there was a preexisting band 3 protein–glycophorin A complex in the human erythrocyte membrane, a point that has been debated for many years because it could not be resolved by cross-linking or ultrastructural studies. With ^{31}P -NMR, Yeagle (1980) has also shown the presence of two phospholipid environments in erythrocyte ghosts: one immobilized, presumably by band 3 proteins, and the second freely diffusing. Elson and Reidler (1979) and Wolf *et al.* (1980) have studied membrane protein diffusion using the FPR technique, which monitors the fluorescence from a membrane probe excited by a laser beam focused to a small spot on the cell surface. Experimentally, after a segment of fluorescence is photochemically destroyed by a brief, intense laser pulse, recovery of the fluorescently labeled membrane component free to diffuse laterally in the membrane region that has been bleached is measured. Both diffusion coefficients and the fraction of the probe free to diffuse in the membrane are calculated. It can be argued that such experiments are susceptible to artifacts caused by thermal effects due to localized membrane heating; however, as discussed by Wolf *et al.* (1980), the measurement of diffusion rates of the Fc receptor for IgE of a rat cell line showed no evidence for photo-induced artifacts. All three of the new biophysical approaches mentioned here should allow us to learn more about how integral membrane proteins live in their hydrophobic microenvironment.

In conclusion, we want to state that, by employing a combination of ultrastructural, biochemical, and biophysical approaches, it should now be possible to definitively localize membrane proteins and determine their structure–function relationship in a wide variety of systems. However, as we have shown with the use of OsO$_4$ as a fixative for thin-section electron microscopy, caution should be exercised with each approach so that the experimenter is aware of what artifacts, if any, are being created.

References

Araki, T. (1979). *FEBS Lett.* **79**, 237–240.

Bayley, H., and Knowles, J. R. (1980). *Biochemistry* **19**, 3883–3892.

Bear, R. S., Palmer, K. J., and Schmitt, R. O. (1941). *J. Cell Comp. Physiol.* **17**, 355–367.

Bennett, V., and Stenbuck, P. J. (1980). *J. Biol. Chem.* **255**, 2540–2548.

Bergman, Y., and Haimovich, J. (1977). *Eur. J. Immunol.* **7**, 413–421.

Blaurock, A. E., and Wilkins, M. H. F. (1969). *Nature (London)* **223**, 906–909.

Bleau, G., Lalumiére, G., Chapdelaine, A., and Roberts, R. D. (1975). *Biochim. Biophys. Acta* **375**, 220–223.

Borochov, H., Abbott, R. E., Schachter, D., and Shinitsky, M. (1979). *Biochemistry* **18**, 251–255.

Bretscher, M. S. (1973). *Science* **181**, 622–629.

Chapman, D., Gomez-Fernandez, J. C., and Goñi, F. N. (1979). *FEBS Lett.* **98**, 211–223.

Corless, J. M. (1972). *Nature (London)* **237**, 229–231.

Criegee, R., Marchand, D., and Wannowius, A. (1942). *Justus Liebigs Ann. Chem.* **550**, 99–133.

Danielli, J. F., and Davson, H. (1935). *J. Cell Comp. Physiol.* **5**, 495–508.

Deetz, J. S., and Behrman, E. J. (1980). *Fed. Proc.* **39**, 2180.

Dodge, J. T., Mitchell, C., and Hanahan, D. J. (1963). *Arch. Biochem. Biophys.* **100**, 119–130.

Eitan, A., Moloney, B., and Livre, A. (1976). *Biochim. Biophys. Acta* **426**, 647–658.

Elson, E. L., and Reidler, J. A. (1979). *J. Supramol. Struct.* **12**, 185–193.

Fairbanks, G., Steck, T. L., and Wallach, D. F. H. (1971). *Biochemistry* **10**, 2606–2617.

Finean, J. B., and Burge, R. E. (1962). *J. Mol. Biol.* **7**, 672–682.

Fossel, E. T., and Solomon, A. K. (1979). *Biochim. Biophys. Acta* **553**, 142–153.

Freedman, R. B. (1979). *Trends Biol. Sci.* **4**, 193–197.

Gerritsen, W. J., Verkley, A. J., Zwaal, R. F. A., and Van Deenen, L. L. M. (1978). *Eur. J. Biochem.* **85**, 255–261.

Gorter, E., and Grendel, F. (1925). *J. Exp. Med.* **41**, 439–443.

Gras, W. J., and Worthington, C. R. (1969). *Proc. Nat. Acad. Sci. USA* **63**, 233–238.

Grinnell, F., Anderson, R. G. W., and Hackenbrock, C. R. (1976). *Biochim. Biophys. Acta* **426**, 772–775.

Gulik-Krzywicki, T. (1975). *Biochim. Biophys. Acta* **415**, 1–28.

Gupta, C. M., Radhakrishnan, R., Gerber, G. E., Olsen, W. L., Quay, S. C., and Khorana, H. G. (1979). *Proc. Nat. Acad. Sci. USA* **76**, 2595–2599.

Hainfeld, J. F., and Steck, T. L. (1977). *J. Supramol. Struc.* **6**, 301–311.

Hake, T. (1965). *Lab. Invest.* **14**, 1208–1211.

Harrel, D., and Morrison, M. (1979). *Arch. Biochem. Biophys.* **193**, 158–168.

Hassell, J., and Hand, A. R. (1974). *J. Histochem. Cytochem.* **22**, 223–239.

Hayat, M. A. (1970). "Principles and Techniques of Electron Microscopy: Biological Applications," Vol. 1. Van Nostrand-Reinhold, New York.

Hirata, F., Toyoshima, J., Axelrod, J. and Waxdal, M. J. (1980). *Proc. Nat. Acad. Sci. USA* **77**, 862–865.

Hong, K., and Hubbell, W. L. (1972). *Proc. Nat. Acad. Sci. USA* **68**, 2617–2621.

Hynes, R. O. (1976). *Biochim. Biophys. Acta* **458**, 73–107.

Ishii, J., and Nakae, T. (1980). *J. Bacteriol.* **142**, 27–31.

Jost, P. C., and Griffith, O. H. (1973). *Arch. Biochem. Biophys.* **159**, 70–81.

Kant, J. A., and Steck, T. L. (1973). *J. Biol. Chem.* **248**, 8457–4864.

Kiehm, D. J., and Ji, T. H. (1977). *J. Biol. Chem.* **252**, 8524–8531.

Kirby, C. J., and Green, C. (1980). *Biochim. Biophys. Acta* **598**, 422–425.

Klausner, R. D., Fishman, M. C., and Karnovsky, M. J. (1979). *Nature (London)* **281**, 82–83.

Korn, E. D. (1967). *J. Cell Biol.* **34**, 627–638.

Korn, E. D., and Weisman, R. A. (1966). *Biochim. Biophys. Acta* **116**, 309–316.

Korn, A. H., Feairheller, S. H., and Filachione, E. M. (1972). *J. Mol. Biol.* **65**, 525–529.

Laggner, P. (1975). *Nature (London)* **255**, 427–428.

Lee, D. R., Schnaitman, C. A., and Pugsley, A. P. (1979). *J. Bacteriol.* **138**, 861–870.

Lesslauer, W. (1980). *Biochim. Biophys. Acta* **600**, 108–116.

Lisak, J. C., Kaufman, H. W., Maupin-Szamier, P., and Pollard, T. D. (1976). *Biol. Bull.* **151**, 418.

Litman, D., Hsu, C. J., and Marchesi, V. T. (1980). *J. Cell Sci.* **42**, 1–22.

Lomant, H. J., and Fairbanks, G. (1976). *J. Mol. Biol.* **104**, 243–261.

Lowry, O. H., Rosebrough, N. J., Farr, A. L., and Randall, R. J. (1951). *J. Biol. Chem.* **193**, 265–275.

Luftig, R. B., Wehrli, E., and McMillan, P. N. (1977). *Life Sci.* **21**, 285–300.

MacLennan, D. H., Seeman, P., Iles, G. H., and Yip, C. C. (1971). *J. Biol. Chem.* **246**, 2702–2710.

Mason, W. T., Fager, R. S., and Abrahamson, E. W. (1974). *Nature (London)* **247**, 188–191.

Maupin-Szamier, P., and Pollard, T. D. (1978). *J. Cell Biol.* **77**, 837–852.

McMillan, P. N., and Luftig, R. B. (1973). *Proc. Nat. Acad. Sci. USA* **70**, 3060–3064.

McMillan, P. N., and Luftig, R. B. (1975). *J. Ultrastruct. Res.* **52**, 243–260.

Monsan, P., Puzo, G., and Mazarguil, H. (1975). *Biochimie* **57**, 1281–1292.

Morel, F. M. M., Baker, R. F., and Wayland, H. (1971). *J. Cell Biol.* **48**, 91–100.

Niehaus, Jr., W. G., and Wold, F. (1970). *Biochim. Biophys. Acta* **196**, 170–175.

Nigg, E. A., Bron, C., Girardet, M., and Cherry, R. J. (1980). *Biochemistry* **19**, 1887–1893.

Oppenheim, J. J., and Rosenstreich, D. L. (1976). "Mitogens in Immunology." Academic Press, New York.

Ouchterlony, Ö. (1949). *Acta Pathol. Microbiol. Scand.* **26**, 507–515.

Packer, L., Mehard, C. W., Meissner, G., Zahler, W. L., and Fleischer, S. (1974). *Biochim. Biophys. Acta* **363**, 159–181.

Parish, G. R. (1975). *J. Microsc.* **104**, 245–256.

Pinder, J. C., Bray, D., and Gratzer, W. B. (1975). *Nature (London)* **258**, 765–766.

Pinto da Silva, P., and Miller, R. G. (1975). *Proc. Nat. Acad. Sci. USA* **72**, 4046–4050.

Pinto da Silva, P., and Nicholson, G. (1974). *Biochim. Biophys. Acta* **363**, 311–319.

Pinto da Silva, P., Kachar, B., Torrisi, M. R., Brown, C., and Parkison, C. (1981). *Science* **213**, 230–233.

Reynolds, J., and Trayer, H. (1971). *J. Biol. Chem.* **246**, 7337–7342.

Richards, R. M., and Knowles, J. R. (1968). *J. Mol. Biol.* **37**, 213–233.

Robertson, J. D. (1957). *J. Biophys. Biochem. Cytol.* **3**, 1043–1047.

Robertson, J. D. (1959). *Biochem. Soc. Symp.* **16**, 3–43.

Robertson, J. D. (1972). *Arch. Intern. Med.* **129**, 202–228.

Röhlich, P. (1976). *Nature (London)* **263**, 789–791.

Rosenbusch, J. P. (1974). *J. Biol. Chem.* **24**, 8019–8029.

Saito, A., Wang, C., and Fleischer, S. (1978). *J. Cell Biol.* **79**, 601–616.

Sauberman, N., Fortier, N. L., Fairbanks, G., O'Connor, R. J., and Snyder, L. N. (1979). *Biochim. Biophys. Acta* **556**, 292–313.

Schmitt, F. O., Bear, R. S., and Clark, G. (1935). *Radiology* **25**, 131–151.

Singer, S. J., and Nicholson, G. L. (1972). *Science* **175**, 720–731.

Sjöstrand, F. S., and Barajas, L. (1968). *J. Ultrastruct. Res.* **25**, 121–155.

Smith, R., and McDonald, B. J. (1979). *Biochim. Biophys. Acta* **554**, 133–147.

Spatz, L., and Strittmatter, P. (1973). *J. Biol. Chem.* **248**, 793–799.

Steck, T. L. (1972). *J. Mol. Biol.* **66**, 295–305.

Steck, T. L. (1974). *J. Cell Biol.* **62**, 1–19.

Steck, T. L. (1978). *J. Supramol. Struct.* **8**, 311–324.

Steven, A. C., ten Heggeler, B., Mulle, R., Kistler, J., and Rosenbusch, J. T. (1977). *J. Cell Biol.* **72**, 292–301.

Stollery, J. G., Boggs, J. M., Moscarello, M. A., and Deber, C. M. (1980). *Biochemistry* **19**, 2391–2396.

Tanford, C. (1973). "The Hydrophobic Effect: Formation of Micelles and Biological Membranes." Wiley, New York.

Tanford, C. (1978). *Science* **200**, **1012–1018.**

Tilney, L. G., and Detmers, P. (1975). *J. Cell. Biol.* **66**, 508–520.

Tourtellote, M. E., and Zupnik, J. S. (1973). *Science* **179**, 84–86.

Tsukita, S., Tsukita, S., and Ishikawa, H. (1980). *J. Cell. Biol.* **85**, 567–576.

Vandeurs, B., and Fuft, J. H. (1979). *J. Ultrastruct. Res.* **68**, 160–172.

Wang, K., and Richards, F. M. (1974). *Israel J. Chem.* **12**, 375–389.

Warren, G. B., Housley, M. D., Metcalfe, J. C., and Birdsall, N. J. M. (1975). *Nature (London)* **255**, 684–687.

Weinstein, R. S., Khodadad, J. K., and Steck, T. L. (1978). *In* "The Red Cell" (T. L. Steck and C. F. Fox, eds.), pp. 413–427. Alan R. Liss, New York.

Wolf, D. E., Edidin, M., and Dragsten, P. R. (1980). *Proc. Nat. Acad. Sci. USA* **77**, 2043–2045.

Wright, J. H. (1902). *J. Med. Res.* **7**, 138–144.

Wu, V. H., and Wisnieski, B. J. (1979) *Proc. Nat. Acad. Sci. USA* **76**, 5460–5464.

Yeagle, P. L. (1980). *Fed. Proc.* **39**, 1762.

Yu, J., and Branton, D. (1976). *Proc. Nat. Acad. Sci. USA* **73**, 3891–3895.

Yu, J., and Goodman, S. R. (1979). *Proc. Nat. Acad. Sci. USA* **76**, 2340–2344.

Yu, J., Fischman, D. A., and Steck, T. L. (1973). *J. Supramol. Struct.* **1**, 233–248.

Chapter 5

Negative Images and the Interpretation of Membrane Structure

K. A. Platt-Aloia and W. W. Thomson

Oh the comfort we feel when the image we see
Fits the model we've drawn in our books to a "T"!
It's easy to say "artifacts? there are none!"
For the image and model agree—we are done!

K. A. Platt-Aloia

Introduction. 171
Preparative Procedures Which Result in a Negative Membrane Image. . . 176
    Freeze-Fixation. 177
    Lipid-Retaining Procedures. 183
    Protein-Nondenaturing Procedures. 185
    Other Procedures Which Sometimes Result in Negative Images. 188
    Summary of Preparative Procedures Which Result in Negative
       Membrane Images. 191
Negative Images in Chloroplast Granal Membranes. 192
Conclusions. 195
References. 197

Introduction

Many physiological and biochemical processes of living organisms are influenced and/or regulated by cellular membranes. Therefore a knowledge of the precise molecular architecture of biological membranes is of paramount importance for an understanding of many cellular functions. Numerous biochemical, biophysical, functional, and structural techniques are available today for the analysis of membrane structure. Most of these techniques are described in other chapters of this series. This chapter concentrates on one specific aspect of the ultrastructural analysis of biological membrane structure; the phenomenon of reversed or "negative" membrane images, as viewed with the transmission electron microscope (Fig. 1).

The normal image of the biological membrane as seen in the electron microscope is frequently described as an electron-dense tripartite (dark–light–dark) "unit membrane" structure (Fig. 2). This image is usually seen in dehydrated, epoxy-embedded tissue which has been fixed either with permanganate or with glutaraldehyde followed by 1% osmium tetroxide. It should be emphasized that the proportion of a membrane that is actually visualized as a tripartite unit membrane image, as opposed to having a globular substructure (Fig. 3), depends on the type of membrane examined as well as on the method of tissue preparation. Specifically, membranes that most commonly exhibit a tripartite structure, at least over small areas of cross section, are the plasmalemma and the tonoplast (plant vacuolar membrane). These membranes have been shown to have a protein-to-lipid ratio of close to 1:1 (Guidotti, 1972). Membranes with higher protein-to-lipid ratios such as mitochondrial cristae (3.2:1 Guidotti, 1972) and thylakoid membranes of plastids (2.3:1 Vernon and Shaw, 1971) more frequently exhibit an electron-dense or globular structure in cross section. There are some preparative techniques, such as fixation with permanganate or ferrocyanide-reduced osmium tetroxide (Karnovsky, 1971), which greatly increase the proportion of unit membrane (tripartite) images, even in mitochondrial cristae and plastid thylakoids (Fig. 4). However these are strong oxidizing agents, and molecular rearrangement of membrane constituents is possible. Thus the significance of the membrane image relative to organization would seem to be low after these methods of preparation. Since much of the biochemical and biophysical data support the presence of a lipid bilayer in biological membranes (Gorter and Grendel, 1925; Tanford, 1978), the tripartite image seen in the electron microscope is frequently interpreted as reflecting a lipid bilayer.

Fig. 1. An electron micrograph of two chloroplasts in a parenchyma cell in the mesocarp of a young developing avocado fruit. The plastid on the right (#1) has a grana–fretwork system with normal, positive-straining membranes and comparatively electron-translucent loculi (L) and A space (A). The plastid on the left (#2), although surrounded by an electron-dense (positive) envelope, has a grana–fretwork system which shows the opposite image to that in the other plastid. The loculus (L) and A spaces (A) are electron-dense whereas the membranes appear electron-translucent by comparison. The stroma (S) is more electron-dense in plastid #2 than in plastid #1. Preparation was by conventional glutaraldehyde followed by 1% OsO_4 postfixation, dehydration with acetone and embedment in epoxy resin. 62,400×. Bar = 0.5 μm.

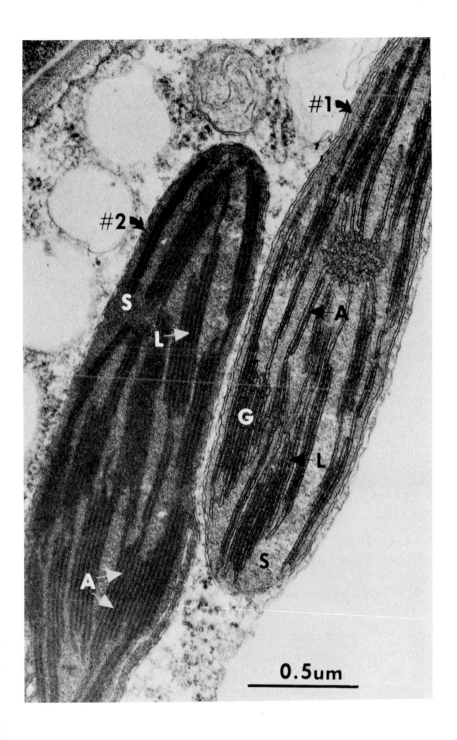

0.5um

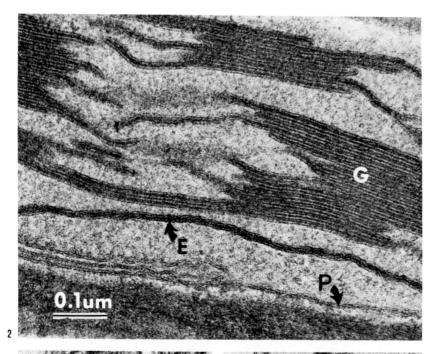

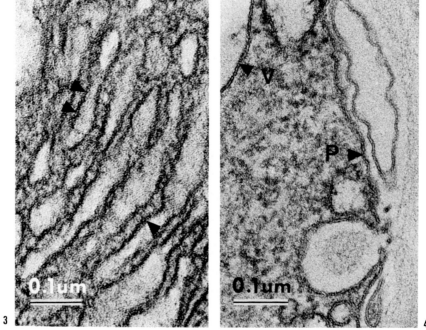

The model of membrane structure that is currently most widely accepted is the "fluid mosaic" model described by Singer and Nicolson (1972). However evidence is accumulating that this generalized model is only that—a structural outline upon which specific elaborations must be made for each membrane type (Sjöstrand, 1980a). Thus it is almost certain that different membranes with such diverse functions as photosynthesis, nerve-impluse propagation, and protein synthesis will have molecular architectures as varied as their functions.

In order to detect and evaluate these sometimes subtle, yet critical, differences at the ultrastructural level, extreme care must be taken to ascertain what molecular rearrangements may occur during preparation of the material. One way to accomplish this is to examine one type of membrane using several different preparative techniques. This is being done by the use of freeze-fracture and freeze-etching techniques, and by the development of methods designed to minimize or eliminate the loss of lipid and/or the denaturation of protein molecules before visualization in the electron microscope (Weibull *et al.*, 1980; Pease and Peterson, 1972; Sjöstrand and Barajas, 1968).

It is well known that many or most of these latter techniques normally result in a change in the electron-density pattern of the membranes, resulting in what have been called negative images. Negative images have also been reported in certain instances in tissue which has been prepared by conventional techniques (see Section III).

Several ideas have been presented in the literature concerning negative images, particularly in regard to how this image pattern may reflect the organization and/or the constitutive nature of membranes. Rarely are all factors analyzed; this has led to considerable confusion and a lack of consistency in terminology. There are many published examples of negative membrane images and in this review we present a relatively comprehensive analysis of the phenomenon, comparing preparative techniques and physiological states of the material, while taking into account what is known about chemical interactions of fixatives and stains with biological molecules.

Fig. 2. Electron micrograph of a portion of a mesophyll cell of a cotyledon of *Sesame* that was fixed with ferrocyanide-reduced osmium tetroxide. All membranes exhibit a strong trilamellar, dark–light–dark unit membrane image. P = plasmalemma, E = chloroplast envelope, G = granum. 147,000×. Bar = 0.1 μm.

Fig. 3. High magnification micrograph of mitochondrial cristae in a salt gland cell of *Tamarix* showing a globular subunit structure of the membranes (arrows). Preparation was as described for Fig. 1. 138,000×. Bar = 0.1 μm.

Fig. 4. High magnification electron micrograph of a portion of a cell from a salt gland in *Tamarix*. The plasmalemma (P) and vesicle (V) membranes have clear tripartite unit membrane images. Preparation as for Fig. 1. 146,000×. Bar = 0.1 μm.

Preparative Procedures Which Result
in a Negative Membrane Image

The conventional preparation of biological material for electron microscopy using glutaraldehyde followed by osmium tetroxide does not preclude major modifications in protein (Lenard and Singer, 1968; McMillan and Luftig, 1978, 1975; Luftig et al., 1977; Sjöstrand and Barajas, 1968; Trump and Ericsson, 1965), extraction of lipid (Ongun, Thomson and Mudd, 1968; Korn and Weisman, 1966; Morgan and Huber, 1962), or molecular rearrangements within membranes (Jost and Griffith, 1973; Moretz et al., 1969a,b). Therefore, other procedures for the preparation of material for electron microscopic studies have been developed (e.g., Weibull et al., 1980; Pease and Peterson, 1972; Sjöstrand and Barajas, 1968). The primary aim in the development of these procedures was to maintain the molecular constituents of the membrane in their native configuration and, at the same time, render the tissue stable enough that thin sections could be made and observed in the electron microscope.

As mentioned previously, these preparative procedures frequently (almost consistently) result in negative membrane images. For the convenience of interpretation and comparison we have divided these techniques into the following categories.

1. Freeze-fixation, including freeze-drying, freeze-substitution, and frozen sectioning or cryoultramicrotomy
2. Lipid-retaining procedures, such as the use of polyglutaraldehyde (GACH; Heckman and Barnett, 1973), glutaraldehyde–urea embedding medium (Pease and Peterson, 1972; Peterson and Pease, 1972), and water-soluble epoxy embedding media (Pease, 1973a).
3. Protein nondenaturing methods (Pease, 1966 a,b; Sjöstrand and Barajas, 1968).
4. Techniques which sometimes, but not always, result in negative images
5. A special membrane system, the grana of chloroplasts, which frequently are shown in negative contrast after conventional preparative techniques.

At the beginning of the first three sections, a brief outline of the basic procedures involved in that category will be described. These descriptions are short outlines and are meant only to differentiate between similar techniques and/or refresh the reader's memory. Major or important modifications of each procedure which are specific to certain studies will be described in the text of each section where appropriate. For more complete explanations, references or reviews on the techniques are given at the beginning of each summary.

FREEZE-FIXATION

The following procedures generally involve rapid freezing of tissues in the presence of cryoprotectants such as glycerol, dimethyl sulfoxide (DMSO) or sucrose. Some studies have indicated that these agents are relatively inert, and do not induce a molecular rearrangement in tissues and membranes (Breathnach *et al.*, 1976). However freeze fracture studies have shown intramembranous particle redistributions after the use of cryoprotectants such as glycerol (Niedermeyer *et al.*, 1977; Pinto da Silva and Miller, 1975). These changes are apparently not overcome or are complicated by further glutaraldehyde-induced changes (Parish, 1975; Pinto da Silva and Miller, 1975; Stolinski *et al.*, 1978). Because of these results, many of the more recent studies employ freezing techniques that avoid cryoprotectants and chemical fixation, and rely instead on very rapid rates of freezing for optimum tissue preservation (D. Goodchild, personal communication; Van Harreveld *et al.*, 1974; Dempsey and Bullivant, 1976a,b; Heuser *et al.*, 1979).

Freeze-Drying

1. Freeze-drying technique (see Rebhun, 1972). This was one of the earliest techniques, other than chemical fixation, used for preparation of biological material for ultrastructural studies (Sjöstrand, 1943). Later improvements in sectioning techniques, and in the electron microscope itself, coupled with the development of a better embedding method for freeze-dried material (Muller, 1957) have made this technique available as a viable alternative to chemical preservation. The technique involves freezing the tissue at rapid rates followed by sublimation of the ice under vacuum or at atmospheric pressure; superior results are usually obtained by the vacuum sublimation method. Frequently, before infiltration of the resin, the dried tissue is fixed (and stained) by exposure to osmium tetroxide vapors. Alternatively the sections of tissue may be stained with osmium tetroxide as well as either uranyl acetate and lead citrate or phosphotungstic acid prior to examination in the electron microscope.

2. Freeze-drying and negative images. Sjöstrand and Baker (1958) used the freeze-drying technique for their early studies on mitochondrial membranes. They achieved successful ultrastructural preservation, but noted that the contrast was such that the membranes appeared as "the negative of that of osmium-fixed material," even when the sections were stained with 1% aqueous osmium tetroxide for 2 hr. They hypothesized that the freeze-drying and embedding may have destroyed the chemical reactivity of the lipids and proteins by extraction and denaturation, respectively. A complete extraction of the membrane components could be ruled out, since electron density and structure were still apparent.

Later in the 1960s (Sjöstrand, 1963; Sjöstrand and Elfvin, 1964), comparisons were made between material fixed in osmium tetroxide or potassium permanganate, and unfixed, freeze-dried tissue. These studies demonstrated the apparent presence of a globular substructure of membranes which was especially evident in the "light line" or "negative pattern" membranes of the freeze-dried material. This substructure in the negative image membranes could also imply an absence of staining rather than a high degree of extraction.

Further improvements in the freeze-drying technique involved an initial brief stabilization of the tissues by cross-linking with glutaraldehyde (1% for 2 min), partial dehydration with ethylene glycol (30% for 3 min), and rapid freezing, followed by drying and infiltrating under vacuum (Sjöstrand and Kretzer, 1975). In this study, sections were stained with saturated uranyl acetate at 60°C, and the membranes appeared in negative contrast, being much less electron dense than the matrix. Sjöstrand and Kretzer pointed out, however, that the membranes were stained, although faintly, and this low affinity of the membranes for the stain was hypothesized to be due to the absence of charged groups in the membrane which are usually present because of the denaturation of proteins caused by conventional preparative procedures (Sjöstrand and Kretzer, 1975).

That extensive extraction of molecules is not the basis for the negative membrane images observed in freeze-dried material is further supported by Terracio et al. (1981). Rapid freezing and vacuum freeze-drying, followed by osmium tetroxide fixation, resulted in positive, electron-dense membrane images; but when osmium was not used, the membranes were not electron dense. In both the osmium-treated and the unosmicated tissue an electron-dense material was visible in the cisternae of the rough endoplasmic reticulum as well as in Golgi vesicles. The retention of substances that are extracted in conventionally prepared material was interpreted as evidence for the stabilization and retention of molecular constituents by freeze-drying (Terracio et al., 1981). Freeze-drying has also been used in electron microscopic microprobe analysis of soluble or diffusible substances such as ions in muscle tissue (Sjöstrom and Thornell, 1975). This and similar studies

(Somlyo *et al.*, 1977, 1979) illustrate the value of freeze-drying for the retention of cellular constituents.

In summary, negative membrane images are frequently seen in freeze-dried material. Although their appearance seems to be associated with the absence of osmium tetroxide in the preparative procedures, there is evidence that the electron-transparent image is not due to substantial extraction of membrane components. Apparently the negative image may simply be a reflection of a lack of osmium and/or uranyl acetate staining of the membrane components. It is still not clear whether the image obtained after the reaction of osmium with cellular membranes is a true reflection of membrane architecture, or whether this image is a result of molecular reorganization and is, therefore, an artifact.

Freeze-Substitution

1. Freeze-substitution technique (see Glauert, 1975; Pease, 1967 a,b, 1973 a,b; Rebhun, 1972). This technique combines the use of physical freezing-fixation with chemical dehydration and infiltration at low ($-70°$ to $-100°C$) temperatures. After rapid freezing the tissue is transferred to either acetone, alcohol, or ethylene glycol for dehydration by substitution for the frozen water. Osmium tetroxide (Dempsey and Bullivant, 1976; Hereward and Northcote, 1972; Malhotra and Van Harrevold, 1965) and/or glutaraldehyde (Pease, 1967 a,b) is often included in the substitution fluid, although occasionally no chemical fixatives are used (Harvey *et al.*, 1976). After several days to a few weeks of substitution, the tissue may be infiltrated with epoxy resin either at low temperatures (Harvey *et al.*, 1976; Lauchli *et al.*, 1970; Pallaghy, 1973) or at room temperature (Hereward and Northcote, 1972; Malhotra and Van Harrevold, 1965; Withers and Davey, 1978). Sections are then cut and may be viewed either unstained or stained with uranyl acetate and/or lead citrate.

2. Freeze-substitution and negative images. As in freeze-dried tissue, the membranes show as a positive image when osmium is included. In an attempt to improve preservation of the fine structure of tissues prepared by the freeze-substitution technique, Pease (1967 a,b) introduced the use of glutaraldehyde after freezing, as well as dehydration with ethylene glycol, and the use of hydroxypropyl methacrylate for embedding. After this procedure all membranes were in negative contrast, and the explanation given was that the lipids may have been extracted by the embedding medium and glycol. Even when osmium tetroxide was included in the 70% ethylene glycol (substitution medium), a similar negative image was obtained. An explanation for this observation was that, since 1,2-glycols form complexes with osmium tetroxide (Milas *et al.*, 1959), it may be that the ethylene glycol sequesters the osmium, thus preventing its reaction with the membranes.

In 1965 Rebhun studied the fine structure of tissues that had been freeze-substituted with osmium tetroxide in acetone after varying degrees of dehydration with sea water, glycerol or DMSO. Tissue frozen without dehydration (cryoprotection) gave positive membrane images as did tissue dehydrated with sea water, DMSO, or 20% glycerol. However samples treated with 100% glycerol had negative membranes. This again, as later postulated by Pease (1967a), could be the result of the reaction of the osmium with glycerol rather than with membrane components. Alternatively the glycerol may be acting as a protectant against osmium-induced denaturation or molecular rearrangement of the membrane (see the discussion on anhydrobiotic organisms at the end of this section).

There have been many other ultrastructural studies employing various freeze-substitution techniques, and negative membrane images are not always seen. In the majority of cases, when the substitution medium is acetone and osmium tetroxide is included, a positive image results (Dempsey and Bullivant, 1976a,b; Hereward and Northcote, 1972; Malhotra and Van Harrevold, 1965; Pallaghy, 1973). When osmium is not included, negative images are seen (Harvey *et al.*, 1976). These observations lead to the conclusion that the osmium, when introduced with acetone, is binding to and preventing extraction of some membrane component if one assumes, a priori, that the positive image is the true image with nothing extracted. This implies that the positive membrane images reflect stabilization of membrane components by osmium, and the negative images are the result of the loss or extraction of membrane due to a lack of fixation or stabilization by osmium. A definitive answer is not presently possible because of conflicting evidence and an obvious shortage of critical information. However, the evidence discussed in the previous section on freeze-drying indicates that the negative image does not necessarily reflect the extraction of membrane components (Sjöstrand and Kretzer, 1975; Sjöstrom and Thornell, 1975; Terracio *et al.*, 1981). In comparison, McMillan and Luftig (1975) have shown that osmium causes a loss of membrane proteins. The argument against membrane extraction is further strengthened by studies on the loss of diffusible substances during preparation by freeze-substitution for elemental analysis. Harvey *et al.* (1976) showed that, even without chemical fixation, less than 4% of the original ion content was lost from tissues prepared for X-ray microanalysis. It is at least consistent to assume that, under similar preparative procedures, the loss of structural components such as membrane lipids or proteins would be minimal.

In a study of freeze-preservation and cell viability, Withers and Davey (1978) found that cells frozen without cryoprotection, or those rapidly frozen in the presence of cryoprotectant (5% DMSO + 10% glycerol) followed by freeze-substitution (OsO_4 in acetone) were either totally disrupted (no cryoprotection), or had positive membrane images (rapidly frozen, with cryoprotectants). Samples frozen by these methods had a viability, upon thawing, of less than 1%. However slow, controlled freezing (1–2°C/min) of cryoprotected cells resulted in 30–70% viability, and freeze-substituted cells treated this way had negative membrane images. This difference in staining after the two freezing regimes is interesting. The higher viability of the slowly frozen cells implies better preservation of cell and membrane structure by this technique. The presence of negative membrane images in this sample may, therefore, be correlated with this superior preservation and may reflect a more natural molecular architecture of the membrane.

Another explanation for the lack of osmium binding in the above situation may relate more directly to the rate of dehydration during freezing and/or to conformational changes in membrane constituents during freezing. It is commonly assumed that rapid freezing eliminates the possibility of molecular rearrangement but slow freezing probably permits the conformational changes of membrane constitutents to be stabilized by glycerol and by glycerol binding to phospholipid head groups (Buckingham and Staehelin, 1969). This stabilization of the membrane polar interface by glycerol could preclude reactivity of osmium with the membrane components. We suggest that the stabilization of the membrane conformations during slow freezing in glycerol also seems to account for the 30–70-fold increase in viability of these cells over those frozen by rapid methods.

An analogous situation occurs with cryptobiotic organisms (tardigrades and nematodes) and seeds. For example, when nematodes are partially dehydrated for three days and then are slowly dried to a level of 2–5% water, rehydration results in close to 100% survival (Crowe and Madin, 1975). During the partial dehydration period the nematodes synthesize large amounts of glycerol and trehalose, both of which interact with membrane polar components, resulting in a stabilization of the membrane in states of maximum water reduction. On the other hand, cryptobiotic organisms that are rapidly dehydrated have a low incidence of survival upon rehydration. This is presumably because without sufficient time for glycerol and trehalose synthesis, and therefore without stabilization of the membranes by these compounds, membrane integrity is lost, and survival upon rehydration is reduced (Crowe *et al.*, 1978; Madin and Crowe, 1975). In this regard it is interesting that Withers and Davey (1978), by using freeze-substitution methods, observed negative membrane images in the cells that had been frozen by a regime that allowed maximum viability.

Ultrastructural studies of dehydrated cryptobiotic organisms and seeds show positive membrane images when aqueous fixatives are used (Crowe *et al.*, 1978; Baird *et al.*, 1979). With dry seeds electron-dense membranes were observed when the primary fixative was nonaqueous, but aqueous postfixation with osmium was used (Thomson, 1979). In comparison, negative images are observed when the dry tissues are fixed nonaqueously with OsO$_4$ vapors (Öpik, 1980). The simplest interpretation is that the electron-dense membrane images are due to a hydration of the tissue with the aqueous fixative, resulting in staining patterns that are typical of normal, hydrated membranes. However, after nonaqueous fixation with osmium vapors, the resulting negative images may be due to insufficient water being present for the reaction of osmium with membrane components (Öpik, 1980). If the mechanism of adaptation to dry conditions in these tissues is protection of the membrane structure by glycerol and/or trehalose (Crowe and Madin, 1975; Madin and Crowe, 1975), then the presence of these protective molecules as well as the absence of water for reactivity effectively eliminates the normal interactions of osmium with the membrane components resulting in the negative membrane images. Further biochemical and physiological studies will have to be done on these systems to verify the presence of any protective substances in the dry seed tissue.

Freeze-Sectioning

1. Freeze-sectioning technique (Cryoultramicrotomy) (see Bernhard and Viron, 1971; Iglesius *et al.*, 1971; and Tokuyasu, 1973). Sectioning tissue while it is still frozen eliminates the need for infiltration with resins. This method is probably the most technically difficult of all electron microscopy preparative procedures and the numerous difficulties in handling fresh, frozen tissue have caused most investigators to use an initial prefixation in glutaraldehyde and/or cryoprotective agents such as dimethyl sulfoxide (DMSO), glycerol, or sucrose (Bernhard and Viron, 1971; Tokuyasu, 1973). Nevertheless the technique is attractive because the use of organic solvents such as acetone or ethanol and the need for infiltration in epoxy resin embedding media is eliminated, reducing the possibility of extraction and molecular rearrangement.

Rapid freezing is normally accomplished by the methods described previously for freeze-drying and freeze-substitution. The tissue is then mounted on a freezing-microtome and sectioned while still frozen. The frozen sections are picked up on coated grids, brought to room temperature, dried, stained, and observed in the electron microscope. The majority of investigators using this technique rely on the use of phosphotungstic acid (PTA) or silicotungstic acid (STA) as negative stains on their sections (Doty *et al.*, 1974; Sjöstrand

and Bernhard, 1976; Vogel, 1976; Williamson, 1978). However "positive" stains such as osmium tetroxide vapors or uranyl acetate and lead citrate have also been used (Bernhard and Leduc, 1967; Bernhard and Viron, 1971; Iglesias *et al.*, 1971; Tokuyasu, 1973).

2. *Frozen sections and negative images.* A globular or granular substructure of membranes is visible after freeze-sectioning and negative staining with PTA or STA (Bernhard and Viron, 1981; Sjöstrand and Bernhard, 1976; Tokuyasu, 1976). When freeze-sectioned tissue is stained with uranyl acetate and lead citrate, the membranes also appear as a negative image (Iglesias *et al.*, 1971). However when osmium is included as an aqueous stain, although membrane staining is faint (Bernhard and Leduc, 1967), the result is a more positive density pattern and may show the trilamellar membrane images seen after conventional preparation (Tokuyasu, 1973). These differences in membrane image are similar to those observed after the preparation of material by freeze-drying and freeze-substitution, and are significant in evaluating the effect of osmium tetroxide on the molecular architecture of membranes. Assuming that rapid freezing negates molecular rearrangements, then the light, but positive, density patterns observed with osmium tetroxide treatment may reflect the normal, in situ distribution of binding sites. Thus these density patterns would be related to the actual organization of the membrane. However the possibility still exists that osmium induces a rearrangement of membrane constituents, even in freeze-dried material.

LIPID-RETAINING PROCEDURES

As alternative procedures for the retention of lipids in tissues during preparation for electron microscopy, techniques have been developed for embedding the tissue in polymerized mixtures of glutaraldehyde and urea (Pease and Peterson, 1972; Peterson and Pease, 1972), glutaraldehyde and carbohydrazide (Heckman and Barnett, 1973), or water-soluble methacrylate embedding media (Leduc *et al.*, 1963; Spaur and Moriarty, 1977). A further advantage of these media, in addition to eliminating the use of lipid solvents, is the fact that they are water-soluble and are therefore more suitable for cytochemical and immunochemical studies (Leduc *et al.*, 1963; Nir and Pease, 1974; Spaur and Moriarty, 1977).

Polyglutaraldehyde Embedding

The technique of glutaraldehyde–urea embedding involves the preliminary fixing of small pieces of tissue in buffered glutaraldehyde, followed by slowly increasing the concentration of glutaraldehyde to a 50% solution (Glauert, 1975). The pH of the solution is kept about pH 5.0 with NaOH. Approximately equimolar urea (0.3 g urea/ml 50% glutaraldehyde) is added, and infiltration is allowed for 15–30 min. The pH is then lowered to pH 4.1–4.3 with saturated oxalic acid to initiate polymerization, which is complete in 1–2 days (Pease and Peterson, 1972). A later modification of this technique included the use of glycol methacrylate with the glutaraldehyde–urea. This method allowed the use of a higher pH (near neutrality), and therefore the retention of proteins in a more natural state (Pease, 1973a). Another polyglutaraldehyde procedure developed by Heckman and Barrnett (1973) combined glutaraldehyde and carbohydrazine (GACH).

Polyglutaraldehyde and negative images

The membrane images observed after polyglutaraldehyde embedment are not true negative images. If osmium vapor is used as a stain, the membranes appear as positive images or as solid, electron-dense lines (Pease, 1973a; Pease and Peterson, 1972). When osmium is not used and sections are stained with uranyl acetate and lead, the membranes appear in negative contrast only after superficial observation. Upon closer examination, narrow electron-dense lines can be seen at both surfaces of the membranes (Heckman and Barrnett, 1973; Pease and Peterson, 1972). This is particularly evident when the glutaraldehyde urea is copolymerized with glycolmethacrylate (Pease, 1973a). The internal, hydrophobic region of the membrane does not stain, although this region appears to be thicker than in conventionally prepared tissues.

Methacrylate-based embedding media

The tissue is fixed in glutaraldehyde, followed by simultaneous dehydration and infiltration with increasing concentrations of methacrylate (Glauert, 1975). Polymerization is achieved with UV light at low temperatures (10°C) (Leduc et al., 1963) or high temperatures (57°C) (Leduc and Holt, 1965). Occasionally osmium tetroxide is used for postfixation (Spaur and Moriarty, 1977). Uranyl acetate and/or lead are normally used for staining.

Methacrylate-Based Embedding and Negative Images

The staining pattern of the membranes of tissues prepared with water-soluble methacrylate embedding media is similar to that just described for polyglutaraldehyde-embedded tissue. The membranes commonly appear in negative contrast (Leduc *et al.*, 1963; Leduc and Holt, 1965); however, with prolonged staining with uranyl acetate and lead, a tripartite image is evident (Dermer, 1973). This latter image is somewhat similar to that obtained with OsO_4 fixation, however the dimensions are different. That is, the interior, light-staining region of the membrane is wider than it is in osmium-fixed tissue and the total membrane thicknesses are often greater (Dermer, 1973). When osmium is used as a postfixative and/or the tissue is dehydrated in ethanol prior to embedding in methacrylate, the membranes appear as positive images (Barsotti *et al.*, 1980; Spaur and Moriarty, 1977).

The interpretations of the membrane images seen in both polyglutaraldehyde- and methacrylate-embedded tissues suggest that the osmium, as well as uranyl acetate and lead, are reacting with proteins or some other component at the surface of the membranes and that the interior lipids are left unstained (Dermer, 1973; Leduc and Holt, 1965). The degree of molecular rearrangement or disruption caused by these methods is unknown, however the decreased reactivity of the membrane components with osmium and uranyl salts indicates fewer reactive sites available than after conventional preparation.

PROTEIN-NONDENATURING PROCEDURES

As mentioned earlier, lipids are a major constituent of biological membranes and the present fluid mosaic model of membrane structure (Singer and Nicolson, 1972) demands that if the structural integrity of the membrane is to be maintained during preparation of material for electron microscopy, then the lipids must be stabilized and preserved. This was the intention of many of the previous techniques of freeze-fixation and polar embedment. However proteins are also important constituents of membranes and, in fact, may outnumber lipid molecules by a ratio as high as, or greater than, 3:1 (Guidotti, 1972). For this reason, and because of the high probability of protein denaturation by conventional preparation techniques (Lenard and Singer, 1968; McMillan and Luftig, 1975), the following protein-retaining procedures were developed:

"Inert" Dehydration

Pease, who developed this technique (Pease, 1966 a,b), considers it to be a physical, rather than a chemical, fixation procedure because it involves the substitution of cellular water with small glycols or glycerol at room temperature with no previous chemical fixation (Pease, 1973b). The basis for the technique is the theory that small glycols and glycerol are not damaging to structured water in the cell and, therefore, should not seriously disturb the native conformation of proteins (Doebbler, 1966; Pease, 1973b).

1. "Inert" dehydration technique (see Pease, 1966 a,b; 1973b). Tissue samples are dehydrated (or substituted) in increasing concentrations of glycol or glycerol (ethylene glycol is preferred in most cases) up to 66%. At this point glutaraldehyde and/or OsO_4 may be used as a fixative to increase lipid retention and electron density, or dehydration may be continued up to 100% glycol. Tissue may then be directly embedded in glycol methacrylate media or, with proper transition chemicals, embedded in epoxy resin mixtures or Vestopal (Pease, 1966 a,b; 1973b).

Ethylene glycol is used in the knife boat, and stains (phosphotungstic acid and uranyl acetate) are dissolved in ethylene glycol as well. This eliminates the extraction of cellular constituents by water (Pease, 1966b).

2. "Inert" dehydration and negative images. The negative membrane images seen in tissue prepared by inert dehydration have been attributed to the more or less complete extraction of lipids (Pease, 1966a, 1973b; Walz, 1979). The reason for this conclusion is the absence of fixative, particularly OsO_4, as well as the solubility of lipids in glycol and methacrylates (Pease, 1966a). Although neutral lipids are apparently lost during this procedure (Cope and Williams, 1968) phospholipid analyses have not been performed either on tissues prepared by this method, or on the dehydrating agent or the plastic, and it is not known to what degree the major membrane lipids are actually extracted. The majority of the micrographs depicted in Pease's articles are negatively stained with phosphotungstic acid, and in most of these the membranes appear rather homogenously white in the areas of direct cross section (Pease, 1966 a,b). However, in regions of tangentially sectioned PTA-stained membranes (Pease, 1966b), and in micrographs of conventionally-stained (uranyl acetate and lead citrate) sections, a light staining is visible, revealing evidence of a globular substructure (Pease, 1966a).

Low Denaturation Embedding

Sjöstrand and Barajas (1968) introduced the technique of low denaturation preparation. The basis for developing a procedure that favors protein stabilization was based on evidence that mitochondrial membranes may have protein rather than lipid subunits as their primary building blocks. This idea was derived mainly from the studies of Fleischer *et al.* (1965), in which they found that even after 90% of the lipid had been extracted, mitochondrial membranes appeared basically unchanged in the elctron microscope. This low denaturation technique, therefore, was developed with the goal of maintaining proteins in their native conformation, in addition to minimizing lipid extraction.

1. Low denaturation technique [see Sjöstrand and Barajas (1968) and Kretzer (1973) for complete details, and Sjöstrand (1980b) and Weibull *et al.* (1980) for recent modifications]. Fixation (actually referred to as "cross-linking") in this procedure is at 0°C with low concentrations (1%) of glutaraldehyde for comparatively short times (1 min for dispersed cells, 30 min for tissue blocks). Dehydration is accomplished by immersion directly into 100% ethylene glycol, also at 0°C (1 min for dispersed cells, 10–30 min for tissue blocks). Samples are then transferred directly to Vestopal or Spurr's resin (1969) for embedding; polymerization is achieved by incubation at 45°C for one week. Thin sections are stained with uranyl acetate.

An alternate method, which makes use of low temperatures in combination with short glutaraldehyde cross-linking and rapid ethylene glycol dehydration has also been used. After cross-linking and partial dehydration, tissue is quick-frozen at $-180°C$, freeze-dried at $-80°C$, and infiltrated, embedded and polymerized in hydroxypropyl methacrylate at $-30°C$. Weibull *et al.* (1980) have also used a new embedding media, Lowacryl HM_2O and K4M which can be polymerized at $-35°C$ with UV light.

The results using all these procedures were essentially the same (Weibull *et al.*, 1980; Sjöstrand, 1978; Sjöstrand and Barajas, 1968). The basic principle of these procedures is to minimize the length of time the tissue is exposed to chemicals which may cause molecular rearrangement, and to keep the tissues at low temperatures to reduce extraction by lowering solubility.

2. Low denaturation procedure and negative images. The negative membrane images apparent after the preparation of tissues by low denaturation techniques are interpreted as being good representations of true membrane ultrastructure (Weibull *et al.*, 1980; Kretzer, 1973; Sjöstrand, 1976, 1977, 1980b; Sjöstrand and Barajas, 1968). Support for this interpretation can be seen in Sjöstrand and Barajas' original study (1968). In one experiment they dehydrated tissue with acetone rather than ethylene glycol—all other treatments were the same. In this sample membranes were more irregular and had a "typical" tripartite image, although they were still lightly stained, probably due to the absence of OsO_4.

Evidence that lipids probably are not extracted by this treatment has been shown by Sjöstrand *et al.* (1978) with dark-field electron microscopic analysis of mitochondrial membranes. This study demonstrated that the mass density of the light-staining cristae is much greater than that of the electron-dense matrix, and that the light image of the membranes prepared by this method is due to a lack of stain interaction with the molecules rather than extraction of the membrane components. An explanation for the difference in staining patterns is that, during conventional preparation, extensive denaturation of proteins by glutaraldehyde (Lenard and Singer, 1968), osmium tetroxide (McMillin and Luftig, 1975), and acetone leads to the exposure of charged groups on the protein molecules (Sjöstrand *et al.*, 1978). These charged sites provide loci for interaction with stains such as uranyl salts and lead. However charged groups are not made available during low denaturation procedures and, as a consequence, the membranes have a very low affinity for stains (Sjöstrand, 1976, 1980b).

Another difference in the membrane image after low denaturation as opposed to conventional preparation is apparent in membrane thickness. For example, in *Chlamydomonas* prepared by low denaturation techniques, the chloroplast membranes are 270Å thick (Kretzer, 1973). However longer exposure to glutaraldehyde (15–30 min compared to 3–6 min), dehydration in acetone, or no fixation at all, resulted in a significant decrease in membrane thickness to 100–210 Å. Again the lack of staining is thought to be due to an absence of charged groups exposed by extraction and denaturation procedures (Kretzer, 1973).

OTHER PROCEDURES WHICH SOMETIMES RESULT IN NEGATIVE IMAGES

In addition to those procedures already discussed, other techniques also result in negative membrane images; some consistently, others only occasionally. Air drying of the tissue with or without fixation has been introduced as a procedure for optimizing lipid retention since it does not require the use of solvents during dehydration. Sjöstrand and Barajas (1968) compared the image of unfixed and fixed, air-dried mitochondria with that of mitochondria prepared by their low denaturing technique. They found that air drying produced negative images, however the membranes were irregular in both arrangement and thickness. If the tissue was cross-linked with glutaraldehyde prior to air drying, preservation was better, and a globular substructure was visible. The average membrane thickness (94Å) was intermediate to that obtained with acetone (50Å) and glycol (150Å) dehydration.

In a series of experiments Thomson (unpublished) fixed leaf tissue by one of two ways: (*a*) with OsO_4 vapor or (*b*) in a 1% solution of OsO_4. The tissue was then air dried at 60°C either immediately after fixation (Fig. 5) or after dehydration in acetone (Fig. 6). The membrane images of the chloroplast grana were of negative contrast in all cases. The only obvious difference between the various preparations was an apparent increase in size of the A component of the grana (see Thomson, 1974) after 1% OsO_4 fixation and complete acetone dehydration before air drying. Similar negative membrane images were reported by Schidlovsky (1962, 1965) in the grana of spinach chloroplasts prepared by air drying. The most logical explanation for the negative contrast of membranes after air drying is, again, a minimal extraction of components which would occur during solvent dehydration. However, as seen in Fig. 6, tissue air dried after acetone dehydration also exhibits negative membrane images. This presents an enigma unless extraction or rearrangement occurs during the replacement of acetone by the embedding media, or air drying reverses some rearrangement which occurs during solvent dehydration.

The use of tannic acid as a fixative in conjunction with glutaraldehyde was introduced by Mizuhira and Futaesaku in 1971. This technique has been effective in increasing contrast, probably because the tannic acid acts as a mordant between osmium and lead (Simionescu and Simionescu, 1967 a,b). Kalina and Pease (1977) have shown that tannic acid also binds to the choline groups of phosphotidylcholine and sphingomyelin, and Gustavson (1949) and Futaesaku *et al.* (1972) suggest that it may interact with positively charged protein groups. In most cases positive membrane images are seen after the use of tannic acid with glutaraldehyde (Kalina and Pease, 1977; Mollenhauer *et al.*, 1977; Saito *et al.*, 1978). However, occasionally, and particularly when plant tissue is used, the membranes appear in negative contrast (Nehls and Schaffner, 1976; Olesen, 1978). This phenomenon is particularly common in the granal membranes of chloroplasts, as we shall discuss in the following section. However it is not uncommon to find that all cellular membranes are in negative contrast (Fig. 7). This is a puzzling observation but it has been suggested that if tannic acid is a mordant, it may protect membrane proteins from denaturation and extraction by osmium tetroxide and dehydrating solvents. It may also further cross-linking and the protection of proteins by glutaraldehyde and possibly osmium (Olesen, 1978; Simionescu and Simionescu, 1976). The distinct subunit type of structure observed in thylakoid membranes after fixation with tannic acid and glutaraldehyde (Olesen , 1978) supports this interpretation. Additionally, similar negative membrane images and particulate substructures have been observed in thylakoids after the treatment of fixed tissue with hot aqueous uranyl acetate before dehydration (Van Stevininck and Van Stevininck, 1975). Again, this image was in-

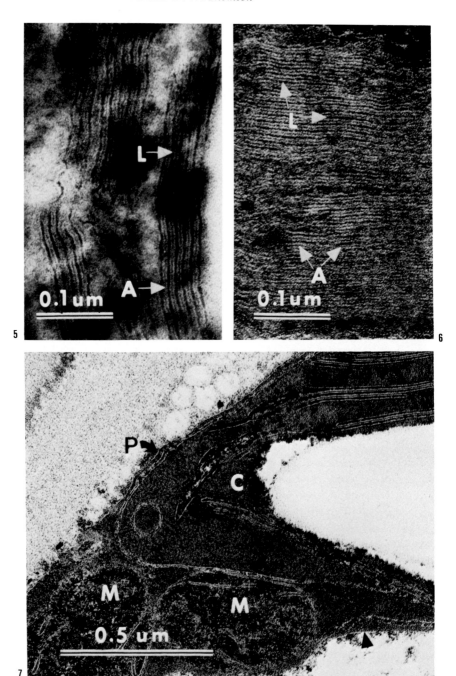

terpreted as due to a stabilizing, mordant effect of the uranyl acetate, which reduced molecular extraction and/or rearrangement during further treatments.

A simpler explanation is that tannic acid binds to the membrane proteins but in so doing reduces the number of available binding sites for the heavy metals. Possibly the only available binding sites are those bound to tannic acid. Thus the apparent negative image results from a major reduction in density and a shift in comparative density patterns (i.e., light-staining membranes) rather than actual negative staining.

SUMMARY OF PREPARATIVE PROCEDURES WHICH RESULT IN NEGATIVE MEMBRANE IMAGES

In reviewing the membrane images obtained by the preparative procedures thus far described, it is apparent that, although a common feature is an apparent electron translucency of the membrane, there is some variability in the image obtained with different techniques. This variation involves the amount of visible substructure and the final thickness of the membranes. Whether these variations are due to differences in the amount of extraction and/or molecular rearrangement by the various techniques, or whether there is a difference in reactivity of the different tissues with heavy metal stains is not certain at this time. It is apparent, however, that almost any preparative technique designed for minimizing molecular rearrangement and extraction results in light-staining or negative membrane images. This indicates that the conventional preparative procedures cause rather extensive conformational changes in membrane architecture, and thus, tissue prepared in this way should be studied with caution.

Fig. 5. Chloroplast grana from a *Phaseolus* leaf which had been fixed in osmium vapors and air dried at 50°C then embedded in epoxy. These membranes appear as negative images with an electron-dense loculus (L) and A space (A). 210,000×. Bar = 0.1 μm.

Fig. 6. Electron micrograph of a chloroplast grana from a *Phaseolus* leaf. The tissue was prepared by fixation over osmium vapors, dehydration in acetone followed by air drying at 50°C, and embeddment in epoxy resin. The loculus (L) and A space (A) are extremely electron-dense and the membranes appear electron translucent or in negative contrast. 207,000×. Bar = 0.1 μm.

Fig. 7. Portion of a cell from a leaf of *Larrea* which had been fixed with 1% tannic acid in glutaraldehyde. The membranes of the mitochondria (M), chloroplast (C), tonoplast (arrowhead), and plasmalemma (P) all appear as negative images against the electron-dense matrix. 84,000×. Bar = 0.5 μm.

Negative Images in Chloroplast Granal Membranes

Negative membrane images have been reported to occur in preparations of the granal membranes of chloroplasts of a wide variety of plants and tissues. In many cases the tissues were immature (Casadoro and Rascio, 1978, 1979 a,b; Damsz and Mikulska, 1976; Platt-Aloia and Thomson, 1977) or specialized for functions other than photosynthesis (Platt-Aloia and Thomson, 1979; Stead and Duckett, 1980; Van Stevininck and Van Stevinick, 1980a). Several interpretations have emerged from these observations, the two most dominant being that the organization of the photosynthetic membranes is incomplete and lacking some necessary osmiophilic component (probably lipid), and that the negative image is really a matter of relative densities because the loculus is highly electron-dense and the membranes appear to be unstained in contrast.

Support for the first idea (incomplete membrane assembly) is derived from the observations that the negatively stained or light-staining membranes occur in young, developing plastids (Fig. 8). As the tissue and plastids mature, the staining of these membranes changes to a normal electron dense pattern (Fig. 9) and the substance in the loculus is lost or decreases in electron density (Casadoro and Rascio, 1978, 1979 a,b; Cran and Possingham, 1974; Platt-Aloia and Thomson, 1977; Rascio and Casadoro, 1979; Stetler and Laetsch, 1969). Proponents of this theory often attribute the electron density of the loculus to an accumulation of lipid, lipoprotein, or other potential membrane components (Salema et al., 1972a). In fact, dissolution of the locular material has been achieved, in some cases, with the use of lipases and/or proteases (Damsz and Mikulska, 1976; Salema and Abreu, 1972).

Contradicting this interpretation are the observations that other characteristics of organization, such as granal stacking, occur and that the crystal-

Fig. 8. Grana from a plastid in a young, developing leaf of *Sesame*. The loculus (L) and A space (A) are electron-dense and the internal membranes appear as negative images. The envelope membranes (arrowheads) stain as positive images. Conventional preparation as for Fig. 1, 102,000×. Bar = 0.1 μm.

Fig. 9. Grana from a plastid in a young, but somewhat more fully developed, sesame leaf than that shown in Fig. 8. The grana–fretwork membranes appear as positive images. L = loculus. Conventional fixation as for Fig. 1. 103,000×. Bar = 0.1 μm.

Fig. 10. Electron micrograph of a portion of a chloroplast from an outer cell in the peel of a Muscat Grape. The loculus (L) is filled with an electron-dense substance and the A space (A) is also electron-dense. The granal membranes show as negative images. The chloroplast envelope membrane (arrowheads) is a positive image. 130,000×. Bar = 0.1 μm.

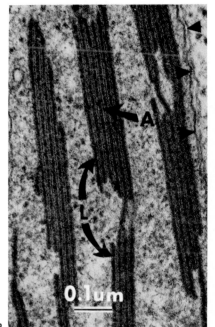

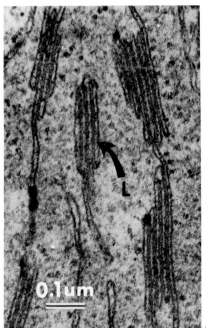

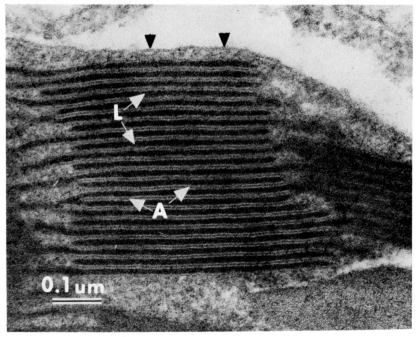

line lattice of the prolamellar bodies still develop (Rascio et al., 1979). Thus it could be argued that if the membranes show a normal degree of secondary organization (stacking and prolamellar body formation) then incomplete assembly of the membranes is not likely. In other words, if some major component of the membrane were lacking such that negative images would result after osmium staining, then intricate processes such as prolamellar body formation and granal stacking would not be possible. This is further substantiated by the fact that no change other than a shift in the electron density pattern occurs during maturation. Although most common in immature tissues, negative images of granal membranes are found in other tissues as well. They have also been described in mature, tannin-containing cells (Fig. 10), in tissue prefixed with tannin (Olesen, 1978), in mature leaves held below their compensation point (Tripodi, 1980), and in plants cultivated in an excess of calcium (Chevalier, 1969). These observations cast doubt on the view that the negative images are due to the lack of essential membrane components (Van Steveninck and Van Steveninck, 1980b).

The second interpretation ascribes the negative images to differentials in the relative contrast or densities between the membrane and the loculus. This interpretation implies that there is a differential reactivity of the osmium with the membrane and the loculus rather than a lack of an essential compositional component in the membrane.

Osmium tetroxide has been shown to react with numerous biological constituents such as unsaturated bonds of fatty acids (Korn, 1966, 1967; Collin et al., 1973; White et al., 1976), charged polar head groups of phospholipids (Hayat, 1970), proteins (Hake, 1965; Nielson and Griffith, 1979), and the hydroxyl groups of o-dihydroxyphenolic compounds (Nielson and Griffith, 1978).

Lead citrate and uranyl acetate, stains commonly used in electron microscopy, both readily combine with reduced OsO_4, and enhance the contrast of membranes and other cellular components. Uranyl salts also react with the phosphate groups of nucleic acids and phospholipids (McLaughlin et al., 1971), as well as with the free amino groups of proteins (Hayat, 1970; Knight, 1977).

Long exposure of leaf tissue to uranyl acetate after fixation with glutaraldehyde and osmium, but before dehydration, results in an increased electron density of the loculus of the grana. Based on this observation is the proposal that the binding of the stain to some component in the loculus such as proteins prevented its subsequent removal during dehydration (Van Stevininck and Van Stevininck, 1975). Similarly, negative images in tissues fixed in the presence of tannin could be explained by a mordant action of the tannin causing binding to components in the loculus resulting in increased electron density, and consequently causing membranes to appear less dense in comparison (Olesen, 1978).

Chloroplasts have been shown to contain enzymes involved in the synthesis and metabolism of phenols, flavanoids and quinones (Bartlett *et al.*, 1972; Kirk and Tilney-Bassett, 1978; Saito, 1974; Sato, 1966; Sharma and Vaidyanathan, 1975). Several of the substrates, intermediates, and products of these pathways are *o*-dihydroxy-substituted phenols which are known to react with osmium tetroxide (Nielson and Griffith, 1978). The presence of these compounds in the loculus of young plastids would provide binding sites for osmium so that further reaction with uranyl acetate could result in highly electron-dense deposits. A shift in the density pattern during chloroplast maturation may reflect a decrease in the accumulation of these products in the loculus resulting in a shift from high electron density to relatively low electron density. If this were the case, the membranes would increase density relative to the loculus and the more typical image pattern would emerge. The same conclusions were reached by Bullivant (1965) and Cope and Williams (1969) ". . . that the membrane is only negative . . . because it has less density than the surroundings . . . [Bullivant, 1965, p. 1193]".

In summary, negative membrane images in chloroplast grana may be the result of an excessive binding of osmium tetroxide and uranyl salts to components in the loculus. This increased binding and enhanced electron density would result in the membranes appearing relatively unstained and negative in contrast. Additionally, the mordant effect of tannins or other phenolic compounds may cross-link membrane constituents, thus resulting in greater retention of the natural molecular configuration of the membrane.

Conclusions

Whether the negative membrane images observed in chloroplast granal membranes and those seen after various specialized preparative techniques are all due to the same, or closely related, phenomena is not presently certain. However reduced molecular rearrangement or extraction has been suggested as the basis for many of the negative membrane images. This suggestion is particularly appropriate when efforts to minimize molecular rearrangement or extraction are made during the preparatory procedures, such as during freeze-drying and freeze-substitution. The interpretation is that if the membrane constituents are not rearranged or extracted, then the so-called negative images or "reverse" image patterns, as well as the common globular subunits, more nearly approximate the true membrane organization. The implication of this interpretation is that "normal" positive images are due to a rearrangement of the membrane constituents. This results in a shift of the binding sites for stains (heavy metals) to new locations and makes more sites available due to the removal of possible blocking components and denaturation of intrinsic proteins.

Many images reported as being negative are not truly so on close examination. In these cases the same density patterns are observed as with positive images except that the density is much less than normally observed. Again, in most instances these reduced density patterns are present when procedures are used to reduce extraction and denaturation of the membrane lipids and proteins. Following the argument in the previous paragraph, this would simply mean that the reduced density is a function of fewer stain binding sites being available due to reduced denaturation and rearrangement.

Differences in electron scattering among different regions of the specimen establishes contrast and density patterns in electron micrographs. The binding of heavy metal stains to biological materials enhances electron scatter. Thus if the stains bind preferentially to certain biological components which have accumulated in particular regions of the cell, then regions will appear in greater positive contrast than adjacent areas. In other words, the sites where these accumulations are large would have a higher density than adjacent regions where the binding of the stains is significantly less. For example, if the locular regions of the grana contain constituents that bind the heavy metals to a greater extent per unit volume than the granal membranes, then the locular regions will appear as a positive image and the membrane will appear negative simply because of the difference in electron scattering. It is not necessary to assume that the membranes appear negative in image because they lack some essential component relative to the final organization of the membrane and that the absence of this component limits the binding of the stains. The membrane may lack some essential final organizational component but this may not be important for the establishment of density patterns. The shift of the locular image from positive to negative and the membrane image from negative to positive could be accounted for by a loss of binding material from the locular regions so that the binding of the heavy metal and the accompanying electron scattering in the membrane significantly exceeds that of the loculus. Similarly, blocking agents (whether endogenous or applied) such as tannic acid, may minimize the binding of the heavy metals to the membrane. This would bring about a negative membrane image due to reduced electron scatter and therefore a lower apparent density of the membrane as compared to adjacent regions where electron scattering remained the same or possibly was increased by the mordant effect of the tannic acid.

References

Baird, L. A. M., Leopold, A. C., Bramlage, W. J., and Webster, B. D. (1979). *Bot. Gaz.* **140**, 371–377.

Barsotti, P., D'Agostino, M., and Marinozzi, V. (1980). *J. Submicrosc. Cytol.* **12**, 233–242.

Bartlett, D. J., Poulton, J. E., and Butt, V. S. (1972). *FEBS Lett.* **23**, 265–267.

Bernhard, W., and Leduc, E. H. (1967). *J. Cell Biol.* **34**, 757–771.

Bernhard, W., and Viron, A. (1971). *J. Cell Biol.* **49**, 731–746.

Breathnach, A. S., Gross, M., Martin, B., and Stolinski, C. (1976). *J. Cell Sci.* **21**, 437–448.

Buckingham, J. H., and Staehelin, L. A. (1969). *J. Microsc.* **90**, 83–106.

Bullivant, S. (1965). *Lab Invest.* **14**, 1178–1195.

Casadoro, G., and Rascio, N. (1978). *J. Ultrastruct. Res.* **65**, 30–35.

Casadoro, G., and Rascio, N. (1979a). *Cytobios* **24**, 157–166.

Casadoro, G., and Rascio, N. (1979b). *J. Ultrastruct. Res.* **69**, 307–315.

Chevalier, S., Baccou, J. C., and Sauvaire, Y. (1969). *C. R. Acad. Sci. Paris* **269**, 1653–1656.

Collin, R., Griffith, W. P., Phillips, F. L., and Skapski, A. C. (1973). *Biochim. Biophys. Acta* **320**, 745–747.

Cope, G. H., and Williams, M. A. (1968). *J. R. Microsc. Soc.* **88**, 259–271.

Cope, G. H., and Williams, M. A. (1969). *J. Microsc.* **90**, 47–60.

Cran, D. G., and Possingham, J. V. (1974). *Ann. Bot.* **38**, 843–847.

Crowe, J. H., and Madin, K. A. C. (1975). *J. Exp. Zool.* **193**, 323–334.

Crowe, J. H., Lambert, D. T., and Crowe, L. M. (1978). *In* "Dry Biological Systems" (J. H. Crowe and J. S. Clegg, eds.), pp. 23–51. Academic Press, New York.

Damsz, B., and Mikulska, E. (1976). *Biochem. Physiol. Pflanzen* **169**, 257–263.

Dempsey, G. P., and Bullivant, S. (1976a). *J. Microsc.* **106**, 251–260.

Dempsey, G. P., and Bullivant, S. (1976b). *J. Microsc.* **106**, 261–271.

Dermer, G. B. (1973). *J. Ultrastruct. Res.* **42**, 221–233.

Doebbler, G. F. (1966). *Cryobiology* **3**, 2–11.

Doty, S. B., Lee, C. W., and Banfield, W. G. (1974). *Histochem. J.* **6**, 383–393.

Fleischer, S., Fleischer, B., and Stoeckenius, W. (1967). *J. Cell Biol.* **32**, 193–208.

Futaesaku, Y., Mizuhira, V., and Nakamura, N. (1972). *Proc. Intern. Congr. Histochem. Cytochem.* **4**, 155–156.

Glauert, A. M. (1975). "Practical Methods in Electron Microscopy," Vol. 3, Part I. North Holland Publ., Amsterdam.

Gorter, E., and Grendel, F. (1925). *J. Exp. Med.* **41**, 439–443.

Guidotti, G. (1972). *Ann. Rev. Biochem.* **41**, 731–752.

Gustavson, H. K. (1949). *In* "Advanc. Protein Chem" **5** (M. L. Anson, J. T. Edsall, and K. Bailey, eds.) pp. 353–421. Academic Press, New York.

Hake, T. (1965). *Lab. Invest.* **14**, 470–474.

Harvey, D. M. R., Hall, J. L., and Flowers, T. J. (1976). *J. Microsc.* **107**, 189–198.

Hayat, M. A. (1970). "Principles and Techniques of Electron Microscopy", Vol. 1. Van Nostrand-Reinhold, New York.

Heckman, C. A., and Barrnett, R. J. (1973). *J. Ultrastruct. Res.* **42**, 156–179.

Hereward, F. V., and Northcote, D. H. (1972). *Exp. Cell Res.* **70**, 73–80.

Heuser, J. E., Reese, T. S., Dennis, M. J., Jan, Y., Jan, L., and Evans, L. (1979). *J. Cell Biol.* **81**, 275–300.

Iglesias, J. R., Bernier, R., and Simard, R. (1971). *J. Ultrastruct. Res.* **36**, 271–289.

Jost, P. C., and Griffith, O. H. (1973). *Arch. Biochem. and Biophys.* **159**, 70–81.

Kalina, M., and Pease, D. C. (1977). *J. Cell Biol.* **74**, 726–741.

Karnovsky, M. J. (1971). *Proc. Ann. Meeting Am. Soc. Cell Biol. 14th* p. 146.

Kirk, J. T. O., and Tilney-Basset, R. A. E. (1978). "The Plastids, Their Chemistry, Structure, Growth, and Inheritance". Elsevier/North Holland Biomedical Press, Amsterdam.

Knight, D. P. (1977). *In* "Practical Methods in Electron Microscopy" (A. M. Glauert, ed.), Vol. 5, Part 1, pp. 26–28. Elsevier/North Holland Biomedical Press, Amsterdam.

Korn, E. D., and Weisman, R. A. (1966). *Biochim. Biophys. Acta* **116**, 309–316.

Kretzer, F. (1973). *J. Ultrastruct. Res.* **44**, 146–178.

Läuchli, A., Spurr, A. R., and Wittkopp, R. W. (1970). *Planta* **95**, 341–350.

Leduc, E. H., and Holt, S. J. (1965). *J. Cell Biol.* **26**, 137–155.

Leduc, E., Marinozzi, V., and Bernhard, W. (1963). *J. R. Microsc. Soc.* **81**, 119–130.

Lenard, J., and Singer, S. J. (1968). *J. Cell Biol.* **37**, 117–121.

Luftig, R. B., Wehrli, E., and McMillan, P. N. (1977). *Life Sci.* **21**, 285–300.

Madin, K. A. C., and Crowe, J. H. (1975). *J. Exp. Zool.* **193**, 335–342.

Malhotra, S. K., and Van Harreveld, A. (1965). *J. Ultrastruct. Res.* **12**, 473–487.

McLaughlin, S. G. A., Szabo, G., and Eisenman, G. (1971). *J. Gen. Physiol.* **58**, 667–687.

McMillan, P. N., and Luftig, R. B. (1973). *Proc. Nat. Acad. Sci. U.S.A.* **70**, 3060–3064.

McMillan, P. N., and Luftig, R. B. (1975). *J. Ultrastruct. Res.* **42**, 243–260.

Mollenhauer, H. H., Morré, D. J., and Hass, B. S. (1977). *J. Ultrastruct. Res.* **61**, 166–171.

Moretz, R. C., Akers, C. K., and Parsons, D. F. (1969a). *Biochim. Biophys. Acta* **193**, 1–11.

Moretz, R. C., Akers, C. K., and Parsons, D. F. (1969b). *Biochim Biophys. Acta.* **193**, 12–21.

Morgan, T. E., and Huber, G. L. (1967). *J. Cell Biol.* **32**, 757–760.

Muller, H. R. (1957). *J. Ultrastruct. Res.* **1**, 109–137.

Nehls, R., and Schaffner, G. (1976). *Cytobiologie* **13**, 285–290.

Niedermeyer, W., Parish, G. R., and Moor, H. (1977). *Protoplasma* **92**, 177–193.

Nielson, A. J., and Griffith, W. P. (1978). *J. Histochem. Cytochem.* **26**, 138–140.

Nir, I., and Pease, D. C. (1974). *J. Histochem. Cytochem.* **22**, 1019–1027.

Olesen, P. (1978). *Biochem. Physiol. Pflanzen* **172**, 319–342.

Öpik, H. (1980). *New Phytol.* **85**, 521–529.

Ongun, A., Thomson, W. W., and Mudd, J. B. (1968). *J. Lipid Res.* **9**, 416–424.

Pallaghy, C. K. (1973). *Aust. J. Biol. Sci.* **26**, 1015–1034.

Parish, G. R. (1975). *J. Microsc.* **104**, 245–256.

Pease, D. C. (1966a). *J. Ultrastruct. Res.* **14**, 356–378.

Pease, D. C. (1966b). *J. Ultrastruct. Res.* **14**, 379–390.

Pease, D. C. (1967a). *J. Ultrastruct. Res.* **21**, 75–97.

Pease, D. C. (1967b). *J. Ultrastruct. Res.* **21**, 98–124.

Pease, D. C. (1973a). *J. Ultrastruct. Res.* **45**, 124–148.

Pease, D. C. (1973b). *In* "Biological Electron Microscopy" (J. K. Koehler, ed.), pp. 35–66. Springer-Verlag, Berlin and New York.

Pease, D. C., and Peterson, R. G. (1972). *J. Ultrastruct. Res.* **41**, 133–159.

Peterson, R. G., and Pease, D. C. (1972). *J. Ultrastruct. Res.* **41**, 115–132.

Pinto da Silva, P., and Miller, R. G. (1975). *Proc. Nat. Acad. Sci. U.S.A.* **72**, 4046–4050.

Platt-Aloia, K. A., and Thomson, W. W. (1977). *New Phytol.* **78**, 599–605.

Platt-Aloia, K. A., and Thomson, W. W. (1979). *New Phytol.* **83**, 793–799.

Rascio, N., and Casadoro, G. (1979). *J. Ultrastruct. Res.* **68**, 325–327.
Rascio, N., Casadoro, G., and DiChio, L. (1979). *Protoplasma* **100**, 45–52.
Rebhun, L. I. (1972). *In* "Principles and Techniques of Electron Microscopy" (M. A. Hayat, ed.), Vol. 2, pp. 3–49. Van Nostrand-Reinhold, New York.
Saito, A., Wang, C. T., and Fleischer, S. (1978). *J. Cell Biol.* **79**, 601–616.
Saito, K. (1974). *Biochem. J.* **144**, 431–432.
Salema, R., and Abreu, I. (1972). *Broteria* **41**, 119–138.
Salema, R., Mesquita, J. F., and Abreu, I. (1972). *J. Submicrosc. Cytol.* **4**, 161–169.
Sato, M. (1966). *Phytochemistry* **5**, 385–389.
Schidlovsky, G. (1962). *In Biologist. Space Syst. Symp.* (J. Robinnette, ed.), pp. 105–130. U.S. Air Force Technical Documentary Rep. No. AMRL-TDR-62-116.
Schidlovsky, G. (1965). *Lab Invest.* **14**, 475–489.
Sharma, H. K., and Vaidyanathan, C. S. (1975). *Phytochemistry* **14**, 2135–2139.
Simionescu, N., and Simionescu, M. (1976a). *J. Cell Biol.* **70**, 608–621.
Simionescu, N., and Simionescu, M. (1976b). *J. Cell Biol.* **70**, 622–633.
Singer, S. J., and Nicolson, G. L. (1972). *Science* **175**, 720–731.
Sjöstrand, F. (1943). *Nature (London)*, **151**, 725–726.
Sjöstrand, F. S. (1963). *Nature (London)* **199**, 1262–1264.
Sjöstrand, F. S. (1976). *J. Ultrastruct. Res.* **55**, 271–280.
Sjöstrand, F. S. (1977). *J. Ultrastruct. Res.* **59**, 292–319.
Sjöstrand, F. S. (1978). *J. Ultrastruct. Res.* **64**, 217–245.
Sjöstrand, F. S. (1979). *J. Ultrastruct. Res.* **69**, 378–420.
Sjöstrand, F. S. (1980a) *Biol. Cellulaire* **39**, 217–220.
Sjöstrand, F. S. (1980b). *J. Ultrastruct. Res.* **72**, 174–188.
Sjöstrand, F. S., and Baker, R. F. (1958). *J. Ultrastruct. Res.* **1**, 239–246.
Sjöstrand, F. S., and Barajas, L. (1968). *J. Ultrastruct. Res.* **25**, 121–155.
Sjöstrand, F. S., and Bernhard, W. (1976). *J. Ultrastruct. Res.* **56**, 233–246.
Sjöstrand, F. S., and Elfvin, L. G. (1964). *J. Ultrastruct. Res.* **10**, 263–292.
Sjöstrand, F. S., and Kretzer, F. (1975). *J. Ultrastruct. Res.* **53**, 1–28.
Sjöstrand, F. S., Dubochet, J., Wurtz, M., and Kellenberger, E. (1978). *J. Ultrastruct. Res.* **65**, 23–29.
Sjöstrom, M., and Thornell, L. E. (1975). *J. Microsc.* **103**, 101–112.
Somlyo, A. V., Shuman, H., and Somlyo, A. P. (1977). *J. Cell. Biol.* **74**, 828–857.
Somlyo, A. P., Somlyo, A. V., and Shuman, H. (1979). *J. Cell Biol.* **81**, 316–335.
Spaur, R. C., and Moriarty, G. C. (1977). *J. Histochem. Cytochem.* **25**, 163–174.
Spurr, A. R. (1969). *J. Ultrastruct. Res.* **26**, 31–43.
Stead, A. D., and Duckett, J. G. (1980). *Ann. Bot.* **46**, 549–555.
Stetler, D. A., and Laetsch, W. M. (1969). *Amer. J. Bot.* **56**, 260–270.
Stolinski, C., Breathnach, A. S., and Bellairs, R. (1978). *J. Microsc.* **112**, 293–299.
Tanford, C. (1978). *Science* **200**, 1012–1018.
Terracio, L. Bankston, P. W., and McAteer, J. A. (1981). *Cryobiology* **18**, 55–71.
Thomson, W. W. (1974). *In* "Dynamics of Plant Cell Ultrastructure" (A. Robards, ed.), pp. 138–177. McGraw Hill. New York.
Thomson, W.W. (1979). *New Phytol.* **82**, 207–212.
Tokuyasu, K. T. (1973). *J. Cell Biol.* **57**, 551–565.
Tokuyasu, K. T. (1976). *J. Ultrastruct. Res.* **55**, 281–287.
Tripodi, G. (1980). *Protoplasma* **103**, 163–168.
Trump, B. F., and Ericsson, J. L. E. (1965). *Lab Invest.* **14**, 507–521.
Van Harreveld, A., Trubatch, J., and Steiner, J. (1974). *J. Microsc.* **100**, 189–198.
VanSteveninck, M. E., and VanSteveninck, R. F. M. (1975). *Protoplasma* **86**, 381–389.

VanSteveninck, M. E., and VanSteveninck, R. F. M. (1980a). *Protoplasma* **103**, 333–342.
VanSteveninck, M. E., and VanSteveninck, R. F. M. (1980b). *Protoplasma* **103**, 343–360.
Vernon, L. P., and Shaw, E. R. (1971). *Methods Enzymol.* **23**, 277–289.
Vogel, F. (1976). *J. Microsc. Biol. Cell.* **26**, 61–64.
Walz, B. (1979). *Protoplasma* **99**, 19–30.
Weibull, C., Carlemalm, E., Villiger, W., Kellenberger, E., Fakan, J., Gautier, A., and Larsson, C. (1980). *J. Ultrastruct. Res.* **73**, 233–244.
White, D. L., Andrews, S. B., Faller, J. W., and Barrnett, R. J. (1976). *Biochim. Biophys. Acta* **436**, 577–592.
Williamson, F. A. (1978). *Int. Congr. Electron Microsc. 9th* **2**, 36–37.
Withers, L. A., and Davey, M. R. (1978). *Protoplasma* **94**, 207–219.

Chapter 6

Interactions of Cytochrome P-450 with Phospholipids and Proteins in the Endoplasmic Reticulum[1]

James R. Trudell, Bernhard Bösterling

Protein–Lipid Interactions of Intrinsic Membrane Proteins. 201
   Choice of Environments in Which to Study Lipid–Protein Interactions 201
   Evidence for the Influence of Phospholipids on Protein Function in
   Reconstituted Systems. 203
   A Review of Techniques for Reconstitution of Cytochrome P-450. 204
Lipid–Protein Interactions of Cytochrome P-450 in Reconstituted
   Vesicles. 207
Recent Studies. 207
Reductive Metabolism of Halothane by Human and Rabbit Cytochrome
   P-450. 229
References. 232

Protein–Lipid Interactions of Intrinsic Membrane Proteins

CHOICE OF ENVIRONMENTS IN WHICH TO STUDY LIPID–PROTEIN INTERACTIONS

Natural Membranes

The native cell membrane offers many obvious advantages for studies of protein–lipid interactions. The proteins occupy their correct position in the

[1]This research was supported by a grant from the National Institute of Occupational Safety and Health (OH 00978) and a stipend to B. Bösterling from the Alexander von Humboldt-Stiftung.

bilayer, all of the major and minor phospholipid constituents are present in the bilayer, the phospholipids have the inside-to-outside ratio of components that is appropriate for the functioning membrane, any transmembrane potentials that may be essential for protein function exist at their correct potential and polarity, the membrane has the appropriate surface charge on the inner and outer surfaces, extrinsic membrane proteins that may function to hold intrinsic membrane proteins into specialized assemblies or control their respective orientation are in their proper location, and the correct electrolyte and nonelectrolyte concentrations exist near the inner and outer surface of the membrane. However, despite these many advantages, the native cell membrane is often resistant to the application of the reductionist techniques of modern science. Spectroscopic techniques usually report the sum of all protein–protein, protein–lipid, and lipid–lipid interactions in the sample. When the researcher wants to study a limited set of protein–lipid interactions of a single protein, it is often necessary to isolate the protein in a highly purified form and then perform the spectroscopy or analytical measurement. In the case of intrinsic membrane proteins, the addition of phospholipids or some other hydrophobic environment is necessary to render the protein in a sufficiently natural form to make spectroscopic observations relevant to the native membrane. There are several classes of reconstitution techniques that have proven to be useful in studies of lipid–protein interactions.

Micelles

Reconstitution of cytochrome *P*-450 into dilauroylphosphatidylcholine micelles has proven to be a major advance in the study of this protein. When reconstituted in these short chain phospholipid micelles, the protein exhibits metabolic activity and reduction by NADPH–cytochrome P-450 reductase (Lu *et al*. 1969). The presence of a single protein and the considerable decrease in the light scattering of micelles as compared to microsomes has allowed the application of a variety of spectroscopic techniques to study the reduction kinetics, binding of substrate, binding of oxygen, and alterations in the spin state of the protein.

Planar Bilayers

Although it would seem to be possible to reconstitute cytochrome *P*-450 into planar bilayers of the type described by Nelson *et al*. (1980) and Schindler and Quast (1980), this experiment has not been accomplished. The main advantage of reconstitutions of proteins into planar bilayers is that the researcher is able to manipulate transmembrane potentials and alter the concentration of solutes opposed to the two surfaces of the bilayer. There is no indication that either of these processes is important to the regulation of cytochrome P-450. The very low molar content of protein in the small planar bilayers has made the application of spectroscopic techniques very difficult.

Phospholipid Bilayer Vesicles

The reconstitution of proteins into phospholipid bilayers offers many advantages. A variety of techniques have been published on the successful reconstitution of functional proteins into vesicles (Kagawa *et al.*, 1973; Hong and Hubbell, 1972). Whereas micelles are thought to have either random or spherically symmetric orientations of the long axes of their components, phospholipid bilayers have an inherently anisotropic parallel orientation of their fatty acid chains. In turn, the parallel orientation of the fatty acid chains results in orientation of intrinsic membrane proteins with respect to the membrane surface. In the case of studies of interactions between two different intrinsic membrane proteins in the same bilayer, the preferred parallel orientation of these two proteins that would occur in a phospholipid bilayer may be very important to the results of the spectroscopic or analytical study.

EVIDENCE FOR THE INFLUENCE OF PHOSPHOLIPIDS ON PROTEIN FUNCTION IN RECONSTITUTED SYSTEMS

Cytochrome P-450 Reconstituted in Micelles

The most striking evidence for the influence of phospholipids on protein function in the case of cytochrome P-450 was a demonstration by Lu *et al.* (1969) that, in the absence of phospholipids or detergent, the protein did not function at all. The series of studies that followed on the conditions for achieving optimal activity in these micelles made a considerable addition to knowledge of the requirement of intrinsic membrane protein for a hydrophobic environment.

Protein Reconstituted in Phospholipid Vesicles

There have been very many demonstrations of the influence of phospholipids on protein function in reconstituted vesicles. For example, in very early studies of reconstitution, Kawaga *et al.* (1973) showed that a mixture of phosphatidylethanolamine with phosphatidylcholine provided greater activity in their reconstituted system. Hesketh *et al.* (1976) demonstrated that calcium ATPase was only active when the reconstituted system contained at least 30 phospholipid molecules per protein molecule. Hubbell *et al.* (1977) demonstrated the importance of phospholipid mixtures and detergents in the reconstitution of rhodopsin into phospholipid vesicles. Bösterling *et al.* (1979) reported the effect of various ratios of phosphatidylcholine to phosphatidylethanolamine as well as phospholipid-to-protein ratios in the activity of their resulting reconstitutions of NADPH–cytochrome *P*-450 reductase and cytochrome *P*-450.

A Review of Techniques for Reconstitution of Cytochrome *P*-450

Micelles

The preparation of pure forms of liver microsomal cytochrome *P*-450 and its associated reductase was followed by reconstitution of its activity by dispersing the solubilized proteins in micelles of deoxycholate and phospholipid (Lu *et al.*, 1969). High turnover numbers in studies of drug metabolism were also obtained in the absence of detergent by the use of dilauroyllecithin in micelle-reconstituted systems (Koop and Coon, 1979). On the other hand, it has been shown that the metabolism of xenobiotics can be catalyzed effectively in pure detergent micelles, such as Triton X-100 (Sugiyama *et al.*, 1979; Kuwahara and Omura, 1980).

The ability to reconstitute monooxygenase activity by the formation of micelles has opened up a new area for the study of the mixed function oxidases. However certain aspects of this detergent–phospholipid dispersion are unlike those of the endoplasmic reticulum. In particular, the ratio of reductase to *P*-450 used to obtain maximum activity in the detergent–phospholipid dispersion (Lu *et al.*, 1969) is up to 50 times that which occurs in the endoplasmic reticulum. Furthermore, due to their aggregational state, it is possible that the cytochrome P-450 and NADPH–cytochrome *P*-450 reductase in the detergent–phospholipid dispersion do not exhibit the same range of protein–lipid and protein–protein interactions, due to lateral and rotational diffusion or transient cluster formation, which are available to proteins in a phospholipid membrane.

These protein–protein and protein–lipid (Stier *et al.*, 1978) interactions may be important to an understanding of the normal hydroxylation function of the mixed function oxidase system as well as to the production of hydrogen peroxide (Nordblom and Coon, 1977; Hildebrandt and Roots, 1975), free radical intermediates (Slater, 1972; Trudell *et al.*, 1981), and activated carcinogens (Weisburger, 1978).

Vesicles

In order to study these protein–protein and protein–lipid interactions, we have prepared a reconstituted system in which the proteins are introduced into the plane of a phospholipid bilayer vesicle and may be able to undergo lateral motion, transient or permanent cluster formation, and rapid vibration contacts. The self-aggregation tendency of the microsomal monoxygenase system was demonstrated by the dissolution of microsomes by sodium cholate and subsequent removal (Mishin *et al.*, 1979). This self-assembly tendency of solubilized membrane proteins and phospholipid is the basis for successful reconstitutions of the purified proteins cytochrome *P*-450 and NADPH–cytochrome *P*-450 reductase in vesicles. Reconstitution into vesicles of pure egg phosphatidylcholine was possible only by means of a high excess of phospholipid (1:40 w:w) (Ingelman-Sundberg and Glaumann, 1977). Lateral mobility of the protein in such membranes was suggested (Taniguchi *et al.*, 1979).

However these techniques appear to be unsuitable for the preparation of nonaggregated reconstituted vesicles with natural phospholipid composition and very high protein–phospholipid ratios which we require for future studies with cytochrome *P*-450 and cytochrome *P*-450 reductase on electron coupling and protein–membrane interactions. Based on knowledge of the structure and composition of liver microsomes (Depierre and Dallner, 1975) we considered the following characteristics to be required for these future studies:

1. A 1:5 ratio of reductase to *P*-450 similar to that found in microsomes.

2. A high enough protein–to-lipid ratio for each vesicle to contain at least one *P*-450 reductase and five *P*-450 proteins. This condition will allow study of electron transfer between *P*-450 reductase and *P*-450 within the same vesicle. A 30 nm diameter vesicle with a 4 nm thick bilayer would require a protein to lipid ratio greater than 1:14 to contain six proteins totaling 3.5×10^5 daltons.

3. The vesicles should contain both PC and phosphatidylethanolamine (PE) because these phospholipids are the two most common in microsomes, where they occur in a 2:1 ratio (Depierre and Dallner, 1975). Mixtures of these phospholipids have previously been shown to be important for optimum protein reconstitution (Kawaga *et al.*, 1973; Hubbell *et al.*, 1977; Hong and Hubbell, 1972; Grant and McConnell, 1974).

4. The vesicles should have a negative surface charge in order to mimic microsomal surface properties as well as to prevent aggregation.

5. The reconstituted vesicles should exhibit an efficient coupling between NADPH oxidation and hydroxylation of substrate.

6. The production of hydrogen peroxide with and without substrate bound to *P*-450 should have the same rate constant as microsomes.

We have accomplished the reconstitution by a technique of solubilization of both proteins and phospholipids in sodium cholate followed by the slow removal of the cholate by dialysis in the presence of glycerol. We have characterized the reconstituted system by gradient centrifugation, electron microscopy, and metabolic activity toward a variety of substrates.

We were able to reconstitute *P*-450 and *P*-450 reductase at a 5:1 mole ratio into PC:PE:PA (2:1:0.06 w:w) bilayer vesicles using a cholate dialysis technique (Kawaga *et al.*, 1973; Hubbell *et al.*, 1977; Hong and Hubbell, 1972; Grant and McConnell, 1974). Vesicles with a protein:phospholipid ratio of either 1:5 or 1:2 (w:w) could be prepared as demonstrated by ultracentrifugation. The 1:5 protein:phospholipd vesicles banded between 1.062 and 1.078 g/ml in a 5–50% glycerol gradient and appeared to be single round closed vesicles of 40–100 nm diameter by electron microscopy. The vesicle with a 1:2 protein:phospholipid ratio banded between 1.090 and 1.097 g/ml and appeared by electron microscopy to be slightly aggregated single vesicles of 40–60 nm diameter.

The density of the band in the density gradient was controlled by the lipid to protein ratio but the width of the band and the diameter of the vesicles were dependent on the duration, temperature, and concentration of cholate treatment at the given protein and lipid concentration. The PC to PE ratio in the vesicles after reconstitution was determined by ^{31}P-NMR spectroscopy, the ratio did not change during reconstitution. When sufficient cholate was used (1.5%) to dissolve all the lipid, the initial ratio of protein to lipid was always maintained in the vesicles following the reconstitution procedure. After dialysis of the mixtures using PC:PE:PA ratios of 2:1:0.06 over 80% of the total lipid and protein are recovered. Up to 90% of these recovered components are found in a single band in the density gradient.

Further experiments demonstrated that PE is essential for the reconstitution of *P*-450 and *P*-450 reductase at high protein:phospholipid ratios. *P*-450 may be reconstituted with PC:PA 1:0.02 (w:w) alone by the slow cholate dialysis technique only when a protein to lipid ratio of 1:10 (w:w) or less is used. When the protein-to-lipid ratio is increased from 1:10 to 1:5 with only PC + PA (Fig. 2f) at a phospholipid concentration of 5–15 mg/ml, a protein–lipid pellet is formed. The inclusion of PE, the second largest component of microsomal phospholipids, along with PC and PA proved to be a satisfactory mixture for the formation of stable vesicles.

The metabolic activity of the vesicle reconstitution and a nonvesicular preparation has been characterized by NADPH utilization and H_2O_2 production with and without the substrates hexobarbital, cyclohexane, aminopyrine, and benzphetamine as well as by the metabolic production of formaldehyde from aminopyrine and benzphetamine. The reconstitution technique produces vesicles of sufficient diameter and protein content (33% by weight) that each may contain at least two reductase and ten or more cytochrome P-450 proteins. This vesicle reconstituted system is similar to microsomes with regard to bilayer structure, phospholipid composition, surface charge, protein:lipid ratio, cytochrome P-450:NADPH–cytochrome P-450 reductase ratio, and enzymatic coupling. Therefore it may be an excellent system in which to study substrate specificity, electron transport, reductive versus oxidative metabolism, and protein–lipid interactions.

Lipid–Protein Interactions of Cytochrome *P*-450 in Reconstituted Vesicles

RECENT STUDIES

Cytochrome P-450 and NADPH–Cytochrome P-450 Reductase Interact with Phospholipids

A study of lipid–protein interactions in reconstituted vesicles must begin with a demonstration that such interactions occur. We measured the order parameter of spin-labeled phosphatidylcholine shown in Fig. 1 with an electron paramagnetic resonance (EPR) spectrometer. In Fig. 2 it is seen that there is a measurable decrease in fluidity of the membrane in the presence of cytochrome *P*-450 and NADPH–cytochrome *P*-450 reductase as compared to protein-free vesicles. Fig. 2 shows the temperature dependence of the order parameter determined by the use of (12,3)-PCSL in vesicles of PC:PE:PA (16:8:1: mol:mol). It can be approximated by a straight line in the temperature range 15–45°C. The presence of cytochrome *P*-450 resulted in a parallel shift of 5–6° at a lipid to protein mole ratio of 300:1.

The demonstration that cytochrome *P*-450 interacted with spin-labeled phospholipids prompted the question of whether there was preferential in-

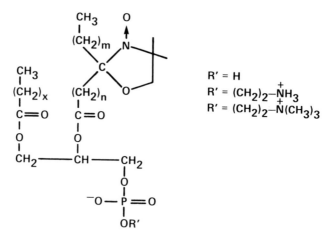

Fig. 1. Structure of spin-labeled phospholipids. Spin-labeled phosphatidylcholines were prepared from egg lysophosphatidylcholine and stearic acid spin-label (Boss *et al.*, 1975) carrying the nitroxide group at C-5 or C-16. Spin-labeled phosphatidylethanolamine and spin-labeled phosphatidic acid were obtained by enzymatic head group exchange of the phosphatidylcholine by phospholipase D (Comfurius and Zwaal, 1977).

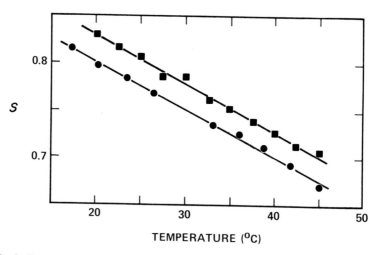

Fig. 2. Temperature dependence of the order parameter S of 16-doxyl phosphatidylcholine in vesicles with (■) and without (●) cytochrome P-450 and NADPH–cytochrome P-450 reductase (5:1 mol:mol) reconstituted with egg phosphatidylcholine:egg phosphatidylethanolamine: dipalmitoylphosphatidic acid (16:8:1 mol:mol:mol) at a lipid-to-protein ratio of 300:1 (mol:mol).

teraction with any particular type of phospholipid. We considered the possibility of chain length of the fatty acid chains, type of head group on the phospholipid, and the charge of the head group.

Preference of Cytochrome P-450 for Negatively Charged Phosphatidic Acid

In a study by Bösterling *et al.* (1981), we described lipid–protein interactions of cytochrome *P*-450 reconstituted in phospholipid vesicles containing a mixture of either phosphatidylcholine or phosphatidylethanolamine with up to 50 mol % phosphatidic acid. Phosphatidic acid has been used in previous studies of lipid–protein interactions in model membranes (Hartmann and Galla, 1978; Sixl and Galla, 1979). The advantage of using a synthetic lipid is the existence of a well-defined lipid phase transition which can be investigated by spectroscopic methods. Mixtures of charged and uncharged phospholipids were prepared such that, at a critical temperature, both fluid and solid phase domains coexist. The mole fraction of each phospholipid in the two domains is different. Large changes in the cooperativity and temperature of the phase separation may be caused by preferential interaction of one of the phospholipids with cytochromes *P*-450 because a change in the mole fraction of the two phospholipids in the gel phase domain will result.

The phase transition curves of mixed membranes containing egg PC and DMPA in different relative concentrations measured by the TEMPO-partitioning technique of McConnell *et al.* (1972) are shown in Fig. 3 in the absence and presence of cytochrome *P*-450. Again, phase transition curves were obtained by measuring TEMPO-partitioning as a function of temperature. No phase transition is observable in pure egg PC membranes; incorporation of cytochrome *P*-450 leads to a decreased fluidity over the whole temperature range. This result is in agreement with measurements of phospholipid spin-labels in the same system described above. Fig. 3 b–d shows the phase transition curves of phospholipid mixtures containing increasing amounts of DMPA. In the absence of cytochrome *P*-450 a clearly visible phase transition is observed between 20 and 40°C. This shows that phosphatidylcholine and phosphatidic acid are not randomly distributed within the membrane but form lateral phase separations. At low temperature, gel phase domains enriched in phosphatidic acid coexist with domains containing mainly phosphatidylcholine so that the phase transition of DMPA is still measurable in the presence of egg PC. The phosphatidic acid domains exhibit a phase transition temperature of about 35°C which is lower than pure DMPA bilayers ($T_m = 47°C$). This finding shows that the phosphatidic acid

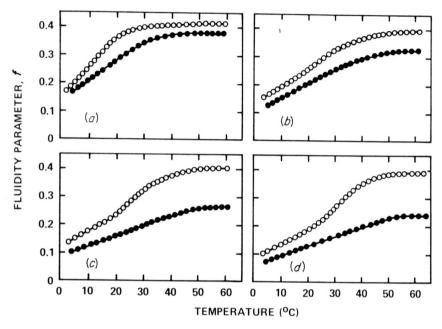

Fig. 3. Phase transition curves of mixtures of egg PC and DMPA in different ratios. Transition curves of preparations without protein (○○○○) are compared to cytochrome P-450 containing vesicles (●●●●). (a) Pure egg PC, lipid-to-protein ratio 300:1 mol:mol; (b) mixture of egg PC and DMPA in a 8:2 ratio (w:w), lipid-to-protein ratio 300:1 mol:mol; (c) mixture of egg PC and DMPA in a 2:1 ratio, lipid-to-protein ratio 180:1 mol:mol; (d) 1:1 mixture of egg PC and DMPA, lipid-to-protein ratio 180:1 mol:mol. From Bösterling *et al.* (1981).

domains contain some egg PC which lowers the phase transition temperature. This is consistent with the results obtained by Galla and Sackmann (1975) in mixed phosphatidic acid–phosphatidylcholine bilayers in which they analyzed the spin exchange interaction when one lipid component was spin-labeled.

In a 1:1 mixture of DMPA and egg PC the phase transition of DMPA disappears in the presence of cytochrome P-450 (Fig. 3d). The phase transition curve in the presence of the protein resembles that of a vesicle containing little DMPA. A possible explanation of this result is that cytochrome P-450 interacts preferentially with the negatively charged DMPA and thereby decreases the amount of free phosphatidic acid to the point where the phosphatidic acid concentration is too low to form a separate phase.

In a mixture of DMPC–egg PA (3:1 mol:mol) we observed the phase transition of DMPC due to a phase separation taking place in the membrane. Again this phase transition is lower than that of pure DMPC. Moreover in this lipid mixture a second domain of lipids melting between 23 and 40°C (Fig. 4a) is observed in the absence of cytochrome *P*-450. Reconstituted vesicles containing cytochrome *P*-450 in a lipid-to-protein ratio of 300:1 mol:mol or less do not exhibit this second higher melting phase but, instead, a sigmoidal melting curve (Fig. 4a) with a 5°C higher phase transition temperature. In accordance with the result from experiments with egg PC and DMPA, we interpret this as preferential binding of egg PA to cytochrome *P*-450 leading to a more pure DMPC phase.

The melting curve of a mixture of DMPC and egg PE at a 3:1 mole ratio has been reported to show no phase separations (Galla and Sackmann, 1975). The phase transition temperature (Fig. 4b) is lowered by about 10°C with respect to pure DMPC and is very broad. By comparison, in the egg PA/DMPC mixture described above (Fig. 4a), the DMPC phase transition was lowered by only 3°C with respect to pure DMPC. The greater depression of T_m gives evidence for the assumption of a random mixture of the uncharged phospholipids in the case of a DMPC–egg PE vesicle. In this case the incorporation of cytochrome *P*-450 increased the phase transition temperature but did not change the shape of the phase transition curve. This suggests that DMPC and egg PE have about the same affinity for cytochrome *P*-450 and preferential removal of free egg PE with the resulting formation of a DMPC gel phase is not observed.

The first indication for a preferential interaction of cytochrome *P*-450 with negatively charged phosphatidic acid was obtained during our reconstitution experiments. It was not possible to obtain a homogeneous vesicle population of the mixed system in the absence of cytochrome *P*-450. Instead we obtained vesicles of phosphatidic acid as well as vesicles with phosphatidylcholine as the main component as was shown by density gradient centrifugation and phase transition curves. However, if vesicles were reconstituted in the presence of cytochrome *P*-450, only one population of vesicles was obtained. Thus, cytochrome *P*-450 mediates in the formation of mixed vesicles. The strong interaction between cytochrome *P*-450 and phosphatidic acid as compared to phosphatidylcholine and phosphatidylethanolamine was shown directly in the EPR spectra of the corresponding spin-labeled lipids. Only with spin-labeled phosphatidic acid did we observe an immobilized component in the presence of cytochrome *P*-450.

In addition to the preferential interaction of cytochrome *P*-450 with phosphatidic acid we also demonstrated strong interaction with phosphatidylcholine and phosphatidylethanolamine. In DMPC vesicles, for example, we observed an increase in phase transition temperature and a broadening of the phase transition. Moreover, with DMPC we observed the appearance of a second high melting phase in the presence of cytochrome *P*-450. These results can be interpreted in terms of a perturbed membrane

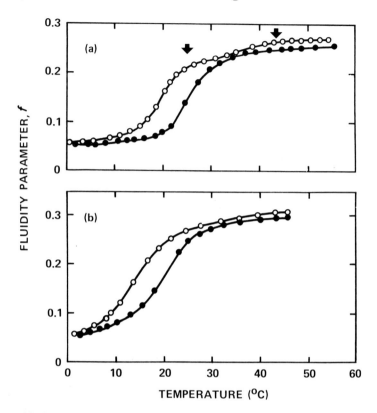

Fig. 4. (a) Phase transition curve of reconstituted mixed vesicles containing DMPC and egg PA in a 3:1 (w:w) ratio without (○○○○) and with cytochrome P-450 (●●●●) at a lipid-to-protein ratio of 300:1 mol:mol. The arrows point to the beginning and the end of the melting of a lipid phase which is only detectable if cytochrome P-450 is not present. (b) Phase transition curve of DMPA–egg PE vesicles (3:1, w:w) in the absence (○○○○) and presence (●●●●) of cytochrome P-450 in a lipid-to-protein ratio of 300:1. Note that the sigmoidal shape of the curve is not changed by the interaction with the cytochrome P-450. From Bösterling *et al.* (1981).

in which the protein strongly interacts with the phospholipids in its immediate surroundings. In the mixed egg PC–DMPA vesicles we observed the disappearance of the DMPA phase transition in the presence of cytochrome P-450. This provides further evidence for a preferential binding of phosphatidic acid to cytochrome P-450.

Most of the binary mixtures of phospholipids used in this study undergo lateral phase separations into domains of gel phase and fluid phase phospholipids. Both of these domains contain a substantial mole fraction of the second lipid component. The mole fraction of the higher melting phospholipid in the gel phase domain affects the cooperativity and temperature of the thermal phase transition. However incorporation of cytochrome *P*-450 leads to a redistribution of the phospholipids in each domain. Charged phospholipids are concentrated in the region surrounding the proteins although they do not necessarily form a lipid halo. This preference for negatively charged lipids is an additional component of the very pronounced lipid–protein interactions between cytochrome *P*-450 and all phospholipids such as phosphatidylcholine and phosphatidylethanolamine.

Phospholipid Transfer between Vesicles: Dependence on Presence of Cytochrome P-450 and Phosphatidylcholine–Phosphatidylethanolamine Ratio

In order to further characterize phosphatidylcholine (PC) vesicle preparations that contain cytochrome *P*-450 or phosphatidylethanolamine (PE) or both, we measured the rate of phospholipid exchange between vesicles (Bösterling and Trudell, 1982a). This technique provides further insight into the dynamics of this two-dimensional three-component system. We measured the rate of transfer of the spin-labeled phospholipid 1-acyl-2-(10-doxyl-stearoyl)-sn-glycero-3-phosphocholine from vesicles containing a high percentage of this spin-labeled phospholipid to acceptor vesicles of various compositions. The rate of transfer was dependent on the lipid composition and on the presence of protein in the acceptor vesicles. Vesicles of high protein-to-lipid ratio, which could be prepared by the use of 33 mol% PE in PC, gave the highest rate of phospholipid transfer and also produced a ^{31}P-NMR spectrum with a chemical shift anisotropy that is not typical of spectra of pure phosphatidylcholine bilayers.

The EPR spectrum of a suspension of vesicles that contains 50 mol % spin-labeled phosphatidylcholine is very broad due to spin–spin exchange broadening. As the spin-labeled phosphatidylcholines are transferred to vesicles of nonspin-labeled phospholipids, the line-width of the EPR spectrum progressively decreases, the intensity increases, and the spectrum becomes identical to that of spin-labeled phospholipid in a phospholipid membrane containing 1 mol % or less of the spin-label. The increasing intensity of the centerline was continuously measured in order to obtain the phospholipid transfer rates. The time course of the increase in the sharp, hyperfine components at 37°C is seen in Fig. 5. A mixture of spin-labeled PC vesicles with vesicles containing cytochrome *P*-450 reconstituted in egg PC–PE (2:1 mol:mol) at a lipid-to-protein ratio of 2:1 (w:w) resulted in a rapid dilution of the spin-label (upper trace) and in the appearance of a single, sharp EPR signal characteristic of anisotropic motion in phospholipid bilayers (Hubbell

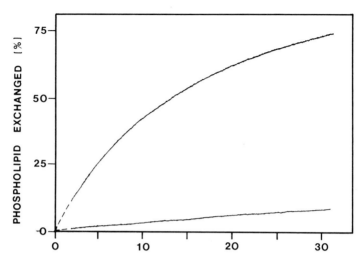

Fig. 5. Time course of the increase in intensity at the maximum hyperfine component measured at 37°C in 0.02 M potassium phosphate buffer pH 7.5 containing 20% glycerol. The upper trace was obtained when cytochrome P-450 PC-PE vesicles (lipid:protein = 2:1, w:w; PC:PE = 2:1, w:w) were added to spin-labeled PC vesicles. The lower trace was obtained when cytochrome P-450 PC vesicles (lipid:protein = 10.1, w:w) were added to the same amount of spin-labeled PC vesicles. The ratio of labeled to unlabeled phospholipid was 1:200 w:w after mixing. From Bösterling and Trudell (1982a).

and McConnell, 1972). The lower trace in Fig. 5 resulted from phospholipid transfer from spin-labeled PC vesicles to vesicles containing cytochrome P-450 reconstituted with only egg PC at a lipid-to-protein ratio of 10:1 (w:w). It can be seen that, at the same total phospholipid concentration, the extent of phospholipid transfer is about one order of magnitude higher with the PE-containing vesicles during the first half hour time period.

Four possible mechanisms for dilution of the spin-labeled phospholipids from the donor vesicles into the large excess of phospholipids in the acceptor vesicles could be considered: (*a*) fusion of donor vesicles with acceptor vesicles; (*b*) transfer of individual monomeric spin-labeled phospholipids in solution at the critical micelle concentration to acceptor vesicles; (*c*) exchange of phospholipids between donor and acceptor vesicles during rapid vibrational contacts; and (*d*) exchange of phospholipids between donor and acceptor vesicles that exist as dimers or higher aggregates.

The possibility that fusion is responsible is unlikely because each fusion of a spin-labeled vesicle with a nonspin-labeled vesicle should reduce the concentration only by a factor of two. Many such fusions would be required to reduce the spin-label concentration below about 10 mol % where spin–spin exchange is diminished enough to begin to decrease the line-width of the EPR spectrum.

A second possible mechanism for the observed dilution of spin-labeled PC would be transfer of individual phospholipid molecules. This mode of transfer is unlikely to be important because of the extremely low monomer concentration of PC. Furthermore, the monomer concentration of spin-labeled PC would be independent of the composition of the acceptor vesicles whereas the observed rate of phospholipid transfer was shown to be very dependent on their composition.

The aggregation of pure PC vesicles is slow because of the dipolar repulsion of PC headgroups and the resulting high energies that are required to bring PC bilayers together within a few Angstroms of each other (Le Neveu *et al.*, 1976). However, in a kinetic study of vesicle aggregation, it has been shown (Kolber and Haynes, 1979), that only vesicles with mole fractions of PE greater than 0.6 aggregate.

The presence of either cytochrome *P*-450 or more than 60 mol % PE in a PC bilayer resulted in an increase in the rate of transfer of spin-labeled PC. However the protein-free phospholipid vesicles containing 30 mol % PE and 40 mol % gave the same rate of phospholipid transfer as pure PC vesicles. The former two vesicle preparations encompass the 33 mol % PE that was used for reconstituting cytochrome *P*-450. Therefore the presence of the protein in a reconstituted vesicle with a PC–PE ratio of 2:1 causes some properties of the membrane to be like those of a vesicle with 70 mol % PE. It is possible that the protrusion of cytochrome *P*-450 from the vesicle's surface in combination with a nonplanar surface may allow direct contact between the spin-labeled PC vesicle and the protein-containing vesicle.

These results support a previous study (Stier *et al.*, 1978) in which reconstitution of cytochrome *P*-450 into a vesicle with a 2:1 mole ratio of phosphatidylcholine–phosphatidylethanolamine and a 2:1 (w:w) protein-to-lipid ratio resulted in a dramatic change in the ^{31}P-NMR chemical shift anisotropy compared to that observed in control vesicles with an identical PC/PE ratio. Similar changes in the ^{31}P-NMR chemical shift anisotropy have been observed in PC/PE vesicles containing greater than 70 mol % PE.

PE is a microsomal lipid known to be involved in the formation of non-bilayer structures: in aqueous suspensions it normally occurs in a hexagonal phase and can only be forced into a bilayer by admixture of an equal quantity of PC (Cullis and DeKruijff, 1978). As a result the ^{31}P-NMR spectra of resuspended microsomal lipids in which the PE–PC ratio is 1:2 retain the typical bilayer shape over the whole temperature range. On the other hand, in suspensions where the PE/PC ratio is greater than 1:1, in addition to the lamellar phase another appears, not truly hexagonal, which allows motional averaging (Cullis and DeKruijff, 1978); these spectra are nearly identical in shape to those of microsomes at higher temperatures.

Electron Transfer between NADPH–Cytochrome P-450 Reductase and Cytochrome P-450 in Reconstituted Vesicles

Knowledge of the mechanism of electron transport from NADPH–cytochrome P-450 reductase to cytochrome P-450 may be necessary for a fundamental understanding of cellular toxicity resulting from drug metabolism. For example, under some conditions, rather than the expected hydroxylation of a substrate, only reduction occurs. The reduction of halocarbons into free radicals or carbenes has been observed (Wolf et al., 1977, 1980; Slater, 1978; Trudell et al., 1981), whereas reductase in the absence of cytochrome P-450 has been shown to directly reduce oxygen to a superoxide anion radical (Bösterling and Trudell, 1981). Increased production of superoxide may be an important consequence of the uncoupling of reductase from cytochrome P-450. Due to the conversion to hydroxyl radicals and the initiation of lipid-peroxidation, the pattern of metabolites of certain substrates (Erickson and Bösterling, 1981) can be expected to be dependent on such a protein–protein interaction.

The modulation of protein–protein interactions by phospholipid can only be examined properly if the proteins are reconstituted in a bilayer with structural similarity to the natural membrane. For the experiments in the present study we have individually reconstituted either cytochrome P-450 or NADPH–cytochrome P-450 reductase or a 1:1 mixture of the two proteins into identical phospholipid vesicles. We have used these vesicle suspensions to test four important questions about electron transfer between these two proteins.

Is a freely diffusible, water soluble molecule responsible for electron transfer from reductase to cytochrome P-450? It is well established that small molecules such as sodium dithionite are capable of reducing cytochrome P-450. Organic peroxides such as cumene hydroperoxide are able to promote the the hydroxylation of substrate by cytochrome P-450 (White and Coon, 1980). It is possible that a small organic peroxide or superoxide anion under oxidative conditions could act as an electron transfer agent between reductase and cytochrome P-450. In order to test this possibility, we compared the benzphetamine N-hydroxylation activity of a mixture of individually reconstituted cytochrome P-450 and reductase with a vesicle suspension containing co-reconstituted cytochrome P-450 reductase.

The results of the first series of experiments would only be interpretable if it were established that protein exchange did not occur between the reductase vesicles and the cytochrome P-450 vesicles, or that these vesicles do not fuse during the time-course of the experiment. To test these two possibilities, we individually reconstituted cytochrome P-450 and reductase into phospholipid vesicles such that the densities of the vesicles were so different that their equilibrium sedimentation position in a linear density gradient was clearly separate. We then allowed mixtures of these individually reconstituted vesicles to equilibrate before they were separated by centrifugation.

A third question was whether the formation of a defined protein–protein complex is necessary for electron transfer or whether a free collision model is a sufficient working hypothesis. We have used magnetic circular dichroism spectroscopy in order to measure whether the association of reductase with cytochrome P-450 results in a specific, long-lived complex.

A fourth question was whether ionic interactions are important in the complex formed between cytochrome P-450 and reductase. We tested this by measuring the effect of ionic strength on the metabolic activity of a suspension of co-reconstituted cytochrome P-450 and reductase vesicles.

The initial goal of this study was to determine whether NADPH–cytochrome P-450 reductase transferred electrons to cytochrome P-450 via a small freely diffusible water soluble molecule or whether contact between the two proteins was necessary for electron transport. Fig. 6 clearly demonstrates that effective electron transport to support benzphetamine N-demethylation occurs only in the vesicles containing co-reconstituted NADPH–cytochrome P-450 reductase and cytochrome P-450. The suspension containing equal concentrations of separately reconstituted proteins had only 8% as much benzphetamine N-demethylation activity. This result strongly suggests that a small electron carrier molecule is not involved in the reduction of cytochrome P-450 in the endoplasmic reticulum.

However the suspension of the two separately reconstituted proteins did have a significantly higher benzphetamine N-demethylation activity than the control suspension containing only reconstituted NADPH–cytochrome P-450 reductase. The possible explanations for metabolic activity in the mixture of vesicles of separately reconstituted proteins include: (*a*) exchange of protein between the two vesicle populations; (*b*) diffusion of two dissimilar vesicles to produce a larger vesicle containing both proteins, and (*c*) transfer of electrons during random collisions of the two separately reconstituted vesicle populations. In order to test for the possibilities of protein exchange or vesicle fusion, cytochrome P-450 and NADPH–cytochrome P-450 reductase were separately reconstituted in phospholipid vesicles at lipid-to-protein ratios of 9:1 and 3:1, respectively.

In a linear glycerol gradient the two vesicle preparations separated cleanly

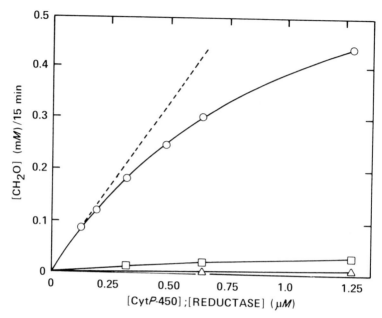

Fig. 6. Benzphetamine N-demethylation activity of vesicles containing either co-reconstituted or separately reconstituted cytochrome P-450 and NADPH–cytochrome P-450 reductase were reconstituted separately or as a 1:1 mixture in phospholipid vesicles. The amount of formaldehyde produced during a 15 min incubation at 30°C with 1 mM benzphetamine was determined as a function of protein concentration in the incubation mixture. The suspension in which the two proteins were co-reconstituted (O–O) shows a high activity that, at higher protein concentrations, falls below the dashed line which is the expected activity extrapolated to infinite dilution for this preparation. In a second set of experiments, vesicle suspensions containing separately reconstituted cytochrome P-450 or NADPH–cytochrome P-450 were mixed 1:1 and thermostatted at 30°C for 20 min. Then NADPH was added, the mixture was incubated for 15 min at 30°C, and the activity was measured as a function of the protein concentration. The N-demethylation activity (□–□) of the mixed vesicle preparation is low but nevertheless significantly higher than a control preparation in which only separately reconstituted NADPH–cytochrome P-450 reductase was incubated with 1 mM benzphetamine and NADPH for 15 min at 30°C (△–△).

with no peak of intermediate buoyant density that would correspond to vesicles containing transferred proteins or fusion between dissimilar vesicles. There was no fraction in the density gradient that exhibited benzphetamine N-demethylation activity greater than that of NADPH–cytochrome P-450 reductase alone. This result suggests that the small activity observed in the suspension of mixed separately reconstituted proteins was due to electron transfer during collision of the vesicles or some small extent of aggregation of the vesicles.

If the NADPH–cytochrome *P*-450 reductase transfers electrons directly to cytochrome *P*-450, it may do so in a preformed complex of considerable lifetime or only during a rapid collision event. In that the magnetic circular dichroism spectrum of cytochrome *P*-450 is a time weighted average of all possible states of its chromophore, it is possible to use this spectroscopic technique to distinguish between the two possibilities described above. The magnetic circular dichroism spectrum of co-reconstituted NADPH–cytochrome *P*-450 reductase and cytochrome *P*-450 is considerably different than that of a mixture containing precisely equal amounts of separately reconstituted proteins and phospholipids. This result suggests that the two proteins are together in a complex for a significant percentage of the time. Moreover the binding of the substrate benzphetamine to the suspension of the co-reconstituted vesicles has a large effect on the chromophore of cytochrome *P*-450. The addition of benzphetamine to a suspension of the separately reconstituted cytochrome *P*-450 did not produce as large an effect in the magnetic circular dichroism spectrum.

The preceding experiments rest on the assumption that the proteins would be incorporated at equal surface area per molecule into both outer and inner bilayers to yield a vesicle with 60% of the proteins in the outer bilayer. This assumption was confirmed by spin-labeling cytochrome *P*-450, reconstituting it into an egg phosphatidylcholine–phosphatidylethanolamine vesicle, adding sodium ascorbate, and measuring the kinetics of reduction of the nitroxide free radical of the spin label. The existence of a two-phase reduction reaction, in which both rates depend linearly on the ascorbic acid concentration, make alternative models unlikely, such as cytochrome *P*-450 being embedded in the center of the membrane.

There are two major requirements that a model for cytochrome *P*-450 reductase association in the endoplasmic reticulum membrane must satisfy. First, there is good evidence presented in this paper and in others (French *et al.*, 1980; Miwa *et al.*, 1979) that reductase and cytochrome *P*-450 transfer electrons in a 1:1 complex. Second, the lower than 1:10 molar ratio of reductase to cytochrome *P*-450 requires that each reductase mlecule be able to reduce many cytochromes *P*-450. In order to fulfill these requirements we would like to propose a model that combines the cluster and random collision models. This model would involve lateral and rotational diffusion of the individual dissociated proteins, cytochrome *P*-450 and reductase, in the membrane to form long-lived complexes of specific orientation. The most simple mechanism would be a reversible association reaction such as

Reductase + Cytochrome *P*-450 ⇌ Reductase–Cytochrome *P*-450 Complex

In that electron transfer by a small molecule was excluded, close juxtaposition of the flavin of the reductase with the porphyrin of cytochrome *P*-450 is required for reduction. This requires that the flavin and porphyrin groups be located near an outer surface of their respective proteins and therefore asymmetric with respect to the axis rotation of the proteins. If both proteins rotate like cylinders about axes that are perpendicular to the membrane surface, then the formation of a stable reductase–cytochrome *P*-450 complex is possible only when both proteins have independently rotated into that orientation that brings the flavin and porphyrin into tangential contact when the proteins collide by lateral diffusion. Only in the case that both proteins are oriented such that the small arc of their 360° axial rotation exposes the electron transfer site to the second protein, would a complex that allows reduction of the porphyrin by the reductase be formed. In all other cases the proteins would diffuse apart.

Lipid–Protein Interactions as Determinants of Activation or Inhibition by Cytochrome b₅ of Cytochrome P-450-mediated oxidations

Liver microsomes are known to contain two, possibly linked, electron transfer systems. NADPH–cytochrome *P*-450 reductase:cytochrome *P*-450 systems are involved in the metabolism of endogenous steroids and fatty acids as well as numerous xenobiotics. NADH–cytochrome b_5 reductase and cytochrome b_5 are components of the stearyl coenzyme A desaturase system (Shimakata, 1972). The two systems do not necessarily function in total independence. For example, a facilitative role for cytochrome b_5 in certain cytochrome *P*-450-mediated reactions has been proposed involving transfer of the second electron for drug oxidations (Cohen and Estabrook, 1971; Hildebrandt and Estabrook, 1971; Correia and Mannering, 1973; Lu *et al.*, 1974; Imai and Sato, 1977; Sugiyama *et al.*, 1979).

Studies aimed at elucidation of the mechanism of cytochrome b_5 effects on cytochrome *P*-450-mediated oxidations using micelle-reconstituted systems of purified proteins have revealed a complex pattern of interactions. Cytochrome b_5 has been reported to have no significant effect on cytochrome *P*-450-catalyzed oxidation of some substrates, but can either inhibit or stimulate electron transfer in the metabolism of other compounds (Lu *et al.*, 1974; Imai and Sato, 1977; Sugiyama *et al.*, 1979; Masters *et al.*, 1981; Morgan *et al.*, 1981; Ingelman-Sundberg and Johansson, 1980). This variability in effects of cytochrome b_5 has been suggested to be due in part to differences in the substrate metabolized or the type of cytochrome *P*-450 used in reconstitution experiments (Sugiyama *et al.*, 1979; Kuwahara and Omura, 1980). However it may also be reflective of differences in the molar ratios of NADPH–cytochrome P-450 reductase, cytochrome b_5 and cytochrome P-450 and/or the ratios of these proteins to phospholipid molecules in the micelle. The molar ratios of NADPH–cytochrome P-450 reductase:cytochrome b_5:cytochrome P-450 found in liver microsomes of phenobarbital-induced rabbits is on the order of 1:4:10 (Rice and Talcott, 1979). In contrast, most studies with micelle-reconstituted systems have involved the addition of 1–5 mol of cytochrome b_5 to a 1:1 molar complex of NADPH–cytochrome P-450 reductase and cytochrome P-450. It might have appeared reasonable to attempt magnification of the effects of cytochrome b_5 on the metabolic activity of cytochrome P-450 by its addition to reconstituted systems in molar excess if its effects were both uniform and linear as a function of concentration. However this does not appear to be the case.

In an investigation by Bösterling *et al.* (1982a), we used reconstituted cytochrome P-450 systems including both dilauroylphosphatidylcholine micelles and phospholipid vesicles to study the effects of cytochrome b_5 on the oxidation of a single substrate, benzphetamine. Variations in the molar ratio of NADPH–cytochrome P-450 reductase:cytochrome b_5:cytochrome P-450 and the ratios of proteins:phospholipids resulted in significant changes of metabolic activity. Depending on the system, cytochrome b_5 could be shown to exert no effect on benzphetamine N-demethylation, to cause almost complete inhibition of substrate oxidation, or to cause a 3-fold higher activity. These results are discussed in terms of a proposed model of lipid–protein interactions relating to electron transfer processes in liver microsomal membranes.

The activity of benzphetamine N-demethylation by micelle-reconstituted systems was determined by measuring the production of formaldehyde at various cytochrome b_5 to cytochrome P-450 LM_2 ratios. A fixed concentration of dilauroylphosphatidylcholine was chosen to correspond closely to that used in other studies (Lu and Levin, 1974; French *et al.*, 1980). Similar experiments were repeated with vesicle-reconstituted systems by the incorporation of detergent-free cytochrome b_5 in the membrane of cytochrome P-450 and cytochrome P-450 reductase-containing phospholipid vesicles. A different activation and inhibition profile was observed. A stimulation of metabolic activity was observed as a function of the addition of cytochrome b_5. Activity was highest for the reconstitutions containing the greatest amount of cytochrome P-450 reductase, and the percentage increase in activity was greatest in those containing the lowest cytochrome P-450 reductase-to-cytochrome P-450 ratio. In contast to micelle-reconstituted systems, the activity in the vesicle-reconstituted systems slowly reached a plateau value at a cytochrome b_5-to-cytochrome P-450 ratio of 1:1, and then declined to a lower value as this ratio was increased to 2:1.

The observed difference in the effect of cytochrome b_5 appears to reflect a difference between the reconstituted systems used. Since all protein-to-protein ratios were comparable, it seemed possible that cytochrome b_5 has a particularly large molar requirement for phospholipids. Thus the occurrence of activation or inactivation could be a consequence of the lipid-to-protein ratio found in the particular reconstituted system. For this reason activity was studied in micelle-reconstituted systems as a function of phospholipid present. Micelles containing cytochrome b_5 exhibited either inhibition, activation, or no effect on activity as a function of the molar ratio of phospholipid to total protein.

Fig. 7 reveals the striking dependence of the increase in activity caused by cytochrome b_5 on the cytochrome P-450 reductase-to-cytochrome P-450 ratio. The ratio of cytochrome b_5 to cytochrome P-450 was 0.5:1, similar to that found in rabbit liver microsomes. The stimulatory ability of cytochrome b_5 is greatest at the low cytochrome P-450 reductase-to-cytochrome P-450 ratios found in microsomes and is lowest at high reductase to cytochrome P-450 ratios employed in other studies on the effect of cytochrome b_5. This dependence was observed in both vesicle-and micelle-reconstituted systems.

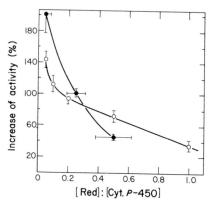

Fig. 7. Dependence of cytochrome b_5 activity increases on the ratio of cytochrome P-450 reductase to cytochrome P-450. Percentage increase of activity of N-demethylation of benzphetamine as compared to equivalent control reconstitutions without cytochrome b_5 as a function of molar ratio of NADPH–cytochrome P-450 reductase to cytochrome P-450 LM_2 in: (●) vesicle-reconstituted systems containing a molar ratio of cytochrome b_5 to cytochrome P-450 of 0.5:1 reconstituted with a 5:1 weight ratio of phospholipid to total protein and (○) micelle-reconstituted systems containing a molar ratio of cytochrome b_5 to cytochrome P-450 of 0.5:1 and 50 mol dilauroylphosphatidylcholine/mol of total protein. The molar ratios in the micelle-reconstituted systems are more accurate because of their simpler preparation. The highest increase of activity is observed at the lower ratios of cytochrome P-450 reductase to cytochrome P-450 which mimic the ratios in the microsomes. From Bösterling et al. (1982a).

Phospholipid requirements could change radically in systems containing three, rather than two, interacting protein components. Therefore this study included an examination of the effects of cytochrome b_5 on substrate metabolism plus its dependence on both phospholipid–protein and protein–protein ratios. Considerations of the molecular structure of cytochrome b_5 and its potential for interactions with phospholipids may furnish a possible explanation for the strong lipid dependence of its inbihitory effects in certain reconstituted systems. Cytochrome b_5 consists of a heme-containing globular component that does not interact with detergents and an elongated "tail" structure capable of interactions with detergent micelles and phospholipid vesicles (Dehlinger *et al.*, 1947; Strittmatter *et al.*, 1972; Visser *et al.*, 1975). The insertion of this hydrophobic segment into the membrane is anticipated to cause reorganization of the protein–phospholipid interactions in the bilayer. Due to the amphipathic structure of cytochrome b_5, an unusually large number of phospholipid molecules would occupy the region under the hydrophilic portion of the protein molecule that is extrinsic to the membrane. Fig. 8 shows such a structural arrangement wherein the hydrophilic portion of the cytochrome b_5 molecule, which has clusters of chraged groups on its surface (Mathews *et al.*, 1972), is lying over the polar head groups of the phospholipids to form a "cap". The distortion of phospholipid structures leading to a change of lipid association with other proteins including cytochrome P-450 is suggested as a plausible explanation for certain inhibitory effects of cytochrome b_5 in reconstituted micelles. The absence of inhibitory effects of cytochrome b_5 in reconstituted vesicles at cytochrome b_5:cytochrome P-450 ratios below unity is expected given the comparatively high phospholipid:protein mole ratio in the bilayer system compared to the micelle.

The apparent high requirement of cytochrome b_5 for phospholipids over that of other protein components in micelle-reconstituted systems demonstrates the need for compensatory changes in the total phospholipid content in such systems as protein–protein ratios are changed. The dependence of activity on mole ratios of components of the endoplasmic reticulum also illustrates the potential for modulation of metabolic activity by changes in the lateral organization with the membrane.

Association of Cytochrome b₅ and Cytochrome P-450
Reductase with Cytochrome P-450 in the Membrane
of Reconstituted Vesicles

In this study by Bösterling and Trudell (1982b) the interaction of cytochrome P-450 and NADPH–cytochrome P-450 reductase was studied in

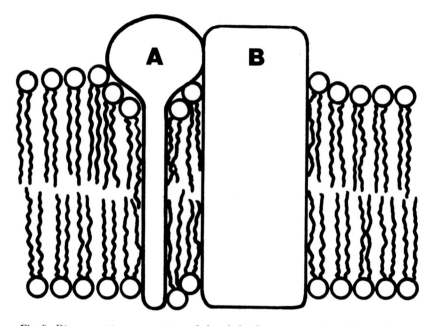

Fig. 8. Diagrammatic representation of phospholipid interactions of cytochrome b_5 (**A**) and another membrane protein (**B**) such as cytochrome *P*-450: The model shows high phospholipid requirement of cytochrome b_5 in its protein–protein interactions for electron transfer. From Bösterling *et al*. (1982a).

vesicle-reconstituted systems. These contained sufficient phospholipid such that no protein–protein interaction would be induced solely to prevent the exposure of hydrophobic protein surfaces to the aqueous environment. Furthermore, cytochrome b_5 was included in order to study a more complete NADPH-dependent electron transport chain. The bilayer of these vesicles was composed of a 2:1 mixture of phosphatidylcholine and phosphatidylethanolamine that was shown to provide functional and structural similarity to microsomes (Bösterling *et al*., 1979; Stier *et al*., 1978). Complex formation in the membrane was studied by magnetic circular dichroism(MCD). MCD has been shown to provide useful information about the electronic structure at the fifth ligand position, the substrate binding site, the oxidation state, and the spin state of cytochrome *P*-450 in microsomes (Dolinger *et al*., 1974) and purified cytochrome *P*-450 in reconstituted systems (Dawson *et al*., 1977; Bösterling and Trudell, 1980). Enzymatic measurements were used to study the stimulatory role of cytochrome b_5 and to obtain information on the electrostatic nature of these protein–protein interactions.

Absorption difference spectroscopy was used to demonstrate an interaction of cytochrome *P*-450 with NADPH–cytochrome *P*-450 reductase as well as with cytochrome b_5. Three different protein–protein interactions were examined in similar reconstituted vesicles: The MCD-difference spectrum in Fig. 9A was obtained by subtracting the sum of the MCD spectra of individually reconstituted reductase and cytochrome P-450 from that of the co-reconstituted preparation. A decrease of 23% of the absolute intensity of the MCD Soret band of cytochrome P-450 was observed. This decrease is similar to the one obtained in micelle-reconstituted systems (French *et al.*, 1980) and demonstrates the existence of a specific protein association in a membrane. The second MCD-difference spectrum (Fig. 9B) shows an interaction in a bilayer between cytochrome b_5 and cytochrome P-450. It was obtained from the MCD-spectra of solutions of equimolar concentrations of cytochrome P-450 vesicles and solubilized cytochrome b_5 before and after mixing and equilibration. It corresponds to a decrease of 13% of the absolute intensity of the Soret band. The spectra in A and B are of very similar shape. The MCD difference spectrum of vesicle co-reconstituted reductase and cytochrome P-450 before and after equilibration with cytochrome b_5 had the same shape but corresponds to a decrease of only 7% of the absolute intensity of the Soret band (not shown). For an interpretation of the difference spectra it is necessary to exclude a change in the MCD spectrum of cytochrome b_5 caused by its incorporation in a membrane. For this purpose the difference spectrum in Fig. 9C has been included which shows an insignificant difference between the MCD spectrum of solubilized cytochrome b_5 and the spectrum of cytochrome b_5 interacting with protein-free vesicles. No significant difference spectrum was obtained before and after mixing vesicle-reconstituted reductase with cytochrome b_5 (Fig. 9D).

N-Demethylation activity with benzphetamine as substrate was used to further characterize the interaction between these membrane proteins. When a reductase vesicle suspension was mixed with a suspension of vesicle co-reconstituted cytochrome b_5 and cytochrome P-450, the activity was 10.6 nmol per min per nmol cytochrome P-450, compared to 6.6 without cytochrome b_5. The incorporation of cytochrome b_5 increased the activity of reductase- and cytochrome P-450-containing vesicles from 47 to 73 nmol CH_2O per min per nmol cytochrome P-450. When 0.3 M KCl containing buffer was used the benzphetamine demethylation activity decreased to 39%, which corresponds well to the percentage of cytochrome P-450 and reductase located on the outer surface of the vesicles. The activity of the remaining enzymes located on the inner monolayer approached zero as KCl diffused inside during a time course of hours. In order to test whether a similar dependence on higher ionic strength exists for the electron flow from reductase through cytochrome b_5 to cytochrome P-450, the same enzymatic activity was measured at 0.3 M KCl with the use of a vesicle-reconstituted system containing the three proteins at equimolar ratios. The difference in specific activity between the two vesicle preparations with and without

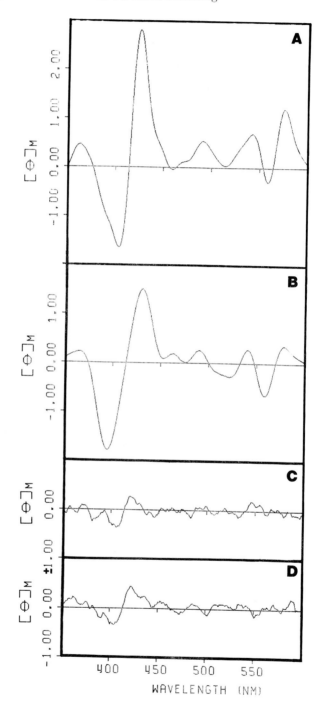

cytochrome b_5 in the absence of KCl is 19.1 nmol CH_2O per min. This difference is due to the activating effect of cytochrome b_5. The residual activity of the complete system of the three proteins following the addition of 0.3 M KCl of 18.7 nmol per min is not significantly different from 19.1. This suggests that the increase in activity produced by cytochrome b_5 at low ionic strength is quantitatively present as residual activity in the presence of 0.3 M KCl.

Studies of enzymatic activities in micelle-reconstituted systems and size determinations of the micelle supported the hypothesis that the observed interaction reflects a specific 1:1 association of these two membrane proteins. An apparent dissociation constant on the order of 0.1 μM was determined (French *et al.*, 1980). On the other hand, such a value could be artifactual because it is derived from micelle-reconstituted systems in which pronounced protein–protein interactions could dominate. There are only about 20 phospholipid molecules per cytochrome *P-450* in such a micelle, which is not even sufficient to surround a protein of molecular weight 50,000 with a single layer of lipids, Furthermore, cytochromes *P-450* themselves are available only as oligomers after purification (French *et al.*, 1980). The dissociation constant of these cytochrome P-450 molecules also has to be on the order of 0.1 μM, since they remain aggregated in dilute solutions and even under the nonequilibrium conditions of gel filtration. For these reasons it is important to demonstrate that the observed protein–protein association reactions are meaningful in that they also occur in the membrane of the endoplasmic reticulum. The present study supports such a projection, in that an association in a membrane would not be expected to occur in the absence of specific contact sites. In the membrane of a vesicle every protein molecule could be surrounded by several phospholipid layers and no protein would be forced to interact with another protein in order to circumvent the exposure of hydrophobic surface areas to water.

The interaction of reductase and cytochrome *P-450* seems to depend on the correct formation of an ionic bond for electron transfer. A similar electrostatic interaction might also exist between cytochrome *P-450* and cytochrome b_5 because at high ionic strength the MCD difference spectrum that resulted from mixing the two proteins disappeared within hours. The

Fig. 9. MCD difference spectra of vesicle-reconstituted systems, obtained by subtraction of MCD spectra which were measured in 0.02 M potassium phosphate buffer pH 7.5 containing 20% glycerol at 20°C. The spectral differences are a result of an association in the membrane of co-reconstituted cytochrome *P-450* and cytochrome *P-450* reductase (**A**) and cytochrome *P-450* with added cytochrome b_5 (**B**). Incorporation of solubilized cytochrome b_5 in pure phospholipid vesicles gave an insignificant MCD-change (**C**). This was also the case following the incorporation of solubilized cytochrome b_5 in cytochrome *P-450* reductase vesicles (**D**). From Bösterling and Trudell (1982b).

most simple mechanism of interaction of the three membrane proteins consistent with the above data would be reversible association reactions between the three possible pairs of different proteins that result in the formation of dimers. Electron transfer from reductase to cytochrome P-450 or cytochrome b_5 or from cytochrome b_5 to cytochrome P-450 would occur during the lifetime of these dimers. The increase in the MCD difference spectra, as well as the alterations in metabolic activity (Bösterling *et al.*, 1982a; Sugiyama *et al.*, 1979; Kuwahara and Omura, 1980) caused by the addition of cytochrome b_5, may be explained either by the formation of a ternary complex, reductase–cytochrome b_5–cytochrome P-450, or by a shift of the association equilibria between the three possible dimers and their monomeric forms.

REDUCTIVE METABOLISM OF HALOTHANE BY HUMAN AND RABBIT CYTOCHROME P-450

The knowledge gained in the previous studies about the factors that control electron transfer and metabolic activity in reconstituted cytochrome P-450 allowed us to attack a problem of considerable physiological importance: the initiation of liver necrosis by halocarbon metabolism. The metabolism of xenobiotics in the liver usually proceeds by the addition of activated oxygen to substrates by cytochrome P-450. However, under conditions of anaerobic incubation *in vitro*, cytochrome P-450 can act as a one or possibly two electron reductant to substrates. If halothane (2-bromo-2-chloro-1,1,1-trifluoroethane) is the substrate, reductive metabolims results in increased binding of metabolites to phospholipids of the endoplasmic reticulum, reduction in content of glutathione, increase in content of conjugated dienes in the fatty acid chains, loss of structural integrity of the endoplasmic reticulum, and liver necrosis. It has often been suggested that this metabolite could be a free radical. In 1961 Butler proposed that the reductive metabolism of another halocarbon, carbon tetrachloride, would result in a free radical metabolite. The binding of a free radical metabolite of halothane to a double bond of a fatty acid chain in a phospholipid would be consistent with the observation of increased conjugation of dienes in the fatty acid chains following reductive metabolism (Wood *et al.*, 1976). Two volatile reductive metabolites of halothane, 2-chloro-1,1,1-trifluoroethane and 2-chloro-1,1-difluoroethylene, have been detected in the expired air of rabbits (Mukai *et al.*, 1975) and human patients (Sharp *et al.*, 1979). We have suggested that the production of a single free radical species, 1-chloro-2,2,2-trifluoroethyl radical, by reduced cytochrome *P*-450 could account for both of these volatile metabolites; hydrogen radical abstraction in the case of the haloethane and the expulsion of a fluorine free radical in the case of the haloethylene (Sharp *et al.*, 1979). The molecular structure of the 1-chloro-2,2,2-trifluoroethyl radical as a major reductive metabolite of halothane is consistent with the following previous studies: A 1:3 stoichiometry between ^{14}C-containing metabolites and fluoride ion in the livers of mice exposed to [^{14}C]halothane (Cohen and Hood, 1969); an approximate 1:1 ratio of [36]Cl:[14]C in the phospholipid extracts of rats exposed under hypoxic conditions to either [[36]Cl]halothane or [^{14}C]halothane (Wood *et al.*, 1976); and an approximate 1:1 ratio of [3]H:[14]C in the $CHCl_3$–MeOH extract of anaerobic incubations of rat liver microsomes with either [^{3}H]halothane or [^{14}C]halothane (Gandolfi *et al.*, 1980).

   In a series of preliminary experiments we found that anaerobic incubations of halothane with liver microsomes produced reactive metabolites that bound at random to double bonds in microsomal phospholipids. However we were unable to isolate a single metabolite-substituted fatty acid in sufficient quantity and purity for structural elucidation by mass spectrometry. In order to circumvent the problem due to the heterogeneity of microsomal phospholipids, we used reconstituted vesicles containing highly purified cytochrome *P*-450, NADPH–cytochrome *P*-450 reductase and cytochrome b_5 (Trudell *et al.*, 1981, 1982a).

   The two most likely reductive metabolites of halothane described above would be predicted to add to a double bond of an unsaturated phospholipid in the following ways. The 1-chloro-2,2,2-trifluoroethyl radical should add to one carbon atom of a double bond and produce a free radical on the adjoining carbon position. This free radical would then abstract a hydrogen radical from another molecule to result in the corresponding substituted and saturated fatty acyl chain. The 2,2,2-trifluorethyl carbene should add across a double bond to form a trifluoromethyl-substituted cyclopropane ring on the fatty acyl chain (Hine, 1962). Therefore the most simple component to add to a reconstituted system as a target for radical or carbene addition would be a straight chain hydrocarbon or a fatty acid with a single double bond. However simple mono-unsaturated small molecules such as hexene or methyl oleate are themselves good substrates for cytochrome *P*-450 and are therefore unsuitable. For this reason we used dioleoylphosphatidylcholine (DOPC) as the only phosphatidylcholine in the reconstituted system since the phospholipid would act both as a potential target for the radical or carbene metabolite and as a structural component of the phospholipid vesicle.

   The anaerobic incubation of 1-[^{14}C]halothane with a suspension of either

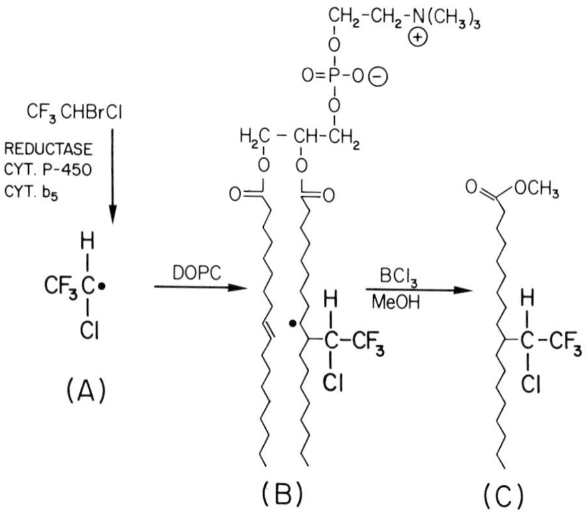

Fig. 10. Halothane is metabolized under anaerobic conditions to form the 1-chloro-2,2,2-trifluoroethyl radical by cytochrome *P*-450 reconstituted in phospholipid vesicles with NADPH cytochrome *P*-450 reductase and cytochrome b_5. (**A**). This radical will add to a double bond of an oleic acid at either the α- or β- position of dioleoylphosphatidylcholine to yield a mixture of four possible isomers of the labeled phosphatidylcholine (**B**). Transesterification of the dioleoylphosphatidylcholine by BCl_3 in methanol yields a mixture of saturated methyl stearates with a 1-chloro-2,2,2-trifluoroethyl group at either the 9- or 10- position (**C**). From Trudell *et al.* (1982a).

human cytochrome *P*-450-HA$_2$ or rabbit cytochrome *P*-450-LM$_2$ reconstituted in phospholipid vesicles with NADPH–cytochrome *P*-450 reductase and cytochrome b_5 (Trudell *et al.*, 1981) resulted in similar binding of radioactive metabolites in terms of dpm/mol phospholipid in the egg phosphatidylethanolamine and dioleoylphosphatidylcholine fractions.

When the dioleoylphosphatidylcholine fraction that was purified by preparative HPLC was subjected to transesterification with BCl_3–MeOH and then applied to a reverse phase HPLC column, a single radioactive peak was obtained. It was subjected to capillary gas chromatography coupled to a mass spectrometer and a mass spectrum was obtained. The molecular structure obtained from the mass spectrum can be explained by the reaction scheme shown in Fig. 10. When halothane is reduced with one electron by cytochrome *P*-450 it can lose a bromide ion and form the 1-chloro-2,2,2-trifluoroethyl radical (**A**). This free radical could then add to either end of the double bond in the two oleic acid chains in dioleoylphosphatidylcholine (**B**). This mixture of four isomers can be transesterified with BCl_3–MeOH to yield methyl oleate in the case of the fatty acid chains that did not react with the free radical, or a mixture of 9- and 10- (1-chloro-2,2,2-trifluoroethyl)-stearate methyl ester.

Acknowledgment

We would like to thank Ms. Betty Hampton for typing this manuscript and Ms. Audrey Stevens for editorial help.

References

Boss, W. F., Kelley, C. J., and Landsberger, F. R. (1975). *Anal. Biochem.* **64**, 289–292.
Bösterling, B., and Trudell, J. R. (1980). In "Microsomes, Drug Oxidation, and Chemical Carcinogenesis" (M. J. Coon, A. H. Conney, R. W., Estabrook, H. V. Gelboin, J. R. Gillette, and P. J. O'Brien, eds.), Vol. 1, pp. 115–118. Academic Press, New York.
Bösterling, B., and Trudell, J. R. (1981). *Biochem. Biophys. Res. Commun.* **98**, 569–575.
Bösterling, B., and Trudell, J. R. (1982a). *Biochim. Biophys. Acta* **689**, 155–160.
Bösterling, B., and Trudell, J. R. (1982b). *J. Biol. Chem.* **257**, 4783–4787.
Bösterling, B., Stier, A., Hildebrandt, A. G., Dawson, J. H., and Trudell, J. R. (1979). *Mol. Pharmacol.* **16**, 332–342.
Bösterling, B., Trudell, J. R., and Galla, H. J. (1981). *Biochim. Biophys. Acta* **643**, 547–556.
Bösterling, B., Trudell, J. R., Trevor, A. J., and Bendix, M. (1982a). *J. Biol. Chem.* **257**, 4375–4380.
Bösterling, B., Trudell, J. R., and Trevor, A. (1982b). *Anesthesiology* **56**, 380–384.
Butler, T. C. (1961). *J. Pharmacol. Exp. Ther.* **134**, 311–319.
Cohen, B. S., and Estrabrook, R. W. (1971). *Arch. Biochim. Biophys.* **143**, 46–53.
Cohen, E. N., and Hood N. (1969). *Anesthesiology* **31**, 553–558.
Comfurius, P., and Zwaal, R. F. A. (1977). *Biochim. Biophys. Acta* **488**, 36–42.
Correia, M. A., and Mannering, G. J. (1973). *Mol. Pharmacol.* **9**, 70–485.
Cullis, P. R., and DeKruijff, B. (1978). *Biochim. Biophys. Acta* **507**, 207–218.
Dawson, J. H., Trudell, J. R., Linder, R. E., Barth, G., Bunnenberg, E., and Djerassi, C. (1977). *Biochemistry* **17**, 33–43.
Dehlinger, P. J., Jost, P. C., and Griffith, O. H. (1974). *Proc. Nat. Acad. Sci. USA* **71**, 2280–2284.
Depierre, J. W., and Dallner, G. (1975). *Biochim. Biophys. Acta* **415**, 411–472.
Dolinger, P. M. *et al.* (1974). *Proc. Nat. Acad. Sci. USA* **71**, 399–403.
Erickson, S. K., and Bösterling, B. (1981). *J. Lipid Res.* **22**, 872–876.
French J. S., Guengerich, F. P., and Coon, M. J. (1980). *J. Biol. Chem.* **255**, 4112–4119.
Galla, H. J., and Sackmann, E. (1975). *Biochim. Biophys. Acta* **401**, 509–529.
Gally, H. -U., Niederberger, W., and Seelig, J. (1975). *Biochemistry* **14**, 3647–3652.
Gandolfi, A. J., R. D. White, I. G. Sipes, and L. R. Pohl. (1980). *J. Pharmacol. Exp. Ther.* **214**, 721–725.

232   James R. Trudell and Bernhard Bösterling

Grant, C. W., and McConnell, H. M. (1974). *Proc. Nat. Acad. Sci. USA* **71**, 4653–4657.
Hartmann, W., and Galla, H. J. (1978). *Biochim. Biophys. Acta* **509**, 474–490.
Haugen, D. A., and Coon, M. J. (1976). *J. Biol. Chem.* **251**, 7929–7939.
Hesketh, T. R. *et al.* (1976). *Biochemistry* **15**, 4145–4151.
Hildebrandt, A., and Estabrook, R. W. (1971). *Arch. Biochim. Biophys.* **143**, 66–79.
Hildebrandt, A. G., and Roots, I. (1975). *Arch. Biochem. Biophys.* **180**, 385–397.
Hine, J. (1962). Physical Organic Chemistry. pp. 434–438. McGraw-Hill, New York.
Hong, K., and Hubbell, W. L. (1972). *Proc. Nat. Acad. Sci. USA* **69**, 2617–2621.
Huang, M. T., West, S., and Lu, A. Y. H. (1976). *J. Biol. Chem.* **251**, 4659–4665.
Hubbell, W. L., Fung, K., Hong, L., and Cheny, Y. S.(1977). *In* "Vertebrate Photoreception"
    (H. B. Barlow, and P. Fatt, eds.). Academic Press, New York.
Imai, Y., and Sato, R. (1974). *Biochem. Biophys. Res. Commun.* **60**, 8–14.
Imai, Y., and Sato, R. (1977). *Biochem. Biophys. Res. Commun.* **75**, 420–426.
Ingelman-Sundberg, M., and Glaumann, H. (1977). *FEBS Lett.* **78**, 72–76.
Ingelman-Sundberg, M., and Johansson, I. (1980). *Biochem. Biophys. Res. Commun.* **97**,
    582–589.
Kagawa, Y., Kandrach, A., and Racker, E. (1973). *J. Biol. Chem.* **248**, 676–684.
Kolber, M. A., and Haynes, D. H. (1979). *J. Membrane Biol.* **48**, 95–114.
Koop, D. R., and Coon, M. J. (1979). *Biochem. Biophys. Res. Commun.* **91**, 1975–1981.
Kuwahara, S., and Omura, T. (1980). *Biochem. Biophys. Res. Commun.* **96**, 1562–1568.
Le Neveu, D. M., Rand, R. P., and Parsegian, V. A. (1976). *Nature (London)* **259**, 601–604.
Lu, A. Y. H., and Levin, W. (1974). *Biochim. Biophys. Acta* **344**, 205–240.
Lu, A. Y. H., Strobel, H. W., and Coon, M. J. (1969). *Biochem. Biophys. Res. Commun.* **36**,
    545–551.
Lu, A. Y. H., West, S. B., Vore, M., Ryan, D., and Levin, W. (1974). *J. Biol. Chem.* **249**,
    6701–6709.
Masters, B. S., Parkhill, L. K., and Okita, R. T. (1981). *Fed. Proc.* **40**, (S)2672.
Mathews, F. S., Levine, M., and Argos, P. (1972) *J. Mol. Biol.* **64**, 449–464.
McConnell, H. M., Wright, K. W., and McFarland, B. (1972). *Biochem. Biophys. Res. Commun.* **47**, 273–279.
Mishin, V. M., Grishanova, A. Y., and Lyakhovick, V. V. (1979). *FEBS Lett.* **104**, 300–302.
Miwa, G. T., West, S. B., Huang, M. T., and Lu, A. Y. H. (1979) *J. Biol. Chem.* **254**,
    5695–5700.
Morgan, E. T., Koop, D. R., and Coon, M. J. (1981). *Fed. Proc.* **40**, (S)2671.
Mukai, S. , Morio, M., Fujii, K. *et al.* (1975). *Anesthesiology* **47**, 392–401.
Nelson, N., Anhold, R., Lindstrom, J., and Montal, M. (1980). *Proc. Nat. Acad. Sci. USA* **77**,
    3056–3061.
Nordblom, G. D., and Coon M. J. (1977). *Arch. Biochem. Biophys.* **180**, 343–347.
Rice, S., and Talcott, R. E. (1979). *Drug Metab. Dispos.* **7**, 260–262.
Schindler, H., and Quast, U. (1980). *Proc. Nat. Acad. Sci. USA* **77**, 3056–3061.
Sharp, J. H., Trudell, J. R., and Cohen, E. N. (1979). *Anesthesiology* **50**, 2–8.
Shimakata, T., Mihara, K., and Sato, R. (1972). *j. Biochem.* **72**, 1163–1174.
Sixl, F., and Galla, H. J. (1979). *Biochim. Biphys. Acta* **557**, 320–330.
Slater, T. F. (1972). *In* "Free Radical Mechanisms in Tissue Injury." Pion Limited, London.
Slater, T. F. (1978). *In* "Biochemical Mechanisms of Liver Injury" (T. F. Slater, ed.), pp.
    27–29, Academic Press, New York.
Stier, A., and Sackmann, E. (1973). *Biochim. Biophys. Acta* **311**, 400–408.
Stier, A., Finch, S. A. E., and Bösterling, B. (1978). *FEBS Lett.* **91**, 109–112.
Strittmatter, P., Rogers, M. J., and Spatz, L. (1972). *J. Biol. Chem.* **247**, 7188–7194.

Strobel, H. W., Lu, A. Y. H., Heidema, J., and Coon, M. J. (1970). *J. Biol. Chem.* **245**, 4851–4854.

Sugiyama, T., Miki, N., and Yamano, T. (1979). *Biochem. Biophys. Res. Commun.* **90**, 715–720.

Taniguchi, H., Imai, Y., Iyanagi, T., and Sato, R. (1979). *Biochim. Biophys. Acta* **550**, 341–356.

Trudell, J. R., Bösterling, B., and Trevor, A. (1981). *Biochem. Biphys. Res. Commun.* **102**, 372–377.

Trudell, J. R., Bösterling, B., and Trevor, R. J. (1982a). *Mol. Pharmacol.* **21**, 710–717.

Van der Hoeven, T. A., and Coon, M. J. (1974). *J. Biol. Chem.* **249**, 6302–6310.

Visser, L., Robinson, N. C., and Tanford, C. (1975). *Biochemistry* **14**, 1194–1199.

Weisburger, E. K. (1978). *Ann. Rev. Pharmacol. Toxicol.* **18**, 395–415.

White, R. E., and Coon, M. J. (1980). *Ann. Rev. Biochem.* **49**, 315–356.

Wolf, C. R., Mansuy, D., Nastainczyk, W., Deutschmann, G., and Ullrich, V. (1977). *Mol. Pharmacol.* **13**, 698–705.

Wolf, C. R., Harrelson, W. G., Nastainczyk, W. M., Philpot, R. M., Kalyanaraman, B., and Mason, R. P. (1980). *Mol. Pharmacol.* **18**, 553–558.

Wood, C. L., Gandolfi, A. J., and Van Dyke, R. A. (1976). *Drug Met. Disp.* **4**, 305–313.

Chapter 7

Membrane Composition, Structure, and Function[1]

George Rouser

Introduction. 236
Steps in the Derivation of Membrane Structure and Packing Principles. . 238
  Sums Analysis of Lipid Class Composition Values. 239
  Derivation of the Packing Principles of Lipids in Membrane
    Compartments. 243
Graphic Analysis and Membrane Structure. 252
  Methods. 252
  General Characteristics of Physical and Biological Systems. 257
  Examples of Variation Ranges for Biological Systems. 263
  The Structural Basis and Significance of the Slope Changes as a Function
    of Temperature. 271
  Matched Levels, Types of Replacements, Membrane Structure, and
    Metabolic Control Mechanisms. 275
Packing of Cholesterol, Gangliosides, and Ceramide Polyhexosides in
    Membranes. 283
References. 285

[1]Abbreviations:1-Anilino-8-napthalene sufonate, ANS; Acidic phospholipids, APL; Ceramide aminoethylphosphonate, CAEP; Gas-liquid chromatography, GLC; Glycolipids cerebroside, CER; Ceramide phosphorylethanolamine, CPE; Digalactosyldiglycerides; DGDG; Diphosphatidyl glycerol, DPG; Intramembraneous particle, IMP; Lysobiphosphatidic acid, LBPA; Monogalactosyldiglycerides, MGDG; N-Acyl phosphatidyl ethanolamine, NAPE; Phosphatidic acid, PA; Phosphatidyl choline, PC; Phosphatidyl ethanolamine, PE; Phosphatidyl glycerol, PG; Phosphatidyl inositol, PI; Phosphatidyl serine, PS; Residual acid phospholipid, RAPL; Sulfolipid, SL; Sphingogomyelin, Sph; Thin layer chromatography, TLC; Total phospholipid, TPL; Total polar lipid, TPol.

Introduction

Membranes are composed of lipid, protein, and water with small amounts of mono- and divalent ions balancing ionic groups of lipids and proteins. It is apparent that membrane proteins are coded for specific interactions that cause each membrane to have its own characteristic enzymes, lipid species, and asymmetrical binding sites. An analysis of the variations in lipid composition values can be expected to show, in a precise and quantitative manner, how protein codes determine membrane structure since lipid interaction with protein is controlled by these codes.

Electron microscopy shows that membranes have a continuous protein coat over the lipid, since an examination of thin membrane sections after lipid extraction shows the same continuous dark outer lines separated by a lighter space that are seen when lipid is present [1, 2]. The continuous dark lines result from protein staining, and the lipid space is between the two protein layers. This general structure is also apparent when the surfaces of membranes are observed with negative stains that disclose small repeating units [3–7]. The small, almost square or rectangular units have, in general, dimensions in the plane of the membrane between 70 and 90 Å. There are no holes left at the surface when lipid is extracted, and membranes exhibit the same stretching characteristics with lipid present or extracted [8]. When membranes are frozen and fractured, they break into inner and outer halves, and the small square or rectangular units visible at the surface of native membranes are seen to be divided into two general types [9]. One, the intramembraneous particle (IMP), passes through the membrane. The IMPs appear to contain lipid since they are not formed if lipid is extracted prior to the fracture [10–12], and the individual small units containing both lipid and protein can be obtained by dissociation of the membrane with a detergent [13]. It thus appears that the IMPs are composed of a central core of lipid with protein around it. The space between IMPs is filled by protein units which appear only on one surface (do not pass through the membrane). The freeze fracture results correlate well with other data showing that some protein functional groups appear on one surface only. With the value of about 50Å^2 for the minimum cross sectional area for a polar lipid molecule, the dimension of about 75Å across the bilayer, and as high as 90 × 90Å for repeating units in the plane of the membrane, it is apparent that lipid occurs as bilayers in small compartments that hold well under 300 molecules. This relatively small number is well within the error range of lipid analysis.

The primary animal membrane lipid classes are quite generally phosphatidyl choline (PC), phosphatidyl ethanolamine (PE), phosphatidyl serine (PS), phosphatidyl inositol (PI), diphosphatidyl glycerol (DPG), and sphingomyelin (Sph). In some invertebrate species, ceramide aminoethyl-phosphonate (CAEP) and ceramide phosphorylethanolamine (CPE) occur in place of sphingomyelin. In the nervous system, the glycolipids cerebroside (Cer) and sulfatide (Sulf) appear mostly as partial replacements for PC and PE, respectively. In addition to the major components, there are a number of minor components: small amounts of ceramide and free fatty acid, acidic phospholipids (APL)—phosphatidic acid (PA), lysobisphosphatidic acid (LBPA), phosphatidyl glycerol (PG), N-acylPE (NAPE), and a number of unidentified components. In a study of human red blood cells using ion exchange column chromatography to concentrate the APL fraction which was then separated by two-dimensional thin layer chromatography (TLC), 14 minor components in addition to PA were found, and the levels were as low as 0.02 % of the total phospholipid [14]. This group of minor components is designated as residual acidic phospholipid (RAPL) in some forms of data analysis.

Most fungi have lipid class compositions similar to those of animal cells [15]. In plants the most characteristic differences are the absence of PS and Sph, the use of mono- and digalactosyldiglycerides (MGDG and DGDG) insetead of Cer, the use of plant sulfolipid (SL) instead of Sulf, and relatively high levels of PG as compared to the levels in animal cells. MGDG and DGDG also occur in some microorganisms, whereas others use primarily PE with a little APL, and others only APL, principally DPG and PG. The types of polar groups of lipids are thus in general quite limited.

With the standard shorthand designations of fatty acids as the number of carbons and the number of cis double bonds as a superscript, the chief saturated fatty acids of all organisms are 14^0, 16^0, and 18^0 with moderately high levels of 12^0 in some yeasts and plants. The chief differences between animals and plants is the use of 20^4, 20^5, 22^5, and 22^6 in animals and the use of 16^2, 16^3, 16^4, 18^3, and 18^4 in plants in addition to 16^1, and 18^2. Fungi in general may use only 16^1 and 18^1, or combine these with the use of 18^2 and in some cases 18^3. Bacterial fatty acids are generally limited to 16^1 and 18^1 in addition to the common saturated acids. In some cases, animal membranes may have significant levels of 20^1, 20^2, 22^2, 22^3 and 22^4, but all of these acids, as well as those of plants, fit into general replacement families. Odd carbon acids are generally absent or occur as very minor components, and iso and anteiso acids with methyl groups on the second and third to last carbon atoms from the methyl end are common only in thermophilic bacteria. Thus fatty acid variations in general follow a relatively simple plan, and most of the differences reflect the ability of a particular species to synthesize particular acids. Double bonds are specified either from the carboxyl end (the delta system) or the methyl end (the omega system), and the most common isomers are the same for all species, i.e., $18^1\Delta^9$, $18^2\Delta^{9,12}$,

$18^3\Delta^{9,12,15}$, $20^4\Delta^{5,8,11,14}$, $22^5\Delta^{4,7,10,13,16}$ (derived from 18^2), $22^5\Delta^{7,10,13,16,19}$ (derived from 18^3), and $22^6\Delta^{4,7,10,13,16,19}$ (derived from 18^3).

The most accurate and precise lipid analysis is based on two-dimensional TLC separation followed by aspiration of the spots and determination of molar amounts—by phosphorous analysis for phospholipids, and an amino group reagent for glycosphingolipids, or a carbohydrate reagent for MGDG and DGDG [16–20]. With quadruplicate analyses, the error for major components is about ±1–2% of the measured value. Although the error increases to ±5–8% for some of the minor components, the error is still in the third significant figure and is thus less than 0.1% of the total. The error for the most minor (trace) components can be reduced to as low as ±1%, if column chromatography is used before TLC separation. Because one-dimensional TLC was used for separations by some investigators, the reported values include various members of the RAPL group with the major lipid classes. Since RAPL varies from values as low as 1–2%, to as high as 15%, this error may be quite large and must be considered in some forms of data analysis.

Adequate separations are generally readily obtained for fatty acids with gas–liquid chromatography (GLC), and peak areas for even the most minor components can be determined with an error of ±0.5% or less. When the fatty acids of a minor lipid class are determined, it is possible to obtain values with significance at 0.001% of the total lipid level. The importance of this type of measurement is apparent from data analyses presented in other sections.

Steps in the Derivation of Membrane Structure and Packing Principles

Lipid class composition values can be analyzed in two ways: by plotting values against each other or against total polar lipid, or by adding, subtracting, multiplying, or dividing values in a search for constant sums or ratios. Since there is no rational basis for multiplication, and subtraction gives essentially the same type of analysis that addition does directly, addition (sums analysis) and division (ratios) are informative. Addition, or sums analysis, proves to be the most basic.

The sequence of steps in deriving the structural features of membranes begins with sums analysis to determine the size and dimensions of the smallest lipid compartments in the smallest repeating units in membranes. The sequence then proceeds through the derivation of packing principles from composition data to the use of graphic analysis in order to determine the size and arrangement of larger repeating units into which the smaller units fit, and the structure of some of the control units of membranes.

SUMS ANALYSIS OF LIPID CLASS COMPOSITION VALUES

Lipid class composition clearly changes under some conditions by a relatively specific replacement of one class by another. The nature of the lipid class replacements is important for Sums Analysis [21]. During development of the flight muscle of the tobacco horn worm [22], DPG increases from 6.8 to 20.3% (Δ = 13.5%), and the increase is mainly by replacement of PC that decreases from 44.8 to 35.9% (Δ = 8.9%). The sum PC + DPG remains relatively constant (51.6 to 56.2%). Changes in yeast growth conditions cause PC to be replaced by PE only when culture density is varied [23], since PC decreased from 44.9 to 26.8% (Δ 18.1%), and PE increased from 12.6 to 32.3% (Δ = 19.7%). In contrast, growth with ethanolamine and choline supplements [24] caused PC to be replaced by PE, PI, and PA (PC = 28.1%, PE + PI + PA =23%). The large decrease of PC for cells grown aerobically (48.8 to 25.8%, Δ − 23%) was also balanced by PE and acidic phospholipids [25].

Replacement between PC and Sph is a major feature of lipids of red blood cells and the lens [26–30), and replacement of both PC and PE by Sph is a prominent feature of the changes with age of the human aorta [31]. Also, Cer replaces PC and Sulf replaces PE in the brain, in which the major changes with age are decreases of PC and PE, and increases of Cer and Sulf [32]. Well-defined lipid class changes are shown by the data for the vernal variety of alfalfa [33]. When grown at 15, 20, and 30°C, the major lipid class changes in the leaves are replacement of MGDG and DGDG by PI and an increase of the pair PG + SL at the expense of the pair PC + PE. This type of replacement is not apparent for leaves of other species [34] since PI is a minor component, and MGDG and DGDG are major components that are replaced by other lipid classes.

Since it is clear that one lipid class may be replaced rather specifically by one other class in one membrane, and by different classes in other membranes, adding lipid class values (sums analysis) to determine whether or not characteristic sums are shown will involve the various possible combinations of the major components. The author's initial analysis included all of the possible sums. It became apparent, however, that the sums of minor components are not consistent, whereas those of major components are. Although the initial search by the author was very tedious, the analysis is very rapid when the general nature of the search is apparent. The approach is illustrated by the values in Tables I and II. Table I shows the major sums of two analyses of membranes with very different lipid class compositions. It is apparent that two closely similar values are obtained for analyses of all membranes, organelles, and organs from animals, plants, and microorganisms. The only qualifications are that the analysis be complete without mixing of lipid classes and extensive autolytic changes, and that one lipid class does not occur at a level above 69.2% of the total, as is the case of PE from *E. coli*.

The results of Sums Analysis of the various types of membranes and organs are summarized in Table III. In all cases the values for lysophospholipids were added to those of the parent lipid since some enzyme degradation is apparent, in particular for membrane preparations. Also, RAPL was considered as a group equivalent to one lipid class. In all cases one of three results was obtained within experimental error: values near 30.8% were associated with those near 69.2%, or values near 38.5% were associated with values near 61.5%, or two sums were near 30.8%, and one was near 38.5%. The values show that there are three different lipid class compartments, two with the same size and the third larger. Also, two compartments are commonly linked together. Since the ratio 30.8/38.5 = 0.800 exactly, it is apparent that the compartment sizes have a 4/5 ratio and that the values to four figures are 30.77% with 69.23% (30.77% + 38.46%) and 38.46% with 61.54% (30.77%

TABLE IA

Sums Analysis of Values between 15 and 85% for Bovine Red Blood Cells

Values	Sums of two	Sums of three	Sums of four
46.2	46.2 + 29.1 = 75.3	46.2 + 29.1 + 3.7 = 79.0	46.2 = 29.1 + 3.7 + 1.8 = 80.8
29.1[a]	46.2 + 19.3 = 65.5	46.2 + 29.1 + 1.8 = 77.1	46.2 + 19.3 + 3.7 + 1.8 = 71.0
19.3	46.2 + 3.7 = 49.9	46.2 + 19.3 + 3.7 = 69.2	29.1 + 19.3 + 3.7 + 1.8 = 53.9
3.7	46.2 + 1.8 = 48.0	46.2 + 19.3 + 1.8 = 67.3	
1.8	29.1 + 19.3 = 48.4	29.1 + 19.3 + 1.8 = 52.1	
	29.1 + 3.7 = 32.8[b]	29.1 + 19.3 + 1.8 = 50.2	
	29.1 + 1.8 = 30.9[c]	19.3 + 3.7 + 1.8 = 24.8	
	19.3 + 3.7 = 23.0		
	19.3 + 1.8 = 21.1		

[a] PE only = 29.1
[b] PE + PI = 32.8.
[c] PE + RAPL = 30.9 Mean = 30.9% (69.1%).

TABLE IB

Sums Analysis of Values between 15 and 85% for Rat Liver Microsomes

Values	Sums of two	Sums of three	Sums of four
65.2	65.2 + 6.4 = 71.6	65.2 + 6.4 + 2.7 = 74.3	65.2 + 6.4 + 2.7 + 2.4 = 76.7
21.8	65.2 + 2.7 = 67.9	65.2 + 6.4 + 1.3 = 72.9	65.2 + 6.4 + 2.7 + 1.3 = 75.6
6.4	65.2 + 2.4 = 67.6	65.2 + 2.7 + 2.4 = 70.3[a]	65.2 + 2.7 + 2.4 + 1.3 = 71.6
2.7	65.2 + 1.3 = 66.5	65.2 + 2.7 + 1.3 = 69.2[b]	21.8 + 6.4 + 2.7 + 2.4 = 33.3
2.4	21.8 + 6.4 = 28.2	65.2 + 2.4 + 1.3 = 68.9[c]	21.8 + 6.4 + 2.7 + 1.3 = 32.2
1.3	21.8 + 2.7 = 24.5	21.8 + 6.4 + 2.7 = 30.9	21.8 + 2.7 + 2.4 + 1.3 = 28.2
.3	21.8 + 2.4 = 24.2	21.8 + 6.4 + 2.4 = 30.6	
	21.8 + 1.3 = 23.1	21.8 + 6.4 + 1.3 = 29.5	

[a] PC + PS + OTHER = 70.3%.
[b] PC + Sph + OTHER = 69.2%.
[c] PC + PS + Sph = 68.9%. Mean near 69% = 69.5%.

TABLE II

Summary of Values for Membrane Sums from 304 Analyses

Membrane	Number of samples	Number near 61.5%	Mean (%)	Range (%)	Number near 69.2%	Mean (%)	Range (%)
Plasma membranes	32	15	61.33	59.5–62.4	27	69.27	68.1–71.3
Viruses	15	11	61.23	60.2–62.3	10	69.07	67.7–70.4
Microsomes	40	31	61.71	60.2–63.0	31	69.32	68.4–71.2
Nuclei	46	34	61.39	60.1–62.6	47	69.16	68.2–70.8
Mitochondria	59	58	61.28	59.0–62.8	16	69.07	68.2–70.3
Retina and rod outer segments	24	27	61.17	60.2–62.6	6	69.15	68.0–70.0
Lens	27	23	61.77	60.0–63.0	13	68.98	68.0–70.2
Parts of the eye	18	12	61.64	60.8–62.5	12	69.49	68.2–70.6
Rough and smooth microsomes	6	4	61.23	60.3–61.8	6	68.00	68.0–69.2
Mitochondrial inner and outer membranes	8	8	60.89	60.3–61.4	5	69.00	68.0–70.7
Brain membranes	29	16	61.12	59.0–63.0	14	69.31	67.3–70.8
Overall values	304	239	61.38	59.0–63.0	187	69.18	67.3–71.3

TABLE III

Sums Analysis Summary of All Values

	Mean near (%)	
Type	30.8	38.5
Whole organ	30.64 (122)	38.42 (93)
Membranes	30.82 (187)	38.62 (239)
Fungi	30.85 (11)	38.60 (9)
Bacterial	31.04 (5)	
Plant leaves	31.03 (28)	38.45 (19)
Overall means	30.78 (353)	38.56 (360)

+ 30.77%). A major reason for the linkage of two compartments is that one class, such as PC in animals, completely fills one compartment and partially fills another. Many analyses give more than one sum near the constant percentage. This is to be expected since values for two or more lipid classes are closely similar in many analyses, and sums of two or more classes are closely similar to the values for major components in some cases. The analyses in Table IV provide a variety of lipid class values that can be used to show that there are no alternatives to the values noted above.

Sums analysis of the values for human brain lipids as a function of age [35] showed the combinations PE + Sulf = 30.79 ±0.56% (mean of 50 values), and PE + Sulf + RAPL = 38.52 ±0.90% (mean of 18 values), to be common.

Sums analysis gives the ratios of compartment sizes but does not fix the number of molecules in the compartments. However the number of molecules can be approximated as shown in Table V from the values for lipids and proteins of membranes. Closely similar results were obtained with the values for red blood cells [36–38] and the Na^+/K^+-ATPase [39, 40], with good general agreement for molecular weights and percentages. The combination of percentages derived from sums analysis and the approximate number of molecules (170–190) fixes the value as 182, and 182 × 0.3077 = 56.00 molecules, whereas 182 × 0.3846 = 70.00 molecules. With each compartment as a bilayer, the dimensions are 56 ÷ 2 = 28 = 4 × 7, and 70 ÷ 2 = 35 = 5 × 7.

These calculations show that the strict requirements for exact whole number values for compartment sizes and bilayer dimensions are met very precisely. It is to be noted that the percentage values obtained by sums analysis are confirmed by the other forms of data analysis described in other sections.

TABLE IV

Membrane Analyses Selected as Most Useful for Testing Alternatives
to the Sums Described in the Text

Type	PC	Sph	PE	PS	PI	Other	R	Sum	(%)
1 Red blood cell	—	46.2	29.1	19.3	3.7	1.8	.9	PE + Other	30.9
2	29.4	24.9	25.9	13.5	1.3	2.0	3.0	PE + Other + R	30.9
3 Semiliki Forrest virus	34.2	26.5	22.8	.8	15.0	—	.7	PE + PS + PI	38.6
4 Sindbis virus	26.2	18.2	35.4	20.3	—	—	—	Sph + PS	38.5
5 Mitochondria	48.1	—	35.5	1.3	.5	14.0	.6	PE + PS + PI + R	37.9
6	43.0	2.9	23.5	.7	4.8	14.4	1.9	PE + PS + PI + R	30.9
7	43.0	5.0	23.0	—	3.0	14.0	1.0	PE + Sph	39.0
								PE + PI + R	38.0
8	40.5	1.6	32.1	3.4	7.8	11.8	2.7	PE + PS + R	38.2
9	40.0	—	37.2	1.0	7.5	12.7	1.3	PE + Other	38.5
10	35.0	2.2	36.7	2.2	4.2	20.0		PE + PS	38.9
11	23.9	—	67.0	1.3	1.2	6.0	.6	PE + PS + PI	69.5
12 Microsomes	65.2	1.3	21.8	2.4	6.4	1.9	1.0	PE + PS + PI	30.6
13	65.1	3.2	16.3	6.7	6.7	.4	1.6	PE + PS + PI	31.3
14	65.6	3.7	18.6	3.3	8.9	—	—	PE + PS + PI	30.8
15	61.3	4.0	23.0	3.5	8.1	—	.1	PE + PI	31.1
16	61.3	3.9	14.6	1.6	7.0	1.4	10.2	PC	61.3
17	59.9	2.9	27.4	3.2	6.5	—	.1	PE + PS + R	30.7
18	59.4	6.3	24.9	2.9	6.5	—	—	PE + Sph	31.2
19	59.1	3.9	22.5	2.7	11.9	—	—	PE + Sph + Other	38.3
20	58.9	3.6	29.3	2.9	3.6	1.7	—	PE + Other	31.0
21	50.8	9.9	23.6	6.0	8.2	1.5	—	PE + PS + Other	31.1
22	38.7	23.5	21.5	9.7	4.7	—	1.9	PE + PS	31.2
23 Nuclei	65.4	5.2	15.7	3.3	6.9	3.3	.2	PE + Sph + PS + PI	31.1
24	41.5	12.7	26.2	7.1	5.2	—	—	PE + PI	31.4
								PE + PI + PS	38.5
25 Retina	51.7	12.7	21.0	9.6	1.6	3.4	—	PE + PS	30.6
26	48.1	4.4	30.0	8.9	4.6	—	4.0	PE + Sph + PI	38.6
27 Lens	24.5	28.0	34.5	13.0	2.5	1.0	.5	PE + PI + Other + R	38.5

DERIVATION OF THE PACKING PRINCIPLES OF LIPIDS IN MEMBRANE COMPARTMENTS

Which lipid species pack into a compartment is determined by codes for both polar groups and fatty acid chains. Aside from the precise nature of the codes, there are major questions concerning the principles of mixed species packing which allow molecules of one type to pack next to molecules of

TABLE V

Calculation of the Number of Phospholipid Molecules
in the Smallest Lipid Compartments

A. From Human Red Blood Cell Values

$100,000 \times 2 = 200,000$ protein through the membrane

$25,000 \times 2 = \underline{\ \ 50,000}$ protein on the inner and outer surfaces

$250,000$ daltons total protein

(note: $200,000/250,000 = 80\%$ through protein)

$250,000 \div 1.65 = 151,515$ molecular weight units $\times 1.3$ for density difference = $196,970$ equivalent molecular weight units of lipid

Lipid mean molecular weight = mean of phospholipid and cholesterol = $770 + 0.88$ $(387) \div 1.88 = 590$ (cholesterol/phospholipid molar ratio = .88)

$196,970 \div 590 = 334$ lipid molecules

$\div 1.88 = 178$ phospholipid molecules

$334 - 178 = 156$ cholesterol molecules

B. Values calculated for rod outer segments and the Na^+/K^+-ATPase from kidney were 182 and 191 molecules, respectively.

C. The 4/5 ratio established by 30.77/38.46 repeats at intervals of 13, but since lipid is arranged as a bilayer, the multiple is 26 and the numbers in the multiple series are $6 \times 26 = 156$, $7 \times 26 = 182$, and $8 \times 26 = 208$. Thus, the correct value is 182 molecules and

$30.77 = 182 \times 0.3077 = 56.00$ molecules

$38.46 = 182 \times 0.3846 = 70.00$ molecules

---

another, and the nature of molecular conformations (relative positions) of the chains of each species. The sums analysis of the combination of lipid class values showing specific replacement of one lipid class by another in one organ or organism, and replacement by other classes in other membranes shows that polar group codes may be combined in a variety of ways to control which lipid classes are replacements for others. The types of chain codes are considered below.

The determination from composition data of whether or not molecules of different lipid species mix and pack side by side is greatly simplified when it is realized that all organisms with similar lipid classes and fatty acids must follow the same general packing principles for the bulk lipid phase in membranes. Thus the data considered previously show the specific class replacements of one membrane to be different from those of another. Sums analysis excludes mixed packing of phospholipid classes with each other because there is no constant principle for mixed packing. Additionally, cholesterol does not pack with any type of phospholipid, since the same constant sums for the polar lipids were found with widely different cholesterol-to-phospholipid ratios. The existence of the chain codes (described below) shows that different species of each lipid class pack in separate compartments since chain codes are possible only if a single species packs in one compartment. Furthermore, the rigid exclusion of position isomers of the coded fatty acids can be explained only if there is no mixed species packing.

Lipid composition data shows that different membranes of an organ may have very different cholesterol-to-phospholipid molar ratios. Mitochondria with ratios as low as 0.03 and plasma membranes with ratios as high as 1.0 represent the common extremes. Thus if mixed packing occurred, it would involve only a small amount of mitochondrial lipid and a large amount of plasma membrane lipid. Such large differences make quantitative checks of the relationship of the cholesterol-to-phospholipid ratio with lipid class and fatty acid composition data relatively simple. The values in Table VI show that the same or closely similar ratios may occur with very different lipid class values and, conversely, that membranes with similar lipid class compositions may have very different ratios. The values in Table VII show that the 20-fold difference in the ratio cannot be explained by differences in the fatty acids of mitochondria and plasma membranes, since these membranes have closely similar fatty acids. Thus no general mixed packing rules are apparent, and it appears that cholesterol packs in a separate space that is coded specifically for cholesterol. Many analyses other than those shown in Tables VI and VII show the same general lack of correlation.

Other observations also exlude cholesterol packing with phospholipids. A fungus unable to synthesize cholesterol was found to grow in its absence (no

TABLE VI

Lipid Analyses Showing the Absence of a Correlation Between Lipid Class Composition and the Cholesterol to Phospholipid Ratio

	TPL (%)							
hl/TPL	PC	Sph	PE	PS	PI	DPG	R	Source
0.51	46.8	24.4	13.0	5.0	11.7	—	—	Hamster kidney PM
0.51	62.1	5.6	18.4	2.8	8.8	2.3	—	Rat muscle ER
0.64	38.5	30.0	15.6	5.2	10.5	—	—	SV5 virus
0.64	16.0	15.7	31.3	15.8	7.1	—	—	Influenza virus
0.63	33.0	5.3	39.9	—	21.8	—	—	Rat intestine PM
0.22	65.9	4.7	17.4	.8	10.7	.4	—	Rabbit muscle ER
0.22	43.6	4.2	21.3	7.5	9.0	8.5	—	Dog heart ER
0.10	58.9	3.6	29.3	2.9	3.6	1.7	—	Rat liver ER
0.10	30.2	13.3	25.5	8.0	1.4	—	1.7	Rat kidney PM
0.81	36.6	18.4	15.4	8.2	7.2	—	7.4	Rat liver PM
0.82	9.8	11.8	39.0	15.0	6.4	—	10.0	Sendai virus
0.83	—	51.0	26.2	14.1	2.9	—	5.8	Bovine red cell

TABLE VII

Cholesterol-to-Phospholipid Ratios of Rat Liver
Plasma Membranes[a] and Mitochondria[b] and Fatty Acid Patterns[c]

	PC		PE		PS		PI		DPG		Sph	
	PM	Mito	PM	Mito	PM	Mito	PM	Mito	PM	Mito	PM	Mito
12°						0.5		0.1		0.7		0.1
X		0.1		0.1		0.9		0.3		1.0		0.6
14°		0.3		0.1		0.6		0.3		1.7		0.6
1		0.1		0.2		1.0		0.3		0.2		0.6
16°	24.8	19.8	21.9	9.8	6.4	8.4	19.7	8.2	11.1	7.7	19	26.6
1	1.4	0.5	0.7	0.4	0.5	1.4	1.9	0.8	3.9	1.9		1.0
16°A		0.2		1.3		0.7		0.9		4.2		0.4
16'A		0.5		2.9		0.2		0.7				0.2
17°	0.7		0.7		0.4							
18°A				1.4				0.1				
18'A		0.2		1.3		0.2		0.5				
18°	26.2	26.6	29.2	28.6	59.8	36.3	46.2	37.9	4.9	3.5	13	23.9
1	11.0	9.7	7.7	6.0	4.4	8.8	16.8	7.8	15.3	10.3	3	9.5
2	19.1	14.0	10.6	6.7	1.6	6.6	5.8	8.9	58.2	65.7	2	11.2
3	0.3				0.4		1.5					
20°						0.4						2.8
1												
2						0.7		0.2		1.9		0.2
3	0.7		1.2		1.1				1.4	0.5		
4	12.9	21.5	19.0	15.2	17.7	13.6	7.5	24.1	1.7			9.9
22°						1.5		0.2			9	3.2
1											1	
5			1.4		0.1	2.1		0.8				4.1
6	2.6	3.8	5.5	21.5	7.2	11.5		5.5	1.3			0.6
23°											11	
1											.4	
24°		0.8		1.5		0.5		0.4			25	0.1
1											12	

[a] Ratio 0.73.

[b] Ratio 0.036.

[c] Note the lack of correlation between the very different cholesterol-to-phospholipid ratios and the generally similar fatty acid patterns.

cholesterol in membranes) and to incorporate cholesterol added to the medium without a significant change in phospholipid class composition [15]. Thus either cholesterol packs equally with all lipid classes or it packs in a separate space. Since it is apparent from other data that cholesterol does not pack equally with all phospholipids, it must therefore pack in a separate space. When human red blood cells are incubated in plasma with a low free-to-esterified cholesterol ratio, they lose about 40% of their cholesterol to plasma without a change in phospholipid class composition [41, 42]. Since the space left can be refilled with cholesterol by incubation of the low-cholesterol cells in normal plasma, it is apparent that it is coded specifically for cholesterol and cannot be entered by any of the plasma phospholipids.

The limited range of variability in the types of membrane lipid polar groups is related to the polar lipid codes and space restrictions. Only myo-inositol and serine are found in polar lipids, even though other similar polyols and threonine are available. The bases are also invariably choline and ethanolamine, and only minor modifications of choline are allowable. The mono- and dimethyl ethanolamines, and the monoethyl dimethyl and diethyl monomethyl (but not the triethyl) analogs of choline enter liver lipids as choline replacements and cure the fatty liver of choline deficiency [43–45], and β-methylcholine can meet the choline requirement for some insects [46]. The analog of choline with sulfur replacing nitrogen (sulfocholine) was also found to cure the fatty liver of choline deficiency [47] and was thus shown to meet the choline code. Later studies established that some diatoms use sulfocholine rather than choline in their membrane lipids [48]. The data thus show that the polar group codes are indeed highly restrictive.

Fatty acid composition data show that some membranes do not have chain codes whereas others have codes specifying particular types of fatty acids. The absence of chain codes is shown by the data for *E. coli* and *A. laidlawii* grown on a variety of fatty acid supplements [49–58]. In both bacteria free replacement among all fatty acids is apparent. The absence of chain codes is also apparent for hamster red blood cells [59], which can be induced to undergo large changes in composition by exposure of the animals to high room temperature for several weeks.

The data suggest at first glance that the various species pack together in a more or less random manner. That this is not the case is shown by the existence of specific chain codes that would not be specific if the species of each lipid class could pack randomly. This preference for nonrandom, like-to-like packing is shown by melting point data for pure lipids in the hydrated state. The *in vitro* conditions that provide the greatest flexibility for chain and molecular conformation adjustments indicate that disaturated species of PC do not mix completely with dioleoyl PC since calorimetry shows the typical melting point of dioleoyl PC when it is mixed with the disaturated species [60].

The simplest chain codes are shown by some fungal mutants. One mutant required an unsaturated fatty acid with a double bond nine carbons from the carboxyl end of the chain (Δ^9) since $14^1\Delta^9$, $16^1\Delta^9$, $18^1\Delta^{9,12}$, and $18^3\Delta^{9,12,15}$ supplements to the growth medium satisfied the requirement, whereas acids with other double bond positions did not [61]. Another mutant required a saturated acid for growth [62]. The requirement was met by both odd and even carbon acids, and composition could be varied from all saturated to 50% unsaturated. Thus it appears that the saturated acid code is on one protein surface with the other surface uncoded and accepting various fatty acids. The involvement of two protein surfaces is apparent from other data. One of the most common animal cell codes is for a saturated acid in one position and a Δ^9 or Δ^5 fatty acid in the other position. The codes are illustrated by the molecular species data [63] for liver PC. On a fat-free diet, $18^2\Delta^{9,12}$ is replaced by $18^1\Delta^9$, and $20^4\Delta^{5,8,11,14}$ is replaced by $20^3\Delta^{5,8,11}$ with 16^0 and 18^0 occupying position one. Although $16^1\Delta^9$ does not appear as a prominent replacement for 18^2 in PC and PE, it is a major replacement in DPG of mitochondria [64, 65]. When the fat-free diet is supplemented with $18^3\Delta^{9,12,15}$, $20^5\Delta^{5,8,11,14,17}$ becomes the replacement for 20^4 and in DPG in particular, 18^3 is a major replacement for 18^2. Thus the data show members of the Δ^9 family except for $14^1\Delta^9$ and the Δ^5 family to be used.

In nervous tissue and the eye, $18^2\Delta^{9,12}$ is a minor component whereas $18^1\Delta^9$ is a major component and 16^1 is present in relatively large amounts in some lipid classes at certain ages. The absence of major replacement between 18^1 and 18^2 is thus attributable to a code that specifies $18^1\Delta^9$.

The data for mouse LM cells cultured with a variety of fatty acid supplements [66] are considered in more detail below in the discussion of replacements with the related changes for liver [67] and *Chlorella sotokiniana* [68].

Other probable animal cell codes are for $22^5\Delta^{4,7,10,13,16}$ ($\omega6$ from $18^2\Delta^{9,12}$), $22^5\Delta^{7,10,13,16,19}$ ($\omega3$ from 18^3) and $22^6\Delta^{4,7,10,13,16,19}$. With the Δ^4 code, 22^5 from 18^2 can replace 22^6, whereas with the $\omega3$ code for 22^6, 22^5 from 18^3 is the replacement. With a Δ^7 code, 22^5 from 18^3 can be replaced in animals by $16^1\Delta^7$ from $18^1\Delta^9$ only. Since animals cannot make replacements to meet the Δ^4 or Δ^7 codes except from 18^2 and 18^3, organs with these codes show symptoms of essential fatty acid deficiency. The retina [69] is a good example since it uses a high level of 22^6, and $18^1\Delta^9$ is the major replacement on a fat-free diet. Since linoleic acid cures the symptoms, the Δ^4 code is indicated. The Δ^4 code is also apparent for rabbit brain PE and PS [70] that have up to 13.4% $22^5\omega6$ and 19.1% 22^6 with only traces of $22^5\omega3$. Boar sperm phospholipids have 34.3–36.4% $22^5\omega6$ and up to 22.9% 22^6 with traces of $22^5\omega3$ [71] so the Δ^4 code is also indicated. In contrast, rat testis and rabbit sperm contain $22^5\omega3$ only [72, 73], and the Δ^7 code is indicated since the $\omega3$ code would include 22^6. Bull, ram, and human sperm contain 22^6 only [73, 74] with low levels of 18^2 and 20^4. Thus the Δ^4 code without conversion of $18^2\omega6$ to $22^5\omega6$ is indicated.

The codes for 22^5 and 22^6 are confined to the 2-position in many animals, but may be on both protein surfaces, particularly in fish muscle [75]. The values for salmon brain and muscle [76] indicate the Δ^4 code since 22^6 and

$22^5\omega^6$ are present. In brain, 18^2 is absent and 18^1 is a major fatty acid with 16^1 representing a minor component. Thus a brain ω^9 code is indicated with $16^1\Delta^9$ being formed by desaturation of $16°$ rather than chain shortening from $18^1\Delta^9$. Fatty acid composition values for various protozoa indicate the ω^3 and ω^6 codes, but are more difficult to evaluate since there is a large uncoded space. The values for *Acanthamoeba* sp. on supplmenets [77] indicate the existence of the ω^6 and ω^9 codes. The values for MGDG fatty acids of the leaves of angiosperms [78], with $16^3\omega^3$ and $18^3\omega^3$ as the major fatty acids, indicate the ω^3 code with the sum $16^3 + 18^3$ as 88.8 to 96.4% of the total. MGDG of *C. vulgaris* [79] appears to use the ω^3 code with $16^4\Delta^{4,7,10,13}$ (ω^3) and $18^3\omega^3$ (38.7% 16^4 + 43.6% = 82.3%) and 18^3 and 18^4 in PC and PE. The Δ^9 code is used by other plants that have high 18^3, and the replacement of $18^1\Delta^9$ and $18^2\Delta^{9,12}$ by $18^3\Delta^{9,12,15}$ during development of plastids in green corn leaves [79] provides a good indication of the Δ^9 code with 18^3 replacing the other Δ^9 acids. The very high values for 18^3 in MGDG and DGDG in some plants without appreciable amounts of the other Δ^9 or ω^3 acids suggests that the Δ^9 code may occur on one side, and the ω^3 code on the other side of the bilayer to make the compartment space specific for $18^3\Delta^{9,12,15}$. This type of coding could also explain the apparent specificity for 22^6 in some fish muscle. It appears that the 18^3 code may be present on one protein surface, as well as both surfaces, since one surface may have the even-carbon saturated acid code. In green corn leaves [80], $18^3\omega^3$ was 93.7% and 80.0% in MGDG and DGDG, respectively; Whereas in SL, $16°$ was 50.2% and 18^3 was 41.0%. Since all of the lipid classes except MGDG have 18^2 (up to 43.0% in PC), the Δ^9 code is indicated. A Δ^{3t} code is indicated by the presence of 20.4% $16^1\Delta^{3t}$ in PG only. The only other trans double bond code apparent is for animal cell spingolipids in which the Δ^4 trans bond is present in sphingosine. The plasmalogen forms of the animal phospholipids with a cis-1 double bond suggests a Δ^1 code.

Some organisms have $18^3\Delta^{6,9,12}$ as well as $18^3\Delta^{9,12,15}$ and the data for *Tetrahymena pyriformis* grown on various supplements [81] indicates the Δ^6 code. Data for bacteria with high levels of iso and anteiso acids [82, 83] strongly indicate a code for a$15°$ in the 2-position since the lowest level on supplements was 68.7% for *B. subtilis* and 68.7% in *Norcardia leishmanii* that also had 65.0% hydroxy a$15°$ in PE.

Animal sphingolipids contain, in general, odd and even carbon saturated and mono-unsaturated acids with variable double bond positions, as well as hydroxy fatty acids. Thus, in addition to the sphingosine code, there appear to be general saturated acid, general mono-unsaturated, and hydroxy fatty acid codes that are met by odd and even carbon acids. The saturated and hydroxy fatty acid codes are apparent for various organisms in glycerolphospholipids. However the monoene code with variable double bond positions appears to be specific for sphingolipids since the general unsaturation code for glycerolphospholipids does not exclude polyunsaturated fatty acids.

The existence of chain codes shows clearly (as noted above) that the packing of species of a lipid class is not random since codes would not be possible if all species could pack side by side. Thus it is apparent that the conformational differences of chain length equivalents prevent mixed species packing. The data for membranes with chain codes show that even members of a replacement family, such as 18^1, 18^2, and 18^3 with the Δ^9 code, do not pack together. If this were the case, that species with conformationally different acids could pack side by side, there would be no reason for the exclusion of other isomers situated in the bulk phase of lipid distant from the coded protein surfaces. The data for all types of organisms show this packing principle. If mixed species packing occurred, isomers of 18^1 other than Δ^9 and 18^2 and 20^4 other than ω^6 could be common, whereas in nature they are rare.

Metabolic production commonly limits some fatty acids as replacements, and unusual acids may be encountered in some tissues. Thus $18^1\Delta^5$ in lung PC [84] and the nonmethylene interrupted acids $20^2\Delta^{5,19}$, $20^3\Delta^{4,11,14}$, and $20^4\Delta^{5,11,14,17}$ in plants [85] can meet the Δ^5 code, and $22^3\omega^9$ and $22^4\omega^9$ of rat red blood cells [86] can meet the ω^9 code. It is to be noted that the Δ^5 and ω^9 codes are also apparent for plasma lipids [87]. All of these chain codes were defined from tables of accurate data derived from 144 publications for animal values, and 286 publications with data for plants and other organisms.

Molecular conformation of polar lipids refers to the different bond angles between polar groups that can cause the fatty acid chains to vary in position and give different molecular lengths. An attempt was made to analyze the melting point data for polar lipids [88–109] to define different conformations, but aside from showing some simple relationships, such as that for the disaturated PC species 12^012^0, 14^014^0, 16^016^0, and 18^018^0, i.e., melting point (°C) = 2 × (melting point in °C of the fatty acid) −84.80, conformation analysis was not possible due to the small number of values available. However analysis of membrane fatty acid composition data provides a good basis for polar lipid conformation changes.

In general fatty acid replacement data shows that unsaturated acids can replace each other as well as replace saturated acids when replacement is not prevented by chain codes. This equivalence for replacement indicates that unsaturated acids are the same length as saturated acids and thus that: 18^1 = 18^2 = 18^3 = 18^0, 20^3 = 20^4 = 20^0, and 22^5 = 22^6 = 22^0. The chain structure variations shown by X-ray diffraction length data are compatible with the equivalence as is the upper length limit for saturated acids of 22^0 22^0 that becomes equivalent to 18^0 22^5, 18^0 22^6, 18^1 22^5, and 18^1 22^6 that are equivalent to 18^0 22^0 = 20^0 20^0.

Organisms in general have rather well-defined fatty acid chain length limits. In animals the lower limit is commonly 14^0 with the shortest species being $16 + 14$. The upper limit is 20^020^0. These limits give the series: $16 + 14$, $16 + 16$, $16 + 18$, $18 + 18$, $18 + 20$, and $20 + 20$. In sphingolipids, the range is 16 to 26 carbons. Since the first four carbons of sphingosine correspond to the glycerol moiety of glycerol phospholipids, the sphingosine chain is equivalent to a 14 carbon acid, and the six species are: $14 + 16$, $14 + 18$, $14 + 20$, $14 + 22$, $14 + 24$, and $14 + 26$. A small amount of 14 carbon acids may be present, and this is correlated with the presence of a 20 carbon analog of sphingosine. The $16 + 14$ to $20 + 20$ [30–40] series is apparent for *A. Laidlawii*, in which growth with 20^0 as a supplement gives greater than 50% incorporation [57]. Thus lipids with both fatty acids being 20^0 (20^020^0) are formed. The lower limit for both *E. coli* and *A. laidlawii* is $16 + 14$ since 14^0 does not go above 50% when the organisms are grown on short chain acid supplements [49–58]. Since all fatty acids appear to replace each other in these organisms without chain codes and mixed packing does not occur, it appears that the different species fill the same compartment space, and that an increase of chain length is balanced by a shift of the chains forward which thus keeps the same space between the polar groups in the bilayer.

The equivalence of different species is shown directly by the data for mycoplasma strain Y [110]. This organism does not oxidize, desaturate, or alter the lengths of chains of fatty acid supplements and has a requirement for an unsaturated fatty acid that is met by elaidic acid $(18^{1t}\Delta^9)$. When grown on 18^{1t}, this acid represents about 97% of the total, and the small amount of 16^0 and 18^0 incorporated was shown to come from albumin required in the medium. When grown with equimolar amounts of 18^{1t} and 10^0, 12^0, 14^0, 16^0, 18^0, or 20^0, about equimolar amounts of 18^{1t} and the saturated acid are incorporated. The sequence is $18^{1t}10^0$ $(=18+10=16+12)$, $18^{1t}12^0$ $(=16+14)$, $18^{1t}14^0$ $(=16+16)$, and $18^{1t}16^0$ $(=18+16)$, $18^{1t}18^0$ $(=18+18)$, and $18^{1t}20^0$ $(=18+20)$. The sequence of six species differs from that of animal cells in that it covers the 28–38 carbon range rather than 30–40 range. Yeast data [25] shows the smallest species to be $16 + 10$, which allows a range of 26–36 carbons.

When the fatty acid values derived from an evaluation of 430 publications containing data for all types of organisms were thoroughly examined, only a few clear exceptions to the 26, 28, or 30 carbon sequences were found in plants [111–113]. In grape-stock seedling stalks with 55% 26^0cp (cyclopropane) in one lipid class, there is clearly some 26^0cp26^0cp $= 26^026^0 = 52$ carbons. The lipid classes of grape stock in general contained some 27 and 28 carbon saturated acids, and high levels of saturated 20 to 24 carbon acids are apparent in glycerolphospholipids that are also seen in orchids [114] and a halophyte [115]. The exceptions fit the sequence beginning with 42 carbons: $20 + 22$, $22 + 22$, $22 + 24$, $24 + 24$, $24 + 26$, $26 + 26$. The presence of longer chain acids was associated with early spring and drought resistant plants which are able to avoid water loss when the air contains little water, as well as with chloride uptake by roots, which was found to be inversely related to the presence of the longer chain acids. This conformational sequence is thus added to or subtracted from the more common plant sequences, and appears to be an adaptation to environmental conditions which would lead to high water loss.

Graphic Analysis and Membrane Structure

METHODS

Graphic analysis is the most generally useful of the various forms of data analysis, and it proved to be the key method for many of the problems involving membrane composition, structure, and function. After many attempts to derive information from data published as plots, it became apparent that the methods for graphic analysis had not been defined adequately. Therefore the rules for correct plotting, line fitting, and quantitative evaluation were derived from studies of model plots and a variety of relationships in physical and biological systems.

The first step in graphic analysis is to make all of the necessary plots. As described previously [21], there are nine ways to plot values for two variables:

A vs. B	$1/A$ vs. B	Log A vs. B
A vs. $1/B$	$1/A$ vs. $1/B$	Log A vs. $1/B$
A vs. Log B	$1/A$ vs. Log B	Log A vs. Log B

It might appear at first glance that there are many more ways to plot, since in addition to N, $1/N$, and Log N, values can be raised to various powers (N^x). However, this is not the case because all exponential relationships are plotted as logs. This is easy to see from the well-known equation for the area of a circle as a function of the size of its radius. The equation $A = \pi R^2$ states that a plot of area against the square of the radius gives a line that passes through the origin and has a slope of π. The equivalent equation is: Log A = Log πR^2 = Log π + Log R^2 = 2 Log R + Log π. This equation states that a plot of Log A against Log R gives a line with a slope of two and an intercept of Log π. It is easy to show the equivalence of the power and log forms of this exponential relationship by entering the same R values into each equation, and plots of log R vs. log A can be made quickly to verify that it is linear.

The second step in graphic analysis is selection of the correct plot. The two primary criteria are that the correct plot gives (a) no slope change or the smallest number of slope changes; (b) all values close to the mean line (no scatter). It is easy to understand that a slope change that can be abolished by plotting in another way does not represent a true structural change. Model plots that are simply lines drawn by the analyst to follow, by definition, any one of the nine functions, and from which values are obtained for plotting with the other eight functions, will show that incorrect plotting causes some linear relationships to be curves and others to be linear with slope changes. Model plots will also show that incorrect plotting introduces scatter that in its most extreme form causes one line to split to two and commonly causes values to move away from the mean line. That a curve is obtained when some linear relationships are plotted incorrectly is easy to show with the equation for the area of a circle since Log R vs Log A gives a line without a slope change and the other eight functions give curves.

Since many physical and all biological relationships give sets of lines rather than one line, the two additional criteria are that the correct plot gives (c) exactly parallel lines; and (d) the smallest number of lines. Parallel lines arise from structural differences and lines are exactly parallel because the structural difference giving more than one line does not involve a change of slope. Slope changes arise from a different type of structural change, and the scatter from incorrect plotting commonly causes line number to increase. Parallel lines are drawn through points by the use of a pair of parallel bars and are confirmed by calculating the precision of the relationship as described below. Criteria a–d are usually sufficient to fix the correct plot for biological relationships. When these leave any doubt, check plots can be used. Another criterion that is usually all that is required, is that the correct plot gives (e) equivalent lines when values for A or B or both variables are plotted as percentage of the maximum values.

Although the author has developed exponential check plots, these are not generally required for biological relationships. It is to be noted, however, that at least one of the three types of root plots ($\sqrt{A}$ vs. B, A vs. $\sqrt{B}$ or $\sqrt{A}$ vs. $\sqrt{B}$) will give an equivalent line with the correct function.

The third step in graphic analysis is the evaluation of the precision of the linear relationships obtained. The equation for the line is calculated and the standard deviation of the ratios of the values found (i.e., listed), to those calculated from the equation (i.e., $F/C \pm$ S.D.), defines the precision. The values for either variable can be used since both give the same result. The ratio should be very near 1.0 exactly, and the standard deviation will match that obtained when repeat determinations, such as quadruplicates, are made for pairs of values. With the common error range for biological systems of $\pm 1\%$, the $F/C \pm$ S.D. is near 1.0 ± 0.010. With physical relationships, error can be as low as 0.02% and thus the standard deviation may be as low as ± 0.0002.

The least squares fit Correlation Coefficient (CC) has been recommended for evaluating linear relationships. However it is not a measure of precision and its use can give rise to incorrect decisions. The CC is a function of the extent to which deviations of values on one side of a line balance those on the other and can thus be very close to 1.0 and indicate a good fit when the $F/C \pm$ S.D. shows a poor fit. A simple example is proved by the atomic numbers and melting points for hydrogen (1, 13.9°), iron (26, 1808°), and molybdenum (42, 2893°). When the values are plotted against each other, they give a reasonably good line to the eye. The equation and CC are: melting point = 70.36 (atomic number) $-$ 46.59 (CC = 0.99988). According to the usual tables of significance, the CC indicates a certainty of over 99%. However the F/C ratio shows that there is no true linear relationship because the calculated values are far from those found in tables: F/C for H = 13.9°/23.77°; Fe = 1808°/1782.71°; Mo = 2893°/2908.42°. The good CC is from a balancing of ($+$) and ($-$) values, i.e., H = $+9.87°$, Mo = $+15.42°$, Fe = $-25.29°$, so that sum of H + Mo deviations of $+25.29°$ matches the Fe $-25.29°$.

The different functions provide different increments for change. There are only six different types of increments for change since, of the nine plots, there are three pairs that differ only in the positions of the variables (A vs. $1/B$ and $1/A$ vs. B; Log A vs. B and A vs. Log B; Log A vs. $1/B$ and $1/A$ vs. Log B). A straight line is obtained when increments for change are exactly balanced and the A vs B function is the only one that gives a constant increment for change. The other eight functions give changing increments (values can increase or decrease with increasing or decreasing increments).

A simple example of the way increments for lines match is provided by the relationship of atomic number to the number of neutrons for helium (2,2), beryllium (4,5) and carbon (6,6). Atomic number increases are 2–4–6, and thus there are increments of two, whereas the number of neutrons increases by 2–5–6 so that the increments are three and one. If the increase in atomic number is expressed as a reciprocal, 2–4–6 becomes 0.5–0.25–0.1667, and the increments then become 0.25 and 0.08333, which are then in the 3/1 ratio, like to the incremental change in neutrons. Thus, the equation for the linear relationship is: Number of neutrons = 8.0 $-$ 12 (1/atomic number). The CC = $1.0 \pm$ zero, and the $F/C \pm$ S.D. = $1.0 \pm$ zero, because all calculated and found values are in exact agreement.

Since each of the functions provides a different type of increment for change, there is in general only one correct plot for a relationship. There are, however, two general types of equivalent plots in addition to the two forms of exponential relationships. Thus, if the A vs. B plot gives a line passing through the origin, exactly equivalent lines will be obtained when the values are plotted as $1/A$ vs. $1/B$ and Log A vs. Log B. The line for the $1/A$ vs. $1/B$ plot passes through the origin and the line for the Log A vs. Log B plot has a slope fo 1.0 exactly. This is apparent from the equations since $A = CB$ is equivalent to $1/A = 1/CB$ and Log A = Log CB = Log C + Log B. The other equivalence is when the $1/A$ vs. B plot gives a line passing through the origin, an equivalent line passing through the origin is obtained with the A vs. $1/B$ plot, and the line for the Log A vs. Log B plot has a slope of -1.0 exactly. The equivalent equations are $1/A = CB$, $A = 1/CB$, Log $1/A$ = Log CB, and since Log $1/A$ = Log 1 $-$ Log A = 0 $-$ Log A, then Log $1/A$ = $-$Log A. The latter equivalence shows why it is not necessary to plot Log $1/A$ or Log $1/B$ since these plots give lines equivalent to Log A and Log B plots, except that the slopes have opposite signs.

Two common mistakes in data analysis have led to errors and a great deal of missed information. One is the concept that it is possible to derive the correct plot for a relationship mathematically. Despite an obvious fact that the increments for change in a biological system are defined by the structural principles underlying a relationship that are not inherent in a general mathematical treatment, the incorrect concept that relationships to temperature for enzyme activities should be plotted Log vs. $1/°K$ in all cases has persisted and given rise to a great deal of confusion and many incorrect conclusions.

The other costly fundamental error made in data analysis has been the assumption that normal ranges of variation for biological systems are about a mean line that passes through the origin on A vs. B plots. That the constant change for A vs. B functions cannot be correct for all relationships is easy to see from such simple observations that body and organ weights of animals do not increase in a constant manner with age. Rather, growth is rapid at earlier ages and slows as the animal approaches maturity. Thus values plotted against age cannot follow the A vs. B function. It is also easy to see that there is no clustering of values about a mean line. Since many relationships are not in even approximate agreement with the two basic assumptions, the evaluations made with them are pseudoquantitative and misleading and commonly give rise to incorrect and/or inadequate conclusions.

A good example of the difference between the standard statistical evaluation of a biological relationship and the correct graphic analysis approach is provided by the values for the volume yield of trees (cubic feet) as a function of the basal area (square feet), for which a detailed description was given for the standard statistical method [123]. The correct plot gives the six line relationship: $1/$volume (cubic feet) $\times$ 10^4 = X $-$ 15.206 Log Area (square feet); where $X = 36.658, 35.460, 35.566, 35.233, 35.517,$ and 35.035 $(F/C =$

0.99986 ± 0.0051). Function was relatively easy to establish since the 1/A vs. Log B plot was the one plot to give only six parallel lines. The value distribution is relatively good with three of twenty values on one range line and five on the other. The values for the area, and the found vs. calculated volumes (F/C), are line 1: 3 values: 110 (2140/2166); 86 (1602/1610); 73 (1370/1365); line 2: 1 only: 79 (1490); line 3: 5 values: 64 (1240/1242); 82 (1560/1559); 84 (1600/1598); 85 (1620/1619); 88 (1680/1681); line 4: 2 values: 75 (1440/1439); 96 (1880/1881); line 5: 4 values: 76 (1500/1507); 80 (1590/1589); 85 (1710/-1696); 93 (1880/1887); line 6: 5 values: 48 (1060/1056); 72 (1460/1472); 76 (1560/1554); 80 (1630/1640); 88 (1840/1829).

The mean slope for a parallel line is determined with some weighting of individual line slopes since the least squares fit is better with widely spaced values and a larger number of values per line. It is generally satisfactory to weight individual slopes on the basis of the ratios for separation of low and high values (e.g., if one is two times that of the other, it is used × 2) and according to the number of values (e.g., lines with two versus ones with five values are used in the 2/5 ratio). The initial slopes ranged from 15.09 to 15.38 with the above values.

The conclusion from graphic analysis principles is that the area-to-volume relationship is like plots of many other biological systems that give six lines due to alternative growth patterns. The values can be plotted to show that they do not vary about a mean line that passes through the origin and that the A vs. B, 1/A vs. 1/B and Log A vs. Log B functions do not give equivalent lines and ranges because the correct plot is Log A vs. 1/B rather than A vs. B. Examples of lines that do pass through the origin are given in other sections.

A handbook of chemistry provides a large amount of data for plotting and several quantitative analyses. A simple way to become familiar with the general rule of linear relationships between variables is to plot the values for the physical properties of the elements: melting points, boiling points, the difference between boiling and melting points, densities and atomic radii against atomic number and weight, and the difference between weight and number, since with the exception of the lanthanides and actinides, triplet lines (values for three elements) are obtained. Lines are obtained for elements in the same groups and series and across groups and series, and quantitative evaluation shows that additional lines judged by eye to be acceptable are rejected because they give F/C errors beyond established measurement error.

The properties of the elements also provide a rapid way to see the value of numerical order analysis, which can be used to show that the components of biological systems follow precise principles similar to those for atomic structure. When the melting and boiling points of the elements are arranged in numerical order, it becomes apparent that values for different elements can be exactly the same, or the same within measurement error, and that many show a common type of increment for change. The most striking feature of melting and boiling points is the large number of values ending in 98 that give the series (in °C); 1098, 1598, 1698, 1798 (two times); 2198, 2398, 2598 (two times), 2898, 2998 (three times), 3098, 3398, 3498, 3598, 3998 (two times), 4098, 4198 (two times), 5098, 5498, 5098, 5898, and 6298. Thus four of 94 melting points and 24 of 93 boiling points form this series, and there are four pairs and one group of three values which are exactly the same. Thus in this series, 10 of 28 (35.7%) are repeat values and 25.8% of all boiling points and 15% of the melting points fall in the series in which differences are by 100°C or multiples of 100°C. There are other series and repeats, and some series show differences of 25°, 50°, and 75°C that fit into the multiples of 100°C series. All of the values indicate that the precise structure principles are followed. When the same numerical order analysis was applied to membrane lipid class values, data for plants and animals as well as human plasma lipids were found to show a high incidence of repeat values and to follow multiples of some particular value for change. Thus this is a rapid way to show uniform principles for biological systems and their similarity to physical systems in general since repeat values are also found for the properties of compounds.

GENERAL CHARACTERISTICS OF PHYSICAL AND BIOLOGICAL SYSTEMS

Although the author was initially concerned mostly with ranges for biological systems, the correct ways to plot relationships as well as their interpretation required plotting values for the physical properties of elements and compounds as a function of weight, temperature, and similar factors. These plots of physical properties disclosed the structural basis for parallel lines and slope changes that were not derivable directly from plots of biological systems, but which clearly follow the same basic structural principles.

When plotted correctly, relationships of physical and biological systems show both differences and similarities. Physical systems give three general types of plots. The least common is one line without a slope change. A more common type is one line with a series of slope changes, and the third, and most common, type is sets of parallel lines without a slope change or up to three slope changes. Since all biological systems plots give sets of lines, they are similar to the most common type for physical systems. Both biological and physical systems are also similar in that they may follow any of the nine functions and the correct plot must be determined for each relationship.

The plots for physical properties of pure substances which show a large number of slope changes, such as the 21 slope changes for the density of water between 0 and 100°C representing a series of structure rearrangements, can be converted to a single line without a slope change, or at most to two lines with three slope changes, when one pure substance is mixed with another. The dramatic difference between the numerous slope changes for the density of pure water, compared to water plus another substance, is illustrated by the relationship to temperature of the solubilities of potassium iodide and calcium hydroxide in water. For example, KI solubility (g/100 g water) = 0.8 (°C) + 128.0, (CC = 1.0; F/C = 1.0 ± zero to three figures), and $Ca(OH)_2$ solubility (g/100 g water) = X − 0.001095°C, where X = 0.1863, and 0.1822 (F/C = 1.0015 ± 0.0079). Since KI gives only one line and $Ca(OH)_2$ two lines and there are no slope changes, the water structure variations giving slope changes are limited in mixed systems. The reason for the absence of many slope changes in the plots of values from biological systems is seen as due to the mixed nature of biological systems.

Line numbers for physical systems are most commonly two or three with a common maximum of six. Biological systems divide into two groups. The first includes growth function parameters for cultured bacterial, fungal, protozoan, and animal cells that most commonly give two or three lines with a maximum of six, which is similar to physical systems. The other is for components and properties of organs of animals and plants, which can give up to 27 lines with the line number increasing in increments of three to give the series 3, 6, 9, 12, 15, 18, 21, 24, 27 (nine types of plots). Thus the ability to show line numbers above six is clearly due to the greater range of structural variation possible when the effects of control factors upon organs are added to the inherent variability of a single type of cell.

The structural basis for the production of parallel lines and slope changes are derivable directly and clearly from the data [124] on the effect of the number of carbon atoms on molecular length (in Angstrom units) for aliphatic carbon chains, determined by X-ray diffraction. Using the fatty acids as an example, the four forms of the terminal group (the free acids, the potassium salts, the acid potassium salts, and the esters) are particularly instructive. The odd and even carbon acid potassium salts give the equation (12–24 carbons): molecular length = 2.5427 (# of carbons) + 4.824 (CC = 0.99993; F/C = 1.0018 ± 0.0025 for one line). In contrast, the odd and even carbon potassium salts give two lines (12–24 carbons), which follow the log–log function: log molecular length = 0.8504 (log # carbons) + 0.5621, 0.5550 (F/C = 1.00005 ± 0.0024). The three line plot for the ethyl esters (16–24 carbons) also follows a different function: log molecular length = 0.01843 (# carbons) + 1.0785, 1.0726, 1.0045 (F/C = 1.000061 ± 0.00150). The plots show that the same chains can adopt different structures and that parallel lines are related to changes of the terminal group.

Plots for free acids show odd and even carbon acid values to fall on separate lines. The two lines formed by each series are designated in the literature as the B and C forms that are obtained by crystallization from different solvents under different conditions such as temperature and rate of evaporation. The longer A forms can be obtained from some acids by pressing the B form between glass plates. The odd carbon acid plot is the easiest to interpret. The equations are: B length = 2.1829 (# of carbons) + 3.05, 3.30, and C length = 2.1829 (# of carbons) + 1.57, 1.96 (mean $F/C = 0.9999 \pm 0.0019$ (B), $F/C = 0.9994 \pm 0.00096$ (C)). Thus the two widely spaced B and C lines are in fact each a pair of closely spaced lines, and there are two types of terminal group angle changes. The differences are clearly limited to the terminal groups, since the slopes of the lines are the same and so the addition of carbon atoms gives a constant effect on bond angles between carbons in the chains. The larger line spacing between the B and C forms is due to bond angle differences between the carboxyl and first methylene carbons, whereas the two closely spaced B and C lines are due to the smaller effects of bond angle variations between the oxygens of the carboxyl groups.

Since the ethyl esters of the acids do not show the odd–even differences, bond angles between the carboxyl and first methylene carbons are the same, and the three lines with wider spacings than those for the acids are attributable to the larger effects of the ethyl group bond angle differences. The potassium salts give two lines with a somewhat wider spacing to the eye than the free acids because the larger potassium ion bond angle differences give greater changes than free acid carboxyl oxygen angle differences.

The reason for the most common maximum number of lines being three, and the absolute maximum being six, is apparent from the plots. The two to three line plots are from a single type of terminal group angle change and the maximum of six arises from two different types of terminal group angle changes. The plots for the acids, as well as those for alcohols show that carbon–carbon bond angles along the chains vary to give bilayer length increases of about 2.000–2.54 Å for a one carbon addition. The acid potassium salts of the fatty acids show the largest angle, which is from the zigzag arrangement seen from the side with all carbon atoms in the same plane when the long axis is viewed from above.

Plots of values for other properties of a homologous series of lipids [124–127] are also instructive. Although all series exhibit plots with parallel lines, some plots of melting point vs. number of carbons in the fatty acid chain show the odd–even difference and a slope change (13 and 14 carbons) which is not seen in other series. The odd–even difference and slope changes are not apparent for the liquid state properties of a lipid series, but parallel lines are also a characteristic for boiling points. When plotted as a function of the number of carbons at pressures between 1 and 760 mm, odd and even fall on one line and the slope varies with pressure: at 1 mm pressure, $(1/BP)10^3 = 4.2813 - 1.6688$ (log # of carbons) [CC = 0.99994; $F/C = 1.0000 \pm 0.0011$], and, at 760 mm pressure: $(1/BP)\ 10^3 = 2.9710 - 1.1322$ (log # carbons) [CC = 0.99991; $F/C = 1.0000 \pm 0.0013$]. When the slopes of the lines versus the number of carbons at each pressure are plotted as a function of pressure, the three lines follow the equation, slope $= X - 0.1817$ log pressure, where $X = 1.6653$ (1,2,572 mm), 1.6556 (4,8,16,256,760 mm), or 1.6412 (32, 64, 128 mm), and $F/C = 0.9996 \pm 0.0025$. Primary amines give similar lines, and the slope plots give: 1/Slope $= 0.10017$ log pressure (mm) $+ 2.2634$ (2, 4, 16, 512 mm), 2.2577 (8, 32, 128, 256 mm), and 2.2497 (1, 64 mm) $F/C = 0.99997 \pm 0.00056$. This is one type of slope plot. The other that also shows parallel lines is made with slopes of lines for relationships that show a series of slope changes such as the density of water between 15 and 100°C. The plot log of density vs. log °K gives a slope change every 5°C and the plots of the slopes give the following four lines: Slope $= 0.002737$ (°C) $+ 0.01812$ (30, 35, 40, 45, 55, 60, 95°C), 0.01580 (25,65,75°C), 0.01339 (20,50,70,80,85°C), and 0.01085 (15,90°C) [$F/C = 1.00043 \pm 0.0036$]. The slope plots are thus a convenient way to summarize the individual lines and show the alternative bond angles at the same time.

The key to understanding the basis for slope changes, and why there are none for some biological relationships, is whether or not a system can produce more than one type of structure change. Thus the plots for the viscosities of benzene and its methyl derivatives as a function of temperature give parallel lines without slope changes because the only type of structure change possible is a change of ring carbon–carbon bond angles. In contrast, the increase of solubility of an aliphatic chain compound in an organic solvent as a function of temperature gives parallel lines due to the changes in terminal group angles. Some of these plots show one slope change, which is the result of a change in the solution of solute molecules, as individual molecules, to the solution of solute molecules as complexes of two or more molecules, thus making it possible for the number of the larger solute molecules to exceed that of the small solvent molecules. The principle is also illustrated by plots for the solubility of salts in water as a function of temperature. Salts such as nitrates, which can show bond angle changes for the negative ion between oxygen molecules, show parallel lines due to the angle changes, as well as slope changes; whereas salts such as sodium chloride which cannot have angle differences show only the slope changes due to the angle changes of water molecules. The angle changes for bonds controlling vesicle permeability can change the permeability of a vesicle to substrate and thus cause a slope change for an enzyme activity as a function of temperature. The slope changes that are commonly found for plots of components of animal organs and organ weights as a function of age are due to rate changes of growth processes.

The overall problem of the structural basis for slope changes and parallel lines, including unambiguous assignments for biological systems, was for a time on a very uncertain basis despite the clear finding with aliphatic homologous series. This was primarily because there was no readily apparent structural basis for the large series of slope changes for systems such as the properties of water as a function of temperature (i.e., parallel lines shown by slope plots exhibiting changes due to a combination of the two types of structure changes), the series of slope changes for the vapor pressure of mercury, the parallel lines seen for the viscosities of group zero elements (the inert gases), as well as the slope changes for various organic compounds. By analogy to the carbon chain homologous series, the findings suggested that substances, including inert gases, associate with each other, and that the bond angles of the complexes can change so that chains of atoms or molecules could show the same types of structure variations apparent for covalently linked carbon chains. It is to be noted that the chemistry handbook values for the viscosities of gases and vapors as a function of temperature provide a useful collection of data that can be plotted to show parallel lines without slope changes. The contrasting one line plots with a series of slope changes are shown by vapor pressure as a function of temperature. The viscosities of helium and argon both give three line plots. The equations for argon are: log viscosity (micropoises) = 0.9121 log °K + 0.1077, 0.0989, and 0.0867 (F/C = 0.99985 ± 0.0054). Hydrogen gives six closely spaced lines.

Direct evidence was obtained for association of atoms and molecules in the gaseous state by analysis of values for the viscosities of gases and vapors as a function of temperature [128]. Numerical order analysis showed a surprising number of exact and near repeat values. Some of the 35 values tabulated for 0°C are shown in Table VIII. The structural similarity of substances structurally unrelated in the conventional sense is shown by the fact that 54.3% of the values are closely similar to at least one other value.

When the values for the viscosities of gases and vapors at 0°C were plotted against weight (atomic or molecular), a maze of lines was obtained with values for very different types of substances giving good lines, such as acetone–methyl bromide–radon: viscosity = 0.8542 (weight) + 22.720 (CC = 0.999996). The weights and found and calculated values (F/C) for viscosity are: 58.01 (72.5/72.3), 94.94 (103.6/103.8), 222 (212.4/212.4). Another example is shown by helium–methane–water: viscosity = 215.39 − 6.958 (weight) (CC = 0.999987). The weights with found and calculated values are: 4.00

TABLE VIII

Viscosity of Gases and Vapors at 0°C

Compound	Viscosity	Compound	Viscosity
Cyanogen	93.5	Acetylene	94.3
Ethyl chloride	93.5	Xenon	210.7
Methyl bromide	103.6	Argon	210.4
Methane	103.5	CO_2	138.0
Water	90.4	HCl	137.0
Methyl ether	90.5	Hydrogen	84.9
Ethylene	90.7	Ethane	84.8
Ethyl ether	68.4	Sulfur dioxide	117.0
Ethyl acetate	68.4	Hydrogen sulfide	116.1
Chloroform	94.4		

(187.6/187.6), 16.04 (103.5/103.8), and 18.02 (90.4/90.2). The numerous lines support the conclusion that atoms and molecules associate in chains that are stable in the gaseous state and can show terminal group and chain angle changes similar to those of aliphatic carbon chains. This type of association also explains why a maze of lines is obtained for the properties of the elements as a function of atomic number and weight across groups and series such as: boron–manganese–copper melting point (°K) = 2508.8 − 39.718 (atomic #) CC = 0.999998: F/C = 1.0 exactly ± 0.00070, and, cobalt-technectium-tungsten: MP(°K) = 40.09 (atomic #) + 686.92 (CC = 0.999998: F/C = 0.99997 ± 0.00074). These are clearly excellent fits with a maximum of ±1°K deviation.

The association of water molecules in chains gives slope changes attributable to angle changes of the chains, and the parallel lines shown by slope plots as due to angle differences of the terminal molecule of the chains which vary when some chain molecule angles change. The same type of explanation is used for the numerous slope changes shown by the vapor pressure vs. temperature plots for elements, such as mercury, and various types of compounds that, like the properties of water, show parallel lines when plots of the slopes of the lines vs. temperature are plotted against the temperatures for slope changes. The parallel lines without slope changes for viscosities of gases and vapors are attributable to angle changes between atoms or molecules of chains that round up in the gas state so that all atoms or molecules in the chains undergo angle changes at the same time, similar to angle changes of carbons in rings, to produce parallel lines.

With parallel lines resulting from bond angle changes, the space between the lines depends upon the differences between the angles, and thus line spacings can be correlated with angle measurements by various methods which, however, have not been studied by the author in sufficient detail to warrant comments. Some preliminary results with the analysis of the number and positions for slope changes do appear worthy of note. The 16 slope changes of water density between 1 and 100°C noted above occur at 5°C intervals, and the viscosity of water gives slope changes at 10°C and vapor pressure at 15°C intervals. The positions are whole number multiples of five that can be seen to be related to the multiples for the melting points of the elements noted above. The multiples of five were also apparent from the plot of the density of aqueous methanol as a function of the weight percent of methanol, that showed the linear ranges on the 1/density vs. % plot of: 2–37%, 38–47%, 48–52%, 53–62%, 63–72%, 73–82%, 83–87%, and 88–91%: $\Delta = 35,10,5,10,10,10,5,5$). The density of water between 4 and 15°C shows slope changes at 2°C intervals (correct plot = Log D vs. °C), and the vapor pressure of mercury plot gives slope changes that are multiples of two. The above changes for salts in water as a function of temperature also follow the multiples of five because they occur at multiples of five from 0 to 95°C.

The vapor pressure of mercury between −38°C (.90° above the melting point), and 1300°C is of special interest in several ways. The temperature change in °K is from 235 to 1573°, which is a 5.69 fold increase. However, the vapor pressure increase is from 1.45×10^{-6} to 6.35×10^5 for a 4.38×10^{11} or 428 billionfold increase. With this very large range, the correct plot clearly must be log vapor pressure, and the function is rather easily established as log vs. 1/°K. The slope changes occur at −30, −14, 2, 34, 62, 98, 116, 146, 168, 218, 244, 290, 334, and 400°C, which exhibit Δ values of 8, 16, 16, 32, 28, 36, 18, 28, 22, 50, 26, 46, 44, 66, and 900°. These are multiples of 2 and 100°, with errors of as low as 0.02% and as high for some of the smaller ranges as 0.27%. The slope changes are difficult to fix by plotting, but can be shown readily by the temperatures at which the found and calculated values begin to deviate more from values below them on another line. Since mercury shows 15 linear periods (14 slope changes), water density 16 slope changes (17 periods), and the range of about 2.00 to 2.54 Å for bond lengths for aliphatic substances as bilayers has a Δ of about 0.03–0.04 Å to give 0.54/0.03 = 18, it appears that there is a maximum of about 17 alternative angles for chain components and that the variations of slope changes follow a limited number of general structural change types.

EXAMPLES OF VARIATION RANGES FOR BIOLOGICAL SYSTEMS

In general, the analysis of published values present the problems of small sample size and retrieval of data from small graphs for replotting. The error of retrieval was generally in the 0.50–1.0% range and at most about 2.0% as judged by the precision of the plots made, and is thus no major problem. Recognition of plots as usually consisting of sets of lines is also no problem since sample sizes of six or more in general are satisfactory to establish the correct plot and more than one line. A sufficiently large number of examples of clear-cut three-line plots was obtained to make it apparent that three is the most common maximum number for relationships.

Enzyme activity plots provide a link between purely physical systems and biological systems. When conditions are chosen that maintain maximum activity, the linear plot will be activity vs. time, substrate etc. When maximum activity is not maintained, one of the other eight functions that provide increments for change which change progressively is followed, and it is necessary to define the correct plot for each relationship since function for an enzyme, or for that matter binding of substances to an enzyme or other protein, can be modified by altering conditions of assay. The plots invariably show more than one line, and may show a slope change. Slope changes may be abolished or caused to appear at a different point by modifying conditions. Although many published plots show a wide range of point distribution, because there are commonly two to three lines and not one line as published, the variations have not previously been recognized as due to alternative structural forms that produce parallel lines, and the obvious range of variation was not explained.

The activity as a function of time for threonine deaminase isolated in crystalline form from $E. coli$ [129] follows the equation: log α ketoglutarate $(\mu M) = X - 0.1416$ (1/time in minutes)10, where $X = 1.7411, 1.7374, 1.7291$ $(F/C = 0.9994 \pm .0031)$. The values for each of the three relatively widely spaced lines show a good distribution over the range. The times with found and calculated substrate values are line 1: 7.0 (3.45/3.46); 18.0 (4.60/4.60); line 2: 9.0 (3.80/3.80); 22.5 (4.75/4.73); 31.5 (4.90/4.93); line 3: 4.5 (2.60/2.60); 13.5 (4.20/4.21); 40.5(4.95/4.94). The time function for the sodium-activated adenosine triphosphatase (Na$^+$/K$^+$-ATPase) of cerebral microsomes [130] as a function of phosphate liberated from ATP is log phosphate $(\mu M) = 0.6004$(log time in minutes) $+ 0.8325, 0.8242, 0.8121$ $(F/C = 1.0015 \pm 0.0086)$. The time and the found vs. calculated phosphate values (μM) for these closely spaced lines are line 1: 1.39 (0.085/0.083); 7.94 (0.241/0.242); 10.00 (0.276/0.278); 12.06 (0.314/0.312); 15.00 (0.356/0.357); 17.71 (0.396/0.395); line 2: 6.00 (0.200/0.200); 20.88 (0.429/0.429); line 3: 4.18 (0.157/0.156); 25.00 (0.465/0.466); 34.00 (0.518/0.521).

When activity is studied as a function of changing conditions such as temperature or the concentrations of substrate, activator, or inhibitor, the activity at each temperature or concentration is best expressed as the slope of the linear relationship. However the common practice of using activities over a constant short period of time shows the general nature of the effects. The activity of turtle bladder Na^+/K^+ ATPase as a function of temperature was plotted correctly [131], but the presence of two lines, log phosphate (μM) liberated/mg protein/hr $= 10.683 - 2.9361$ ($1/°K$)10^3, and $10.627 - 2.9361$ ($1/°K$)10^3 ($F/C = 0.9990 \pm 0.0075$) was not recognized. As one line, the error is increased from 0.75 to 5.88%. The distribution of values is good, and the temperature and found vs. calculated P_i values are line 1: 288.4 (3.19/3.17); 306.5 (12.55/12.66); line 2: 296.0 (5.10/5.12); 311.9 (16.50/16.37); 319.5 (27.20/27.36). The temperature function varies as shown by the correct plot for the values for chick heart Na^+/K^+ ATPase [132], which is, log phosphate (μM)/mg protein/hr $= 0.04598$ (°C) $+ 0.2046$, 0.0980 ($F/C = 1.0002 \pm 0.0146$). The values for temperature (in °C) and found vs. calculated Pi values are line 1: 0° (1.6/1.6); 20° (13.3/13.3); 25° (28.8/28.6); 30° (38.1/38.4); line 2: 15° (6.0/6.1); 35° (52.1/51.0). The value distribution was interpreted by the authors as showing slope changes rather than parallel lines.

The activity of rabbit muscle microsomal calcium ATPase (the calcium pump) as a function of temperature [133] gives five lines: log phosphate (μM) $= 28.21$ (log °K) $- 67.89$, 67.95, 68.00, 68.02, 68.04 ($F/C = 0.9961 \pm 0.021$). The somewhat larger error is due to the greater range covered for phosphate release. Although the published values clearly show a wide range of variability, only one line was drawn through the center of the range. Plots for the activity as a function of temperature in other publications showed a slope change that could be abolished by sonication. Since the preparations were from the same source, it is apparent that the methods of preparation of the Na^+/K^+-ATPase and the assay conditions can product slope changes that are due to permeability changes to the substrate (ATP) since the active site is on the inner surface of the vesicles.

The data in one paper [134] for calcium uptake and ATP hydrolysis by skeletal muscle microsomes is of interest because the uptake plot gives six lines: log calcium uptake (nM)/mg protein/min. $= X - 4.9089$ ($1/°K$)10^3, where $X = 19.710$, 19.561, 19.655, 19.493, 19.610, and 19.446 ($F/C = 1.0052 \pm 0.0266$). The error is due to the very large range of 62–6501 nM calcium. The plot was interpreted as showing slope changes by the authors, but the simple rule for line fitting described in this chapter, which is to assign slope changes only when all parallel lines show it, is not followed and there is clearly no slope change. The value distribution is good except for the first line with only one value on it. The temperature and the found vs. calculated values for calcium are line 1: 303.0° (2307); line 2: 299.7° (1907/1879); 292.9° (759/787); 288.1° (425/413); 282.7° (200/196); line 3: 307.0° (4226/4195); 295.0° (929/933); 285.7° (269/269); line 4: 298.7° (1390/-1337); 279.8° (100/104); line 5: 309.4° (4246); line 6: 314.2° (6501/6621); 312.5° (5584/5464); 277.4° (62/59).

The correct ATP hydrolysis plot showed five lines with a slope change, in contrast to other plots showing no slope change, and the interpretation that the slope change is due to the differences in conditions and involves a permeability change is supported by the absence of a slope change for calcium uptake and the disappearance of a slope change for ATP hydrolysis after sonication [135].

The relationship to substrate with the log–log functions is illustrated by the activity of *R. capsulata* glutamine synthetase [136]. The two line plot is: log velocity = 0.2153 log NH_4Cl (mM) × 10 − 0.1386, 0.1522 (F/C = 0.9992 ± 0.0057). The values on the widely spaced lines are for the concentration of ammonium chloride (mM), and the found vs. calculated velocities: line 1: 2.5 (0.145/0.145); 4.0 (0.160/0.161); 5.0 (0.170/0.169); line 2: 0.5 (0.100/0.0996); 1.0 (0.115/0.116); 10.0 (0.190/0.190). The values were published as A vs. B and 1/A vs. 1/B plots, and the only plot to give parallel lines without a slope change is log vs. log.

The relationship of activity to the concentration of an activator is illustrated by the data for the activation of *M. sporium* methanol dehydrogenase by ammonium chloride [137] that follows the equation: % maximum activity = 97.79 log NH_4Cl (μM) − 30.20, 51.07 (F/C = 1.0004 ± 0.0068). The NH_4Cl values with the found vs. calculated activity values are line 1: 1.0 (43.5/43.1); 15 (60.0/60.4); line 2: 5 (17.4/17.3); 20 (76.0/76.2); 25 (85/85.7); 30 (94/93.4); 35 (100/99.9).

The oxygen consumption of yeast as a function of temperature [138] provides an example of the activity of a membrane enzyme system *in situ*. The three line plot is: oxygen uptake (mm/min) = 3.253 (°K) − 895, 899, and 910 (F/C = 1.0014 ± 0.012). The constant increment function arises from the use of conditions that maintain maximum rate. The values for temperature and the oxygen found vs. calculated are line 1: 305.7° (101/100); 280.5° (17.7/-18.0); line 2: 301° (80.5/80.6); 292.0° (50.8/51.3); 289.1° (42.5/41.8); 285.9° (31.2/31.4); 283.4° (23.2/23.3); line 3: with one value only (296.8°: 64.5).

The yeast oxygen uptake values are of interest to compare with the data published in 1910 [139] for the relationship of percentage saturation of human hemoglobin to oxygen tension (mm). Values for the effect of different salts on the relationship were presented. The 10 values for binding of NaCl give the three line plot: log % saturation = X − 0.6702 (1/oxygen tension)10, where X = 2.1108, 2.0922, 2.0642 (F/C = 1.0014 ± 0.0093). The value distribution for the lines is relatively good, and for oxygen tension vs. found and calculated % saturation are line 1: 10 (27.5/27.6); 20 (60/59.7); 25 (69.5/69.6); line 2: 30 (75/73.9); 35 (79.5/79.5); 40 (83/84.1); line 3: 15(41/-41.4); 50 (85.5/85.2); 60 (91/89.6); 100 (98.5/98.4).

The values in other salts follow the A vs. 1/B function and the slopes of the 2–3 line plots are different. In Na_2HPO_4, the % saturation = 104.8, 103.9,

$103.1 - 35.67(1/O_2)10$ $(F/C = 1.0001 \pm 0.0059)$. In $NaHCO_3$, the % saturation $= 107.2$, $106.6 - 55.66(1/O_2)10$ $(F/C = 1.0007 \pm 0.0049)$. In Ringer's solution, the % saturation $= 108.9$, 106.4 $104.6 - 72.89(1/O_2)10$ $(F/C = 1.0002 \pm 0.0047)$. The slopes give the ratio $72.9/55.7/35.7 = 1/0.76/0.49 = 4/3/2$, so that it is apparent that chain bond angles of heme vary in a precise way when the overall structure is similar, as is apparent from the following of a single function. In contrast, the log function for NaCl shows another overall type of structure. Bond angle variations of the binding site produce two to three lines and ring bond angle changes produce slope differences much like the angle changes for aliphatic chains noted previously.

Values for the binding of substances to membrane sites also show two to three lines. Values for the rate of glucose binding (pM/mg protein/2 min) to the isolated renal brush border [140] as a function of glucose concentration (μM) give the two lines: velocity $= 0.8356$ (log glucose [μM]) $+ 0.0723$, 0.0274 $(F/C = 0.999 \pm 0.021)$. The rates and the glucose found vs. calculated values are line 1: 0.64 (0.57/0.56); 1.28 (.96/1.00); 10.11 (5.68/5.65); 114.9 (42.6/42.7); line 2: 5.32 (2.92/2.95); 26.8 (11.5/11.4).

The binding of calcium to isolated sarcoplasmic reticulum vesicles as a function of total calcium concentration [141] is of interest because the relationships for bound-to-total, free-to-total, and free-to-bound must match exactly. In the presence of $CaCl_2$ only, the equations for the three lines are: bound $Ca^{2+} = 0.8092$ (total Ca^{2+}) $- 0.024$, 0.195, 0.613, $(F/C = 1.0019 \pm 0.0054)$. When NaCl (100 mM) is added, the relationship is: log bound $Ca^{2+} = 0.8105$ log (total Ca^{2+}) $- 0.2742$, 0.3281, 0.3510 $(F/C = 1.0001 \pm 0.0103)$. When $MgCl_2$ (100 mM) is added, the relationship is: log Bound $Ca^{2+} = 0.8820$ log (Total Ca^{2+}) $- 0.3096$, 0.2796, 0.2557 $(F/C = 0.99998 \pm 0.0090)$. It is to be noted that calcium uptake and ATP hydrolysis by the vesicles give four to five lines, and sets of parallel lines are apparent from some published plots, such as the values of ATP hydrolysis as a function of temperature [133], which do not show a slope change.

When the components of cultured cells as a function of culture time are determined, they give linear relationships that generally show a slope change before the cells enter the stationary phase, while some show an additional slope change in the rapid growth phase. The functions vary and must be determined for each set of conditions and each type of component, and two to three lines are usually found. Illustrations for major types of components are the relationships for dry weight, DNA, RNA, and proteins. The dry weight of *C. lipolytica* [142] grown at 17°C follows: log dry weight $\times 10 = 1.5086$ (log time [hrs]) $- 0.9547$, and 0.9192 $(F/C = 0.999 \pm 0.0100)$. There are thus two major alternative levels for water and total solids. The value distribution on the lines alternates in such a way that it is apparent that there are two lines and the times, with found and calculated dry weight values, are line 1: 17.28 (.90/.89); 34.40 (2.48/2.51); line 2: 10.40 (0.38/0.38); 24.90 (1.40/1.42); 43.30 (3.27/3.27); 60.00 (5.38/5.34). Growth under other conditions gave different functions with slope changes at different times.

With the amount of DNA (mg/ml) as a measure of growth of *B. subtilis* spores as a function of time [143], the three line relationship is: log DNA (mg/ml) = 3.205 log time (min) − 5.002, 4.977, 4.958. The 15 values distribute fairly well over the lines as can be seen by comparing the times and found vs. calculated DNA values; line 1: 105 (33/33); 123 (55/55); 132 (69/69); line 2: 75 (11/10.8); 95 (23/23); 100 (27/27); 130 (62/62.9); line 3: 50 (2.8/2.8); 60 (5.0/5.0); 70 (8.0/8.1); 85 (15/15); 110 (35/34.6); 140 (75/75); 150 (95/94); 158 (110/111).

The rate of biosynthesis of major groups of components can be defined by the rate of incorporation of specific isotope labeled precursors, as was the case for a study of *M. xanthus* [144] in which the incorporation of valine into protein, uridine into RNA, thymidine into DNA, and diaminopimelic acid into murein, were determined. The plots for valine and uridine are of particular interest. Both follow the constant increment A vs. B function, and for valine the three lines are: $(counts/min)10^{-3} = 2.40$ (time [hrs]) − 0.32, 0.16, and 0.12 $(F/C = 1.0024 \pm 0.019)$. The uridine incorporation equations also show three lines: $(CPM)10^{-3} = 0.674$ (time [hrs]) − 0.014, 0.048, and 0.097 $(F/C = 0.992 \pm 0.022)$. The values for each relationship are good illustrations of sets of three lines since they can be plotted directly without conversions. For valine the lines with the found and calculated CPM values are line 1: 1.0 (2.1/2.06); 1.5 (3.2/3.25); 4.0 (9.2/9.2); line 2: 0.5 (1.0/1.0); 3.0 (7.0/7.0); line 3: 2.0 (4.7/4.7); 3.5 (8.4/8.2). The uridine values are line 1: 1.0 (0.65/0.66); 1.5 (1.01/0.99); line 2: 3.0 (2.00/2.01); line 3: 0.5 (0.24/0.25); 3.5 (2.27/2.27).

When alternative levels are established by replacement, line number is reduced when the sum of the components is plotted. The sum of the valine and uridine incorporation values gives one line: (uridine + valine CPM) $10^{-3} = 3.095$ (time [hrs]) − 0.3214 $(CC = 0.99982: F/C = 1.0023 \pm 0.022)$. The times and the found to calculated values are: 0.5 (1.24/1.19); 1.0 (2.75/2.76); 1.5 (4.21/4.33); 2.0 (6.00/5.91); 3.0 (9.00/9.05); 3.5 (10.67/10.63). The alternative levels in this case are established by shunting of energy for biosynthesis between the two pathways. This is a general mechanism that causes all cell components to vary in a precisely related way even when there are no common components, as is discussed in more detail later.

Many studies have been made of the effect of growth temperature on composition and, in particular, fatty acid changes of membrane lipids. The data for *E. coli* [145] show a large increase of 16^0 and smaller increases of 14^0, 17^0, and 19^0 cyclopropyl acids with a decrease of 18^1 and almost no change in 16^1, as temperature is increased. The sum of the acids that increase gives the two line relationship: % acids up = 0.776 (°C) + 19.02, and 17.31 (F/C = 0.998 ± 0.0037). The values provide another, easy to plot example of widely spaced parallel lines, and the temperature and found vs. calculated percentage values are line 1: 10^0 (26.6/26.8); 15^0 (30.6/30.7); 20^0 (34.7/34.5); 35^0 (46.2/46.2); line 2: 25^0 (36.9/36.9); 30^0 (40.5/40.6); 40^0 (48.2/5=48.3).

When grown at temperatures between 25 and 40°C, A. *laidlawii* also shows an increase in the percentage of 16^0, but the range is only 36.9–40.8% [146]. Despite this small range, the values give the two widely spaced lines: % 16^0 = 0.2157 (°C) + 32.36, and 32.14 (F/C = 1.0 exactly ± zero). All values fit perfectly to the three figures reported. The temperature and the found vs. calculated values are line 1: 20° (36.9/36.9); 30° (39.0/39.0); 35° (40.1/40.1); line 2: 25° (37.5/37.5); 40° (40.8/40.8).

The effects of temperature on membrane properties is illustrated by the changes in the contraction rate of the water vacuole of *Amoeba proteus* [147]. The three line plot is: log rate (μm^3/sec) = 0.0460 °C) + 0.9735, 0.9370, 0.8900, (F/C = 0.9968 ± 0.0167). Although only one value establishes the center line between 5 and 30°, the distribution is good and is typical of plots made with only six values: line 1: 15° (45.9/46.1); 25° (133.2/132.9); line 2: 20° (72.0); line 3: 5° (13.1/13.2); 10° (22.2/22.4); 30° (190.7/186.3). The value for 35°C is not on the lines and thus there is a slope change at about 30°C.

Comparisons of physical and biological systems that are not under control by specific external regulatory factors, and thus respond directly to changing conditions, show that the same basic structure principles are followed for bond angle variations. Thus the variations of oxygen bond angles of formic acid (only one carbon atom), give the three line relationship of viscosity to temperature between 10 and 100°C: log viscosity (dynes/cm^2)10^3 = X − 5.106 (log °K), where X = 13.869, 13.846, and 13.830 (F/C = 1.0023 ± 0.0085). These three line plots are also found for carboxyl groups of long chain fatty acids and carboxyl groups of membrane proteins, such as those of skeletal muscle microsomes which cause calcium binding to show three lines. Bond angle shifts of membrane components as a whole give three lines, as shown by the water vacuole contraction rate of *Amoeba proteus*.

In the final analysis, the choice of examples among multicellular organisms to document and illustrate the principles of sets of lines and the way line numbers vary was rather simple. The values for lung lipid classes (Table IX) can be used to make the simple millimole lipid class vs. millimole total phospholipid plots, since the lines pass through the origin. This also makes them plot in equivalent ways as 1/lipid class vs. 1/TPL, and to give sets of parallel lines plotted by log vs. log. Since values for new born dogs and those 20 and 90 days of age were available to compare with those from adult dogs,

TABLE IX

Lipid Composition of Human and Animal Lungs[a]

Lipid	Human			Dog (Beagle)														
				Newborn					20 Days		90 Days		Adult					
	1	2	3	4	5	6	7	8	9	10	11	12	13	14	15	16	17	18
TPL	0.424	2.28	1.70	1.86	2.01	2.18	2.31	2.55	1.74	1.94	2.33	2.40	1.12	1.22	1.60	1.77	1.92	2.03
PC	0.208	0.869	0.975	1.058	1.130	1.220	1.208	1.355	0.981	0.760	1.021	1.134	0.487	0.521	0.648	0.620	0.849	0.889
PE	0.073	0.387	0.280	0.320	0.347	0.421	0.421	0.460	0.225	0.457	0.509	0.478	0.214	0.235	0.325	0.345	0.348	0.400
Sph	0.049	0.293	0.183	0.221	0.240	0.230	0.286	0.295	0.234	0.333	0.369	0.339	0.184	0.203	0.293	0.315	0.275	0.333
PS	0.029	0.170	0.111	0.133	0.145	0.149	0.169	0.189	0.119	0.186	0.238	0.219	0.097	0.113	0.152	0.186	0.165	0.181
PI	0.014	0.074	0.020	0.022	0.065	0.064	0.029	0.077	0.021	0.020	0.065	0.067	0.028	0.031	0.042	0.032	0.058	0.065
DPG	0.004	0.037	0.010	0.013	0.018	0.015	0.021	0.020	0.010	0.020	0.023	0.021	0.010	0.011	0.016	0.023	0.023	0.022
RAPL	0.047	0.449	0.116	0.089	0.069	0.159	0.172	0.154	0.151	0.166	0.100	0.140	0.100	0.106	0.124	0.249	0.202	0.140

Lipid	Adult dogs									Rat					Mouse	Bovine	Frog
	19	20	21	22	23	24	25	26	27	28	29	30	31	32	33	34	35
TPL	2.07	2.14	2.23	2.28	2.28	2.34	2.37	2.42	2.60	1.67	1.68	1.88	1.90	1.94	2.08	1.56	0.910
PC	0.946	0.907	0.966	0.942	1.031	0.943	1.045	1.166	1.136	0.746	0.763	0.858	0.895	0.959	1.012	0.633	0.408
PE	0.373	0.394	0.447	0.426	0.410	0.431	0.462	0.428	0.510	0.367	0.371	0.414	0.416	0.419	0.452	0.340	0.204
Sph	0.315	0.347	0.357	0.369	0.315	0.349	0.386	0.336	0.421	0.171	0.167	0.189	0.184	0.204	0.202	0.257	0.109
PS	0.178	0.188	0.196	0.221	0.194	0.208	0.211	0.215	0.239	0.151	0.159	0.168	0.167	0.181	0.161	0.152	0.086
PI	0.062	0.058	0.071	0.064	0.066	0.068	0.078	0.065	0.081	0.063	0.067	0.069	0.082	0.080	0.077	0.054	0.037
DPG	0.021	0.021	0.022	0.021	0.023	0.021	0.024	0.019	0.023	0.019	0.018	0.024	0.022	0.012	0.017	0.015	0.009
RAPL	0.175	0.225	0.171	0.237	0.241	0.320	0.164	0.191	0.190	0.151	0.130	0.161	0.134	0.085	0.160	0.113	0.057

[a] Values expressed as millimoles/100 gm fresh weight.

human, and other animal species, the differences noted for many components of young animals which change to the adult levels during the first few
weeks of life are illustrated, as well as the nature of species variation. The PC
vs. TPL plot shows nine lines for all but the six newborn dogs, and one 20
day old dog that forms a separate range as a group of three lines. The PE vs.
TPL plot also gives nine lines plus three as a separate range for two newborn
and one 20 day old dog. The Sph vs. TPL plot shows a group of nine lines
plus two groups of three lines whereas the PS vs. TPL plot shows a group of
nine plus a group of six lines. The 18 line maximum is shown by the plot of
the sum of the minor acidic phospholipids (RAPL). Plots of sums can be
made to illustrate the way line numbers vary, as was described previously.

The values for skeletal muscle of vertebrates and invertebrates [118] can
be plotted to show that the vertebrate and invertebrate values for PC and PE
plotted against TPL fall on the same lines that pass through the origin. The
values reported for the polar lipids of 20 plant species [34] also provide
excellent examples since the correct plot is, like the lung and skeletal muscle
plots, simply lipid class (millimoles) vs. TPL (millimoles), and the formation
of lines passing through the origin by values from diverse species is readily
apparent [see also 116–119].

The principle of line number variation as groups of three up to a maximum
of 27 lines was shown with plots of mouse (C57 black) organ and body
weights as a function of age (102 values each) all of which gave 18 lines,
mouse and human brain lipid and water values (32 mouse and 64 human
whole brain lipid values and 102 water values for mice), as well as values for
heart and liver for which samples sizes were large enough to establish maximum lines numbers. In addition, a large series of samples for human plasma
lipids showed not only that the same general types of line formations were
obtained, but that large sample sizes, e.g., over 350 for the log PC vs. log
TPL plot (which shows only 15 lines), do not show additional lines with large
sample sizes. The general rule, therefore, seems to be that sample sizes of
three times the number of lines, at most, establish the maximum line
number.

THE STRUCTURAL BASIS AND SIGNIFICANCE OF THE SLOPE CHANGES AS A FUNCTION OF TEMPERATURE

The concept that lipids in membranes must be in the liquid crystalline
state to function, and that slope changes seen in plots of enzyme activities
and probe mobilities in membrane lipids vs. temperature are due to lipid
melting points, has served as the basis for many studies. The concept ap-

pears to provide an explanation for the ability of some animals to reduce body temperature to as low as 1°C during hibernation and for the sensitivity to cold of some plants. The idea that unsaturated fatty acids with low melting points are required to maintain fluid carbon chains was dealt a lethal blow when studies of bacterial and fungal mutants showed that growth was obtained on fatty acid supplements that caused membrane lipids to contain all or mostly saturated fatty acids. The values for *A. laidlawii B.* on various supplements [146] are good illustrations.

The keys to analyzing the literature for the temperature plots are knowing how to plot and fit lines correctly (which eliminates slope changes caused by incorrect plotting), and recognizing the fact that probes with polar groups can detect structure changes in both polar and hydrocarbon regions of the membrane, and the fact that calorimetry can detect both types of structural changes.

As noted above, it is apparent from the data for skeletal muscle microsomal Ca^{2+}-ATPase activity, that plots may or may not show a slope change with vesicles prepared from the same source. These slope changes represent differences in permeability to ATP due to the use of different experimental conditions, and they can be abolished by sonication [135], which does not alter pure lipid melting points. The data from one paper [96] illustrates the need for correct plotting, and the fact that skeletal muscle microsomal ATPase activity slope changes are not due to lipid melting points. The plots presented were all log vs. $1/°K$ following the widespread belief that this function is always correct. The plot for dioleyl PC vesicles with the probe tempo (2,2,6,6 -tetramethylpiperidine-1-oxyl) showed a slope change that shifted in position as a function of lipid concentration at about 27°C. Both the shift in the slope change, and the finding that the melting point is detected at about $-20°C$ by calorimetry, are seen to be the result of incorrect plotting. The correct plot for DOPC: $\alpha = 0.04123$ (°K) -10.607 (CC = 0.9998: F/C 1.002 ± 0.016). The temperature and the found vs. calculated values are: 325.2° (2.80/2.80); 312.5° (2.30/2.28); 301.2° (1.80/1.81); 292.8° 1.45/1.47); 284.1° (1.10/1.11); 276.2° (.80/.78). The spin label probe motion parameter thus follows the constant increment A vs B function in vesicles of this lipid. The probe in the microsomal vesicles follows a different function without a slope change: log $\alpha = 0.01628$ (°K) $- 4.397$ (CC $- 0.9991 : F/C - 1.0003 \pm 0.018$), with temperature and F/C values: 313.0° (0.500/0.499); 306.7° (0.400/0.394); 300.3° (0.300/0.310); 293.3° (0.240/0.238); 288.2° (0.200/0.197); 282.5° (0.158/0.159). Still another function is followed by the motion parameter in lipid extracted from the membranes: $\alpha = 27.28$ (log °K) $- 67.68$ (CC $= 0.9997 : F/C = 1.002 \pm 0.017$). Because the plots in lipids do not show slope changes when made correctly, whereas those for enzyme activity do, it is apparent that the slope changes are not due to lipid melting points. This conclusion is consistent with the plot that shows slope changes for vesicles reconstituted with DOPC after removal of the native lipid.

The broad peaks obtained by calorimetry for animal cell membranes have been accepted by many as representing lipid melting points. The failure to observe a slope change for mitochondrial membranes with the fluorescence of the aromatic hydrocarbon perylene as the probe [498] shows, however, that the calorimetry peak for these membranes is due to other structural changes since perylene detects lipid melting points. Since some spin label probes with polar groups show one slope change with the mitochondrial membranes, it appears that some probes of this type can detect other structure changes. That the structure changes are of a general type that affects all types of lipids is shown by the probes showing only one slope change despite the fact that they contain many different species of lipid that, as pure lipids, have a wide range of melting points. The observation that a slope change is present when yeast cells are grown on 16^0 with a nitroxyl stearate probe that is not observed with its cholesterol derivative [62], is easily explained. It is apparent that the small amount of probe (nitroxyl stearate) used could not prevent a major structure change of the membrane and the slope change is due to a general type of structural change similar to that found with the amoeba water vacuole, which was noted previously. This structural change is detectable with the stearate probe because the nitroxyl group can enter the polar group region which is not possible with the cholesterol derivative.

Probe motion parameters in pure isolated lipids and in membrane lipids comomonly give a maximum of three lines. A good example with 14 values is the fluorescene of pyrene in dilauroyl PC vesicles [94]. The ratio of the fluorescence of the eximer (associated molecules) to monomer gives: $I_E/I_M = 0.01426$ (°K) $+ 3.6653$, 3.6846, 3.6409 ($F/C = 0.9998 \pm 0.0030$). The values for the lines are line 1: 1° (0.243/0.244); 3° (0.272/0.272); 5.8° (0.314/0.313); 40° (0.800/0.799); line 2: 8.7° (0.347/0.346); 24.2° (0.566/0.568); 26.8° (0.605/0.605); 30° (0.652/0.651); 35° (0.723/0.722); line 3: 11.8° (0.384/0.386); 14.6° (0.426/.426); 17.7° (0.471/0.470); 21° (0.519/0.517); 45° (0.855/0.858). The absence of a slope change between 1° and 45°C is in keeping with the melting point of 0°C by calorimetry. A good example of a three line plot with a nitroxyl spin label is the motion parameter in heated skeletal muscle microsome vesicles [149] that gives: $\log t_0 = 0.9163$ (1/°K)$10^3 - 2.2811$, 2.3101, 2.3239 ($F/C = 0.9998 \pm 0.0070$). The eleven values of temperature and F/C from 4.7 to 59.9°C are line 1: 24.2° (6.35/6.32); 48.9° (3.65/3.67); line 2: 4.7° (9.64/9.74); 9.1° (8.65/8.64); 13.8° (7.75/7.66); 29.6° (5.21/5.21); 52.3° (3.19/3.21); 59.9° (2.77/2.76); line 3: 18.5° (6.58/6.58); 35.1° (4.42/4.46); 40.2° (4.02/3.99).

When a pure lipid vesicle shows a melting point, both spin label and fluorescent probes will show a slope change of either the connected or disconnected type. When the lines at the slope change connect, the only structure change is for the carbon chains coming closer together, whereas disconnected lines show an additional change of the structure of the chains. With both types of changes, line number may differ in the two regions. With pyrene fluorescence in $16°$ $16'$ PC vesicles [94], there is a connected type of slope change at 26.7°C with two lines from 12.5 to 26.7°C and three lines from 26.7 to 45.0°C: 12.5–26.7°, $\log I_E/I_M = X - 1.0625 \, (1/°K)10^3$, where X = 4.4132, and 4.4061 (F/C = 1.00045 ± 0.0029); and 26.7–45.0°, $\log I_E/I_M = X - 0.4910 \, (1/°K)10^3$, where X = 2.5113, 2.5063, and 2.4996 (F/C = 0.99998 ± 0.0029). The two lines of the lower temperature region connect with the two upper lines of the higher temperature region. With 12-nitroxyl stearate in $16°18'$PC vesicles [97], there is a slope change at about 16.8°C in keeping with calorimetry and one of the three lines from 3.1 to 16.8°C connects with the one line from 16.8 to 40.7°C: long $t_0 = 1.5110 \, (1/°K)10^3 - 3.8916$ (F/C = 1.00014 ± 0.0036; CC = 0.99987). The slope change for pyrene in $14°14°$ PC vesicles [94] is disconnected, and with the values published, the lower period ends at 21.3°C and the upper begins at 23.5°C. This type of slope change is also seen with melting points of saturated fatty acids as a function of the number of carbons in the chains.

When the $14°14°$ PC vesicles are prepared with 20 mol% cholesterol [94], the connected slope change is at 14.6°C, in keeping with general melting point values that show mixtures to have lower melting points, and there is one line from 3.0 to 14.6°C and three lines from 14.6 to 36.5°C.

The probe data show that the carbon–carbon bond angles of fused rings vary in the same general way as those of aliphatic chains and one ring substances such as benzene. This is also seen with the fluorescence of 1-anilino-8-napthalene sufonate (ANS) as shown by the data for its fluorescence in the presence of egg PC vesicles [150]. The correct plot, which does not have a slope change, is: $\log$ polarization = $0.7434 \, (1/°K)10^3 - 1.2882$, 1.2937, and 1.3009 ($F/C$ = 0.9989 ± 0.0043). The eleven value distribution over the lines is good and thus documents a three line plot over the range 10 to 60°C; line 1: 10° (0.2173/0.2176); 20° (0.1773/0.1771); 35° (0.1330/0.1332); 40° (0.1205/0.1219); line 2: 30° (0.1443/0.1442); 45° (0.1108/0.1105); 60° (0.0864/0.0867); line 3: 15° (0.1908/0.1903); 25° (0.1551/0.1559); 50° (0.1001/0.0999); 55° (0.0924/0.0922).

Since calorimetry shows a slope change for this type of lipid vesicle, and ANS in contact with $16°16°$ PC vesicles shows a slope change at 40°C in agreement with calorimetry, it appears that the egg PC polar groups do not change at the melting point, whereas those of $16°16°$PC do, since ANS detects polar group changes only.

MATCHED LEVELS, TYPES OF REPLACEMENTS, MEMBRANE STRUCTURE, AND METABOLIC CONTROL MECHANISMS

The alternative levels for all cell and organ components are exactly matched because all levels change together in reponse to varying conditions. This exact matching is shown by the rather remarkable features of plots. Lipid values for whole cells are a composite of values for individual membranes that have different relative amounts of lipid classes, but a plot of whole cell values gives small line numbers because all levels vary together in an exactly matched way. This matching is even more dramatic for whole organ values. Brain is composed of neurons, glial cells, and blood vessels, and each general type consists of a variety of subgroups that differ in size, shape, and function. Analysis of each type of cell after separation from the other types shows them to have large composition differences, as do the individual major types of membranes. Despite these differences and large regional variations, values for whole brain components plotted against age or each other show line numbers that vary from three to eighteen in most cases, with a maximum for water content vs. age being twenty-seven lines.

An interesting and important example of the matched and additive nature of organ lipid values was obtained in a study in the author's laboratory of the total phospholipid and phospholipid class composition of fruit flies (*Drosophila*). Due to their small size the whole organism was used, and values for controls as well as mutants were obtained for pools of many insects of each group. The two control groups were compared to morphological mutants (no eyes, no antennae), five chromosomal abnormalities, and five mutants that shake when exposed to ether (shaker mutants). Some of the abnormal flies were found to have low TPL. Plots of the values for the lipid classes showed log vs. log to be correct, and values gave six lines for PE and PC vs. TPL. The additive nature of cell organ values was thus clear. The six PE vs. TPL (millimoles/100 gm fresh weight) lines are: log PE (mM) = 1.0638 (log TPL, mM) − 0.2513, 0.2712, 0.2598, 0.2746, 0.2677, and 0.2808 (F/C = 1.0005 ± 0.0027), with the low mean error of 0.27%. The value distribution for control and abnormal flies with found vs. calculated values for PE are line 1: shaker, 3.004 (1.815/1.808); XXY chromosome, 2.601 (1.554/1.549); triploid, 2.831 (1.688/1.696); line 2: shaker, 3.015 (1.781/1.777); no eyes, 2.803 (1.653/-1.647); and 2.769 (1.616/1.623); line 3: no antennae, 2.720 (1.568/1.567); haploid for chromosome IV, 2.911 (1.682/1.682); line 4: control, 2.928 (1.680/1.681); shaker, 3.217 (1.855/1.854); triploid for chromosome IV, 2.706 (1.545/1.543); line 5: only one shaker value, 3.123 (1.786); line 6: control, 3.311 (1.874/1.872); shaker, 2.013 (1.102/1.103).

Since all levels for components are exactly matched, the values for one organ component can generally be plotted against age or the values for another component without a change in line number. Thus if one component gives three lines and another six lines when plotted against age, the plot of values for the two components against each other will show six lines, that is the larger number for the versus age plots. Six lines will also be obtained if both components give six lines plotted against age. The ratio of two components will also give the same line number as the individual plots, and sums of values for two components will not show a change in the number unless there is replacement between the two components.

In one sense, the matched alternative levels for all components are always the result of replacement since the control of energy use by different metabolic pathways causes some to increase and others to decrease. Alternative levels may also be established at various precursor levels. The balance between oxidation of acetate and its conversion to lipids is important, and when regulation is abnormal as it is in the "carbohydrate sensitive" human, carbohydrate is converted to lipid to a greater extent and all plasma lipids levels rise. The shifts of metabolism may be at the next level in lipid metabolism which involves conversion of carbon precursors to cholesterol or fatty acid, and fatty acids are in turn shifted to varying formation of triglycerides and phospholipids. The next steps for phospholipids are the shifting for example between CDP choline and CDP ethanolamine, that can cause PC and PE levels to be inversely related, as shown for yeast [23]. Another alternative may be the distribution of choline between PC and Sph, which is common for animal organs. Various phospholipids can also be converted to others by terminal group exchange reaction, as well as by membrane protein–protein interaction codes that cause proteins with different lipid class binding specificities to replace each other and thus to cause lipid class replacements to be the result of protein shifting rather than shifts of lipid metabolism.

One of the simplest types of replacements is shown by the effects of supplements of culture media when the cells do not have codes specifying particular fatty acids, as in the case for mouse LM cells [66]. When grown in medium without fatty acid supplements, the cells have 16^0, 16^1, 18^0, and 18^1 as major acids with small amounts of 14^0 and 20^1 and only 1.2% 15^0 and 0.4% 17^0 and 17^1. When grown with odd carbon supplements at different levels, odd carbon acids replace other acids and in particular 18^1. When plots of the percentage values for total odd carbon acids are made against the percentage values for other acids, reduction in line number is obtained with the sum 18^1 and 20^1 (which arises from the conversion of 18^1 to 20^1). This results in two main lines with one value representing the less favored third alternative level: percentage $18^1 + 20^1 = X - 69.09(\%$ odd carbon acids), where $X = 66.35, 65.71, 64.80$ ($F/C = 0.9998 \pm 0.0035$). The lines with percentage odd and found vs. calculated for percentage $18^1 + 20^1$ followed by the acid used as the supplement are line 1: 20.3 $(52.4/52.3)15^0$; 36.7 $(41.2/41.0)15^0$; 37.8 $(40.1/40.2)19^0$; 4.3 $(63.2/63.4)18^{1t}$; line 2: (one only) 51.4 $(30.2)19^0$; line 3: 20.5 $(50.9/50.7)17^0$; 29.1 $(44.6/44.8)17^0$; 19.8 $(51.3/51.2)19^0$; 21.5 $(49.8/50.0)21^0$; 1.0 $(64.2/64.2)18^1$. The values for 18^1 and 18^{1t} supplements fall on the odd carbon supplement lines, whereas those for even carbon saturated and 18^3 supplements do not.

The fatty acids of *Chlorella sorokiniana* show large changes as a function of growth temperature [68]. This organism synthesizes 16^2, 16^3, 18^2, and 18^3 in addition to 16^0, 16^1, 18^0, and 18^1 of *E. coli* and *A. laidlawii*. As growth temperature is increased from 14 to 38°C at 4° intervals, plots for individual acids show parallel lines and slope changes. The increase of 16^0 is similar to that for *E. coli* and is from 21.7 to 40.7%. There is almost no change in the values for 16^1 and 18^1, but there are large changes for 16^2, 16^3, 18^2 and 18^3. With 16^2 and 18^2 going down to 22°C and then up and 16^3 and 18^3 going up to 22°C and then down. When sums are made, the acids divide into three families: $16^0 + 18^0$, $16^1 + 16^2 + 16^3$ and $18^1 + 18^2 + 18^3$. The equations for the two major families give three and two levels: % $16^0 + 18^0 = 1.0261$ (°C) $+ 7.89$, 7.42, 6.99, and % $18^1 + 18^2 + 18^3 = 64.43$, $64.07 - 0.7919$ (°C). The three lines for $16^0 + 18^0$ are reduced to two lines that exactly match the $18^1 + 18^2 + 18^3$ values when added to $16^1 + 16^2 + 16^3$, which shows a small decrease with increase of temperature. Thus it is a relatively simple matter to show that the major temperature effects are on the rate of conversion of saturated to unsaturated acids and the conversion of two to three double bond acids.

Plots of human blood plasma lipid values gave results closely similar to those found with other types of plots, and in addition illustrate two important features. Since serial samples can be obtained from one subject over varying periods of time, and diet and other conditions varied, the way individual subjects vary with individual metabolic patterns can be defined. Line numbers established with serial samples were found to be from three to eighteen, with the increase by groups of three lines as seen for organ lipid values and other organ component plots. The basic plots were found to be the molar values for each phospholipid class against total phospholipid and the values for total cholesterol (TC), triglyceride (TG), and total phospholipid (TPL) against their sum as total lipids plotted log vs. log (μM/ml). The sums of two components show a reduction in range width and the plot TC + TG vs. TL gives some dramatic reductions in range width and line number. Although this sum shows line number reduction for all normal and pathological values, the most dramatic reduction is seen when the plots of TC vs. TL, TG vs. TL, and TPL vs. TL give larger line numbers. This is the case with values from hyperlipidemic subjects with the type IV pattern that is characterized by elevations of all lipids with a relatively greater increase of TG. With 16 values from one subject [151], the TC vs. TL plot shows a wide range, but 10 of the 16 values clearly form lines, and the TG vs. TL plot shows 13 of 16 values on lines, with the TPL vs. TL plot showing 15 of the 16 values on lines. Thus, despite the relatively wide ranges, formation of lines is easy to see. The TC + TG vs. TL plot shows three closely spaced lines. The spacing is so close that the range shows little error when treated as one line: log TL = 0.921 (log TC + TG) + 0.208 (values as μM/ml) (CC = 0.9992 *F/C* = 0.9996 ± 0.011). The slopes for all subjects are invariably close to 0.922 and give three to six lines. Total line number for all normal subjects is 12, and some pathological values give lines with different intercepts on the higher TC + TG side of the range. Since values for hyperlipidemics are high and on the same lines with the lowest values in cases of acanthocytosis, the range for TL is 1.80 to 120.9 μM/ml.

The large reduction in range width and line number for the plasma TC + TG vs. TL plot is an excellent illustration of the way graphic analysis can show an important feature of a biological relationship that is not at all apparent from a table of values. The finding also illustrates alternative levels based upon direction of carbon precursors to cholesterol and fatty acid synthesis.

Analysis of brain lipid data gives similar results when sums of percentage values and plots of millimole values are used to define replacements in contrast to the findings with plasma lipids for which only millimole plots show the nature of replacements. The difference is due to codes for brain lipids that direct replacement limited to particular types of compartments that give constant percentage values for sums. On the other hand plasma lipoprotein particles, which do not have an interaction code, show a changing percentage of TC + TG. Data for 64 samples of whole brain, and 11 values for regions of 4 of the brains, gave four groups by sums analysis of percentage total polar lipid (TPoL) values. One group of 50 values showed the sum (PE + Sulf) to be 30.79 ± 0.56% TPoL, that is clearly very close to the 30.77% value derived for for the size of one membrane compartment by sums analysis of membrane and organ values. The second group of 18 samples that gave PE + Sulf % above 30.77% showed the sum PE + Sulf + RAPL to be: 38.52 ± 0.75% TPoL. This is also in good agreement with the 38.46% value of a compartment size derived from general sums analysis. Of the remaining seven samples, five with PE + Sulf values below 30.77% appear to fit the sum PE + Sulf + part of RAPL = near 30.77%, and the other two values appear to be in slightly greater error than the other 68 samples.

Human brain lipids change throughout life. This was apparent from the examination of the tables of values for representative samples of whole brain

[120,121]. When plotted as a function of age, values for total lipid and all lipid classes show a rapid rise from birth to 1.58 years conceptual age where there is a slope change. After this point the increase is less rapid to 50.1 years for the low lipid side of the normal range and 68.4 years in the high lipid side, after which values decrease. As total lipid increases the relative amounts of cerebroside (Cer), sulfatide (Sulf), and sphingomyelin (Sph) increase, whereas the relative amounts of Pc and PE decrease, with only small changes for PS and the sum of the minor acidic phospholipids (RAPL). The changes are due to an increase of myelin which contains more Cer, Sulf, and Sph than other membranes. The large increase of Cer is clearly matched by the large decrease of PC so that Cer replaces PC in the sense that, in myelin, Cer enters space into which PC fits in membranes of neurons. Analysis of the data as sums of percent of the TPoL and plots of millimolar values against those for TPoL that is the sum of TPL and Cer + Sulf (total glycolipid), showed that PE is replaced by Sulf [120].

The brain lipid values illustrate the exact matching of glial and neuronal membrane systems and show how cholesterol and polar lipids are related. Since the characteristic sums for compartments are obtained with percentage TPoL values, which do not include cholesterol, the polar group codes limit replacements to polar lipid classes. This is confirmed by the failure of the TL vs. age plot (log vs. log) to show a smaller line number than the cholesterol vs. age plot (also log vs. log), which would be found if the alternative levels for cholesterol were achieved by replacement of polar lipids. Thus, despite the fact that cholesterol levels reflect differences in metabolic conversion of precursors to the cholesterol vs. polar lipid pathways, the metabolic replacement is not apparent since lipid class codes determine the alternative lipid class levels, as is the case for other organs, determined from the results of sums analysis.

An informative example of code replacement in plants is provided by the data for alfalfa leaf lipid class changes as a function of temperature [33]. The vernal variety, when grown at temperatures of 15, 20, and 30°C, showed large changes of lipid class composition that are similar to those for human brain in that they involve replacement between phospholipids and glycolipids as well as phospholipid classes. The largest changes, as growth temperature was increased, were for PI (4.0, 11.3, and 38.1%) that are matched by decreases of MGDG (28.5, 26.5, and 14.4%) and DGDG (27.6, 24.0, and 8.7%). The sums for PI + MGDG + DGDG at 15, 20, and 30°C were 60.1%, 61.8%, and 61.2% for a mean of 61.0 ± 0.86%, which is in agreement within measurement error, with the value 61.54% derived from general sums analysis. Plots of the percentage TPoL values for PG (4.5, 7.5, 11.3%) and SL (6.0, 9.1, 15.9%) increase with temperature, match the decreases of

PC (16.7, 12.6, 7.6%) and PE (12.7, 9.0, and 4.0%), and show linear relationships. One is: % PC = 22.686 − 1.337(%PG) (CC = 0.99994; F/C = 0.9999 ± 0.0040). The close correspondence is easy to see with the found vs. calculated PC values: 16.7/16.7; 12.6/12.7; and 7.6/7.6. The sum PC + SL is relatively constant (22.7, 21.7, 23.5%) as is the sum PE + PG (17.2, 16.5, 15.3%). Another excellent line is: % PC = 33.32 −21.47 (log % SL) (CC = 0.9997, F/C = 1.001 ± 0.010), and the perfect fit line: % PE = 28.71 −20.57 (log % SL) (CC = 1.0 exactly, F/C = 1.0 exactly ± zero). Another good line is % PG = 16.06 (log % SL) −7.957 (CC = 0.99998, F/C = 0.9997 ± 0.0076). This shows that all of the relationships among the classes that replace each other are linear and that the changes of SL are exponential. These changes illustrate how graphic and sums analysis together can provide the details of lipid replacements under changing conditions.

The lipid classes of human aorta and the lens of eyes of some species show large changes with age that consist of an increase of Sph, that in the lens is mostly a replacement for PC, whereas in aorta, Sph replaces all of the other phospholipids [31]. There is also an inverse relationship between PC and Sph that gives a linear relationship for the percentage PC plotted against log of percentage Sph for red blood cells of several species, with PC varying from zero in cattle, sheep, and goats to 51.4% in rat cells. The range for lens shows species differences from less than 5% PC to about 50% PC [29,30], and plots of percentage PC vs. percentage Sph for various species show a linear relationship for vertebrates, including the cod fish. Values for humans and rats fall on both range lines with cod and bovine values. Rabbit and monkey values as well as rat and bovine values fall on intermediate lines. The range lines are: % PC = 52.43 − 0.8484 (%SPh) [F/C = 1.0 ex ± 0.003], and 44.81 − 0.8484 (%SPh) [F/C = 1.0053 ± 0.0111]. The values on range line 1 for percentage Sph followed by the found vs. calculated values for percentage PC are: human, 56.7 (4.3/4.3); 57.8 (3.4/3.4); rat, 9.0 (45.0/44.8); cod, 5.0 (48.0/48.2). The corresponding values on the other range line are: human, 47.0 (5.0/4.9); bovine, 24.0 (24.5/24.4); rat, 15.5 (31.5/31.7); and calf, 14.1 (32.9/32.8). The plot slopes show that species differ in the extent to which choline is used as PC or Sph, and, in human lens, there are changes with age so that the percentage Sph rises from 35 at 2.6 years to 67 at 83 years.

The changes of organ weights with age are a function of the effect of regulatory factors that relate the components of organs to each other. Plots of organ weights as a function of age show how the sums of values for all components change relative to those of other organs. Organ weight plots present one of the more difficult problems in graphic analysis because the correct function for each organ must be determined and ranges are relatively broad. Plots for several species showed that different organs may follow different functions and show slope changes at different ages. The most informative plots were those done with values from 102 mice (C57 black), which showed different functions for different organs, but 18 lines were obtained for each organ and for body weight plotted against age. Thus, in the highest tier of regulation, only certain organ weight combinations are used and the exact additive nature of organ weights is apparent from the body weight plots.

The translation of line number variations to membrane structure features appears to be fairly clear in some respects. Thus the "groups of three" principle is assignable to bond angle variations of one control factor system acting at one site on the membrane surface, and each additional group of three lines is attributable to the addition of a site for another control factor system. With the maximum of 27 lines, the number of sites becomes nine as one dimension of the membrane arrangement. Since the maximum number of lines can be established with 1.5 to 3.0 times as many samples as there are lines, and there is in general no strong favoring of particular lines, the factors appear to act in sequence and each additional factor can activate only if the units preceeding it in the sequence are activated. The presence or absence of any one factor in the sequence can produce any particular line number with about equal frequency as other numbers.

The translation of line spacing for lipid plots into membrane structure features also follows some clear-cut principles. The smallest reproducible line spacing is the value for filling one compartment in one small repeating unit and thus the number of small units that come together as large units can be calculated. Larger line spacings are multiples of the smallest spacings, but their analysis to date has not disclosed any pattern attributable to reproducible membrane structure features.

The search for small, reproducible, line spacings showed a common small spacing to be almost exactly 0.10% of the total membrane lines. This was apparent for a number of the minor components of several organs. As an example, the PS values for 10 dog heart samples as percentage of the TPL were 2.3, 2.6, 2.7 (five times), 2.8 (two times), and 3.6%. The 2.6–2.7–2.8% series with heavy repeating of 2.7 shows the 0.10% change. The same type of result was obtained for PI and Sph. The PI values were: 3.6, 3.7 (two times), 3.8 (two times), 4.1 (two times), 4.2 (two times), and 4.3%. The Sph values were: 3.7, 3.8, 3.9, 4.3 (three times), 4.6, 4.9, and 5.2%. The same spacing was found for lung DPG. Since DPG is a double lipid, it cannot fit into a compartment with an odd number of molecules in both dimensions and it must thus fit into the 4×7 units that account for 30.77% of the total. Thus the approximate number of small units is $30.77/0.10 = 308$. Since this number is not divisible by 9 to give a whole number, the nearest value of 306/9 = 34 is in closest agreement. This gives 30.77/306 = 0.10056% as the exact increment for change for the smallest compartments and 38.46/306 = 0.1256% as the increment for the larger compartments.

Two other smaller increments were apparent for the trace components of membrane lipids. One series that is apparent from human red cell values [14] gives about 0.02% as the smallest values for a series, and the mean of about 0.021 % was obtained from several trace component values of organs. The search for even smaller increments was made with fatty acid data for human brain lipids. From the analysis of the minor fatty acids of minor phospholipids, a large "scale-up" factor ($\times$ 10^4) was obtained. A very favorable plot was for PI, 20^1 that gave 0.00175% as the line spacing when 20^1 molar values were plotted against TPoL molar values. Since this represents only one of two acids in the PI molecule, the value for a lipid class becomes $0.00175 \times 2 = 0.00350\%$. These smaller increments are attributable to the larger units, giving the near 0.10%, coming together in groups. If so, the smaller increments must have whole number relationships to one of larger increments, and this is the case since 0.1256/0.021 = 5.98 (6.0) and 0.1256/0.00350 = 35.89 = 36. It thus appears that there are a maximum of 36 large units in the group of large units, and that the arrangement is 6 $\times$ 6 since the 0.021% Δ is correct for one row of units in the 6 $\times$ 6 arrangment.

A search for tests of the general applicability of the 9 $\times$ 34 arrangement of small units in a large unit gave two general types of checks. One was the length of the fibers formed by stretching red blood cell membranes, which is considered later and is in good agreement with the 9 $\times$ 34 arrangement. The overall view of membrane structure is that lipids pack into one of three compartments that hold either 56 or 70 molecules of polar lipid. The two compartments holding 56 molecules are designated as "box" units and are formed by the membrane protein that passes through membranes and gives rise to intramembraneous particles by freeze–fracture electron microscopy. The single compartment that contains 70 molecules is composed of protein that appears on one side of the membrane only, and can thus be designated as a "sandwich" unit since lipid is between the protein layers. The "box" and "sandwich" units combine to form the smallest repeating units seen by electron microscopy (70 $\times$ 90Å). These small units combine in a 9 $\times$ 34 arrangement to give larger units composed of 306 small units, and the larger units are arranged in groups of 36 as 6 $\times$ 6, or 35 as 5 $\times$ 7. Bilayers appear to be parallel rather than perpendicular to the plane of the membrane since there is a continuous protein coat. Lipid–protein interaction is through both polar groups and carbon chains; that is possible with sandwich units if bilayers are parallel to the membrane surface [21].

Packing of Cholesterol, Gangliosides, and Ceramide Polyhexosides in Membranes

Cholesterol does not pack in the same space with any of the polar lipids, as shown by sums analysis and other forms of data analysis (Section II). Sums analysis also indicates that ceramide polyhexosides and gangliosides pack in separate spaces rather than mixed with polar lipids. The only information available for the analysis of ganglioside compartment size was the fatty acid composition of the total gangliosides of human brain as a function of age [122]. Plots of the values for minor acids gave clear cut line spacings that were multiples of four and five times 0.0035% (0.014% and 0.019%), and a few spacings that suggested 0.003–0.004%, but these were not clear cut. The plots suggest that gangliosides pack in 70 molecule compartments, although the spacing may only reflect the sites for receptors in the control unit.

A different approach is required to determined the compartment sizes for cholesterol. The dimensions of the large units into which the compartments fit are clear for brain and probably for other organs as $306 = 9 \times 34$. One of the fundamental values is the cholesterol to phospholipid molar ratio. Since electron microscopy does not show units of different sizes that can be correlated with the amount of cholesterol in membranes, it appears that the repeating units containing cholesterol are the same size as those for polar lipids. This is to be expected on the basis of general packing principles that dictate either the same size or whole number multiples of the polar lipid size. It thus appears that one dimension of the cholesterol compartments is fixed since four cholesterol molecules packing hydroxyl group to hydroxyl and side chain to side chain, with overlapping chains and with the hydroxyl groups of the two outer cholesterol molecules facing outward as for the polar groups of phospholipids, are required to give a length similar to that of a polar lipid bilayer.

With one dimension of the cholesterol compartments as four molecules, a series of possible sizes can be established. Thus, $4 \times 4 \times 4 = 64$, $4 \times 5 \times 4 = 80$, $3 \times 7 \times 4 = 84$, $4 \times 8 \times 4 = 128$, etc., are possible sizes. The cholesterol isotope exchange values for human red blood cells show about 40% to be exchangeable, and about 40% of the total cholesterol can be removed from the membrane by incubation in plasma with a low free-to-esterified cholesterol ratio [41]. There are thus at least two different types of cholesterol compartments. When ratios of the values for possible sizes are determined, it is seen that $84/(84 + 128) = 39.6\%$. One possibility is that there are two compartments, $84 = 3 \times 7 \times 4$ and $128 = 4 \times 8 \times 4$, or that the 128 molecules could be two compartments of 64 ($4 \times 4 \times 4$). Several other ratios also give values near 40% for xchangeable cholesterol, and so it is necessary to check the fit of sizes to cholesterol-to-phospholipid molar ratios.

The most common cholesterol-to-phospholipid ratio for human red blood cells is about 0.89%. With the 306 large unit size and 182 phospholipid molecules per unit, $306 \times 182 \times 0.89 = 49,566$ cholesterol molecules. With compartments in each cholesterol unit being 84 and 128, the total number of compartments becomes $49,566/212 = 233.80 = 234$ compartments. The dimensions 18×17 mean that the number of rows becomes $233.80/34 = 6.88 = 7$ rows. Thus there is a good fit to 34 rows. The whole row calculations for other sizes that give 39–40% for exchangeable cholesterol exclude $96 + 144$ and $64 + 96$, but $72 + 112$ gives $14.97 = 15$ rows for 17×18, and thus is not excluded.

The range of cholesterol-to-phospholipid molar ratios reported for membranes is 0.03 to 1.49. Since the differences in ratios must represent whole rows of cholesterol units, one row of 18 units (17×18) represents a ratio of $18 \times 212/306 \times 182 = 0.069$. With 9×34 rather than 18×17, the value is 0.035%. To obtain good fits to the various ratios reported, it was necessary to use three combinations of compartment sizes (i.e. $84 + 84$, $84 + 128$, and $128 + 128$). The lowest ratio is for $9 \times 34 = 306$ and $9 \times (84 + 84)/55,692 = 0.027 = 0.03$. The highest ratio is for 18 rows in the 18×17 arrangement since $18 \times 18 \times (128 + 128)/55,692 = 1.489 = 1.49$. The fits of alternatives from the red cell exchange data were not as good as the fits with the three combinations noted above. Using 72 and 112, which give 39% exchangeable and fit the red cell values as noted above, the combination of $112 + 112$ gives 20.6 rows for the ratio of 1.49, and is thus excluded.

A further check on the red cell cholesterol compartment sizes is possible with the size of the large unit composed of cholesterol and phospholipid units. The part of the small repeating unit in human red cell membranes with protein passing through the membranes gives intramembranous particles 85 Å $\times$ 85 Å [10]. With the 9×34 dimension and 34 rows of phospholipid plus 26 rows of cholesterol units, the length in one dimension becomes 60×85 Å $= 5100$ Å for the 9×34 arrangement. The value with the 9×34 arrangement is in good agreement with the range of 4000–5000 Å for the lengths of fibers formed from human red cell membranes when broken by stretching [9]. Each small repeating unit is composed of a compartment with protein which does not pass through the membrane and which is one-half the size in one dimension of those compartments which have protein passing through the membrane (85 $\times$ 42.5 Å. Thus the dimensions of each unit are about 85 $\times$ 128 Å. The value 128 Å is in the range of 100–200 Å for the widths of the fibers produced by stretching the membranes, and the range suggests that cleavage occurs at different points to give about 85, 128, 170, and 212 Å widths. The good general agreement of the red cell compartment sizes with the various red cell values indicates that the sizes are correct and that the arrangement is $9 \times 34 = 306$ with the 85 Å dimension for the small units in the 34 across dimension for the large units. This arrangement gives an increment for the cholesterol-to-phospholipid ratio of 0.034 per row that gives the series 0.887 (0.89), 0.853 (0.85), and 0.819 (0.82) that is in good agreement with the variations of the ratio for human cells.

References

1. S. Fleischer, B. Fleischer, and W. Stoeckenius, *J. Cell Biol.* **32**, 193–208 (1967).
2. L. Napolitano, F. Lebaron, and J. Scaletti, *J. Cell Biol.* **34**, 817–826 (1967).
3. R. B. Park and J. Biggins, *Science 144*, 1009–1011 (1964).
4. F. L. Crane, J. W. Sniles, Jr., K. S. Prezbindowski, F. J. Ruzicka, and F. F. Sun, *in* "Regulation of Function of Biological Membranes" (E. J. Jarnefelt, ed.), Vol. 11, Amsterdam, pp. 21–56. Elsevier, 1968.
5. R. J. Baskin, *J. Cell Biol.* **48**, 49–60 (1971).
6. E. Nickel and L. T. Potter, *Brain Res.* **57**, 508–517 (1973).
7. G. Moll, *Bioenergetics* **6**, 41–44 (1974).
8. W. M. Wong and P. H. Geil, *J. Supramol. Struct.* **3**, 401–414 (1975).
9. V. T. Marchesi, R. L. Jackson, J. P. Segrest, and I. Kahane, *Fed. Proc.* **32**, 1833–1837 (1973).
10. L. Packer, *Bioenergetics* **3**, 115–127 (1972).
11. A. Forge and J. W. Costerton, *Can. J. Microbiol.* **19**, 1056–1057 (1973).
12. W. M. Hess, D. J. Weber, and J. V. Allen, *Can. J. Biol.* **51**, 1685–1688 (1973).
13. D. H. MacLennan, P. Seaman, G. H. Iles, and C. C. Yip, *J. Biol. Chem.* **246**, 2702–2710 (1971).
14. J. D. Turner and G. Rouser, *Anal. Biochem.* **38**, 423–436 (1970).
15. J. W. Hendrix and G. Rouser, *Mycologia* **68**, 354–361 (1976).
16. G. Rouser, G. Kritchevsky, D. Heller and E. Lieber, *J. Am. Oil Chemists' Soc.* **40**, 425–454 (1963).
17. G. Rouser, A. N. Siakotos, and S. Fleischer, *Lipids* **1**, 85–86 (1966).
18. A. Yamamoto and G. Rouser, *Lipids* **5**, 442–444 (1970).
19. G. Rouser, G. Kritchevsky, and A. Yamamoto, *in* "Lipid Chromatographic Analysis" (G. V. Marinetti, ed.), Vol. I, pp. 99–162. Dekker, New York, 1967.
20. G. Rouser, G. Kritchevsky, A. Yamamoto, G. Simon, C. Galli, and A. J. Bauman, *Methods Enzymol.* **14**, 272–317 (1969).
21. G. Rouser, *in* "Biochemical Effects of Environmental Pollutants" (S. D. Lee, ed.), pp. 141–202. Ann Arbor Science Publ., Ann Arbor, Michigan, 1977.
22. S. H. Chan and R. L. Lester, *Biochim. Biophys. Acta* **210**, 180–181 (1970).
23. K. Hunter and A. H. Rose, *Biochim. Biophys. Acta* **260**, 633–639 (1972).

24. J. A. Ratcliffe, G. F. ssacks, G. E. Wheeler, and A. H. Rose, *J. Gen. Microbiol.* **76**, 445–449 (1973).

25. D. Jollow, G. M. Kellerman, and A. W. Linane, *J. Cell Biol.* **37**, 221–230 (1968).

26. R. E. Anderson, *Exp. Eye Res.* **10**, 339–344 (1970).

27. R. E. Anderson, *Biochim. Biophys. Acta* **187**, 345–353 (1969).

28. B. Plazonnet, P. Tronche, P. Bastide, and J. Komer, *C.R. Soc. Biol.* **163**, 398–399 (1969).

29. R. M. Broekhuyse and J. H. Veerkamp, *Biochim. Biophys. Acta* **152**, 316–324 (1968).

30. R. M. Broekhuyse, *Biochim. Biophys. Acta* **187**, 354–365 (1969).

31. G. Rouser and R. D. Solomon, *Lipids* **4**, 232–234 (1969).

32. G. Rouser, G. Kritchevsky, A. Yamamoto, and C. F. Baxter, *Adv. Lipid Res.* **10**, 261–360 (1972).

33. P. J. C. Kuiper, *Plant Physiol.* **45**, 684–686 (1970).

34. P. G. Roughan and R. D. Batt, *Phytochemistry* **8**, 363–369 (1969).

35. G. Rouser, unpublished.

36. R. L. Juliano and A. Rothstein, *Biochim. Biophys. Acta* **249**, 227–235 (1971).

37. T. L. Steck and J. Yu, *J. Supramol. Struct.* **1**, 220–232 (1973).

38. J. T. Hoogeveen, R. Juliano, J. Coleman, and A. Rothstein, *J. Membrane Biol.* **3**, 156–172 (1970).

39. P. L. Jorgensen, in "Role of Membranes in Secretory Processes" (L. Bolis, R. D. Keynes, and W. Wilbrandt, eds.), pp. 247–255. American Elsevier, 1972.

40. L. E. Hokin, J. L. Dahl, J. D. Dixon, J. F. Hackney, and J. F. Perdue, *J. Biol. Chem.* **248**, 2593–2605 (1973).

41. J. R. Murphy, *J. Lab. Clin. Med.* **60**, 86–109 (1962).

42. C. F. Reed, *J. Clin. Invest.* **47**, 749–760 (1968).

43. C. S. McArthur, C. C. Lucas, and C. H. Best, *Biochem. J.* **41**, 612 (1947).

44. O. E. Bell, Jr. and D. R. Shrength, *Arch. Biochem. Biophys.* **123**, 462–467 (1968).

45. H. J. Mersmann and D. R. Strength, *Fed. Proc.* **24**, 477 (1965).

46. R. G. Bridges, J. Ricketts, and J. T. Cox, *J. Insect Physiol.* **11**, 225 (1965).

47. G. A. Maw and V. DuVignaud, *J. Biol. Chem.* **176**, 1029 (1948).

48. R. Anderson, B. P. Livermore, M. Kates, and B. E. Volcani, *Biochim. Biophys. Acta* **528**, 77–88 (1978).

49. R. D. Mavis and P. R. Vagelos, *J. Biol. Chem.* **247**, 652–659 (1972).

50. E. Schecter, L. Letellier, and T. Gulik-Krzywicki, *Eur. J. Biochem.* **49**, 61–76 (1974).

51. D. F. Silbert, *Biochemistry* **9**, 3631–3640 (1970).

52. I. R. Baacham and D. F. Silbert, *J. Biol. Chem.* **248**, 5310–5318 (1973).

53. M. Esfahani, M. Barnes, and S. J. Wakil, *Proc. Nat. Acad. Sci. USA* **64**, 1057–1064 (1969).

54. R. M. McElhaney, *J. Mol. Biol.* **84**, 145–147 (1974).

55. R. N. McElhaney, J. DeGier, E. C. M. Van Der Neut-Kok, *Biochim. Biophys. Acta* **298**, 500–512 (1973).

56. J. C. Romijn, I. M. G. Van Goldie, R. N. McElhaney, L. L. M. Van Deenen, *Biochim. Biophys. Acta* **280**, 22–33 (1972).

57. L. Huang, S. K. Lorsch, G. G. Smith, and A. Huang, *FEBS Lett.* **43**, 1–5 (1974).

58. P. W. DeKruff, M. Van Duck, R. W. Goldbach, R. M. Demel and L. L. M. Van Deenen, *Biochim. Biophys. Acta* **330**, 269–282 (1973).

59. P. J. C. Kuiper, A. Livne, and N. Meyerstein, *Biochim. Biophys. Acta* **248**, 300–305 (1971).

60. M. C. Phillips and H. Hauser, *Chem. Phys. Lipids* **8**, 127–133 (1972).

61. B. J. Wisnieski, A. D. Keith, and M. R. Resnick, *J. Bacteriol.* **101**, 160–165 (1970).

62. S. A. Henry and A. D. Keith, *Chem. Phys. Lipids* **7**, 245–265 (1971).

63. L. M. G. Van Golde, W. A. Pieterson, and L. L. M. Van Deenen, *Biochim. Biophys. Acta* **152**, 84–95 (1968).
64. A. Yamamoto, M. Isozaki, K. Hirayama, and Y. Sakai, *J. Lipid Res.* **6**, 295–300 (1965).
65. M. A. Williams, R. C. Stancliff, L. Packer, and A. D. Keith, *Biochim. Biophys. Acta* **267**, 444–456 (1972).
66. R. E. Williams, B. J. Wishieski, H. G. Rittenhouse, and C. F. Fox, *Biochemistry* **13**, 1969–1977 (1974).
67. H. Brockerhoff, R. J. Hoyle, and P. C. Hwang, *Biochim. Biophys. Acta* **144**, 541–548 (1967).
68. G. W. Patterson, *Lipids* **5**, 597–600 (1970).
69. R. E. Anderson and M. B. Maude, *Arch. Biochem. Biophys.* **151**, 270–276 (1972).
70. A. Hamberger and L. Svennerholm, *J. Neurochem.* **18**, 1821–1829 (1971).
71. L. A. Johnson, V. G. Pursel, and R. J. Gerrits, *J. Anim. Sci.* **35**, 398–403 (1972).
72. T. W. Keenan, S. E. Nyquist, and H. H. Mollenhauer, *Biochim. Biophys. Acta* **270**, 433–443 (1972).
73. A. Poulos, A. Darin-Bennett, and I. G. White, *Comp. Biochem. Physiol.* **46B**, 544–549 (1973).
74. A. Poulos, J. K. Voglmayr, and I. G. White, *Biochim. Biophys. Acta* **306**, 194–202 (1973).
75. D. B. Menzel and H. S. Olcott, *Biochim. Biophys. Acta* **84**: 133–139 (1964).
76. E. M. Kreps, M. A. Cheboxareva, and V. N. Akulin, *Comp. Biochem. Physiol.* **31**, 419–430 (1969).
77. E. D. Korn, *J. Biol. Chem.* **239**, 396–400 (1964).
78. R. Jamieson and E. H. Reed, *Phytochemistry* **101**, 1837–1843 (1971).
79. R. M. Leech, M. G. Rumsby, and W. W. Thompson, *Plant Physiol.* **52**, 240–245 (1973).
80. O. Hirayama and T. Suzuki, *Agr. Biol. Chem.* **32**, 549–554 (1968).
81. R. M. Lees and E. D. Korn, *Biochemistry* **5**, 1475–1481 (1966).
82. T. Kaneda, *Biochim. Biophys. Acta* **270**, 32–39 (1972).
83. I. Yano, Y. Furukawa, and M. Kusunose, *Biochim. Biophys. Acta* **202**, 189–191 (1970).
84. R. J. King, J. Rush, and J. A. Clements, *J. Appl. Physiol.* **35**, 778–781 (1973).
85. J. L. Gellerman and H. Schlenk, *Experientia* **19**, 522–525 (1963).
86. B. L. Walker, *Arch. Biochem. Biophys.* **114**, 465–471 (1966).
87. B. L. Walker, *J. Nutr.* **92**, 23–29 (1967).
89. M. C. Phillips, Ladbrooke, B. D., and D. Chapman, *Biochim. Biophys. Acta* **196**, 35–44 (1970).
90. M. C. Phillips, H. Hauser, and F. Paltauf, *Chem. Phys. Lipids* **8**, 127–133 (1972).
91. P. H. J. Vergvergaert, A. J. Verkleij, P. F. Elbers, and L. L. M. Van Deenen, *Biochim. Biophys. Acta* **311**, 320–329 (1973).
92. A. J. Shimshick and H. M. McConnell, *Biochemistry* **12**, 2351–2360 (1973).
93. C. W. M. Grant, S. H. W. Wu, and H. M. McConnell, *Biochim. Biophys. Acta* **363**, 151–158 (1974).
94. A. K. Soutar, H. J. Pownall, A. S. Hu, and L. C. Smith, *Biochemistry* **13**, 2828–2836 (1974).
95. B. deKruyff, R. A. Demel, and L. L. M. Van Deenen, *Biochim. Biophys. Acta* **255**, 331–347 (1972).
96. A. G. Lee, N. J. M. Birdsall, J. C. Metcalf, P. A. Toon, and G. B. Warren, *Biochemistry* **13**, 3699–3705 (1974).
97. S. Eletr and A. D. Keith, *Proc. Nat. Acad. Sci. USA* **69**, 1353–1357 (1972).
98. B. deKruyff, R. A. Demel, A. J. Slotboom, and L. L. M. Van Deenen, *Biochim. Biophys. Acta* **307**, 1–19 (1973).
99. W. Stoffel and H. D. Pruss, *Hoppe-Seylers Z. Physiol. Chem.* **350**, 1385–1393 (1969).

100. D. Chapman, R. M. Williams, and B. D. Ladbrooke, *Chem. Phys. Lipids* 1, 445 (1967).
101. K. Jacobson and D. Papahadjopoulos, *Biochemistry* 14, 152–161 (1975).
102. H. K. Kimelberg and D. Papahadjopoulos, *J. Biol. Chem.* 49, 1071–1080 (1974).
103. A. J. Shimshick, W. Kleeman, W. C. Hubbell, and H. M. McConnell, *J. Supramol. Struct.* 1, 285–294 (1973).
104. P. Overath, H. U. Schairer, and W. Stoffel, *Proc. Nat. Acad. Sci. USA* 67, 606–612 (1970).
105. D. Chapman, *in "Proteids of Biological Fluids" (H. Peeters, ed.), pp. 165–173. Pergamon, Oxford, 1974.*
106. *F. Francis and S. H. Piper, J. Am. Chem. Soc.* 61, 577–581 (1939).
107. J. C. Smith, *J. Chem. Soc.* 625–627 (1936).
108. F. D. Gunstone and I. A. Ismail, *Chem. Phys. Lipids* 1, 209–224 (1967).
109. P. G. Barton and F. D. Gunstone, *J. Biol. Chem.* 250, 4470–4476 (1975).
110. A. Rodwell, *Science* 160, 1350–1351 (1968).
111. P. J. C. Kuiper and B. Stuiver, *Plant PUysiol.* 49, 307–309 (1972).
112. P. J. C. Kuiper, *Plant Physiol.* 43, 1367–1371 (1968).
113. A. Kylin, P. J. C. Kuiper, and G. Hansson, *Plant Physiol.* 261, 271–278 (1972).
114. R. Crotean and I. S. Fagerson, *Phytochemistry* 8, 2219–2222 (1969).
115. J. D. Weete, W. G. Rivers, and D. J. Weber, *Phytochemistry* 9, 2041–2045 (1970).
116. C. F. Baxter, G. Rouser, and G. Simon, *Lipids* 4, 243–244 (1969).
117. G. Rouser, G. Simon, and G. Kritchevsky, *Lipids* 4, 599–606 (1969).
118. G. Simon and G. Rouser, *Lipids* 4, 607–614 (1969).
119. S. Adachi, T. Ishibe, M. Isozaki, A. Yamamoto, T. Kakiuchi, and Y. Shingi, *J. Jpn. Soc. Gastroent.* 67, 332–342 (1970).
120. G. Rouser, A. Yamamoto, and G. Kritchevsky, *Arch. Int. Med.* 127, 1105–1121 (1971).
121. G. Rouser, A. Yamamoto, and G. Kritchevsky, *Adv. Exp. Med. Biol.* 13, pp. 91–109 (1971).
122. G. Rouser and A. Yamamoto, *J. Neurochem.* 19, 2697–2698 (1972).
123. F. Freese, "Elementary Forest Sampling," Agriculture Handbook No. 232, U.S. Dept. Agriculture, p. 36. U.S. Govt. Printing Office, Washington, D.C., 1962.
124. R. W. Ralston, "Fatty Acids and Their Derivatives." Wiley, New York, 1948.
125. G. Egloff, (ed.), "Physical Constants of Hydrocarbons," Vol. 1. Van Nostrand-Reinhold, New York, 1939.
126. K. S. Markley, *"Fatty Acids: Their Chemistry and Physical Properties,"* Wiley (Interscience), New York, 1947.
127. E. S. Latton, *in* "Fatty Acids: Their Chemistry, Properties, Production and Uses" (K. S. Warkley, ed), Part 4, pp. 2584–2636. Wiley (Interscience), New York, 1967.
128. N. A. Lange, "Handbook of Chemistry," 10th ed. McGraw-Hill, New York, 1969.
129. Y. Shizuta, A. Kurosawa, T. Tanabe, K. Inowe, and O. Hiyashi, *J. Biol. Chem.* 218, 1213–1219 (1973).
130. P. D. Swanson, H. F. Bradford, and H. McIlwain, *Biochem J.* 92, 235–247 (1964).
131. Y. E. Shamoo, and W. A. Brodsky, *Biochim. Biophys. Acta* 203, 111–123 (1970).
132. N. Sperelakis and E. C. Lee, *Biochim. Biophys. Acta* 233, 562–579 (1971).
133. A. Martonosi, *Biochim. Biophys. Acta* 150, 694–704 (1968).
134. G. Inesi, M. Millman and S. Eletr, *J. Mol. Biol.* 81, 483–504 (1973).
135. V. M. C. Madeira, W. C. Atunes-Madeira, and P. Cervalus, *Biochem. Biophys. Res. Commun.* 58, 897–904 (1974).
136. B. C. Johansson and H. Gest, *J. Bacterial.* 128, 683–688 (1976).
137. R. N. Patel and A. Felix, *J. Bacterial.* 128, 413–424 (1976).

138. S. Eletr, M. A. Williams, T. Watkins, and A. D. Keith, *Biochim. Biophys. Acta* **339**, 190–201 (1974).
139. A. V. Hill, *Proc. Physiol. Soc. (London), January 22,* (1910).
140. R. J. Chertok and S. Lake, *Biochim. Biophys. Acta* **339**, 202–209 (1974).
141. H. A. Bertrand, E. J. Masoro, T. Ohnishi, and B. P. Yu, *Biochemistry* **10**, 3679–3685 (1971).
142. H. Arthur and K. Watson, *J. Bacterial.* **128**, 56–68 (1976).
143. A. Keynan, A. A. Berns, G. Dunn, M. Young, and J. Mandelstan, *J. Bacterial.* **128**, 8–14 (1976).
144. A. Kim Chi and E. Rosenberg, *J. Bacterial.* **128**, 69–79 (1976).
145. H. G. Marr and J. C. Ingraham, *J. Bacterial.* **84**, 1260–1267 (1962).
146. R. M. McElhaney, *J. Mol. Biol.* **84**, 145–147 (1974).
147. K. Ahmad and P. Couillard, *J. Protozool.* **21**, 330–338 (1974).
148. B. Rudy and C. Gitler, *Biochim. Biophys. Acta* **288**, 231–236 (1972).
149. S. Eletr and G. Ines, *Biochim. Biophys. Acta* **290**, 178–185 (1972).
150. C. Lussan and J. F. Faucon, *FEBS Lett.* **19**, 186–188 (1971).
151. R. H. Furman, R. P. Palmer, K. La Rshom, and L. N. Norcia, *Am. J. Clin. Nutr.* **9**, 73–102 (1961).

Chapter **8**

Mechanoelastic Properties of Biological Membranes[1]

J. D. Brailsford

Introduction. 291
Special Problems of Biconcave Membranes. 292
    Definition of Terms. 296
    Structural Requirements and Observed Properties. 300
    Physical Models. 301
    Possible Sources of Bending Elasticity. 302
Calculation of Elastic Strain Energy. 311
    Biconcave Shape. 312
    Other Shapes. 314
Conclusion. 317
References. 318

Introduction

In this chapter we shall consider mainly the membrane of the human red blood cell and use relatively simple arguments concerning its physical properties. This biological membrane has long been recognized as the most convenient one to study as it is readily available and uncomplicated by cytoplasmic structure. The latter characteristic, however, implies that the external equilibrium shape of the red cell is the direct result of the physical properties of its membrane. This is because the content of the cell, being

[1]Funding was provided by the Department of Pathology and Laboratory Medicine, Loma Linda University, Loma Linda, CA 92354, and the Educational Foundation of America.

Membrane Fluidity in Biology, Vol. 1
Concepts of Membrane Structure

liquid, can not account for the morphological behavior of the cell, even with the assistance of surface tension. Nor would the membrane be able to do so if it were also purely liquid in nature. Thus in discussing membrane fluidity we are confronted at the outset by an enigma. The red cell membrane must have a structure that enables it to behave like a solid. Moreover this structure must also be sufficiently complicated to account for the ability of the cell to transform from its normal biconcave shape into various crenated forms and cup-shaped stomatocytes such as, for example, those shown in Fig. 1. The whole intriguing range of shapes into which the red cell membrane is capable of transforming, under the influence of a variety of chemical agents, was described more than thirty years ago by Ponder (1948) and has since been beautifully illustrated by Bessis (1974).

Most of the arguments presented below depend upon a considerable background of mathematical analysis, but, since the requisite information is available in the literature spanning the last decade, only the conclusions will be stated and references given, with sufficient explanation to bind the discussion into a coherent whole. The very simplicity of the arguments gives them great force so that they should not be ignored in the overall picture of membrane structure, provided that the limitations of applying conclusions arrived at from a study of the red cell to biological membranes in general are kept in mind.

Special Problems of Biconcave Membranes

Our starting point in this deductive exercise is the smooth and curious biconcave shape adopted by the normal human red cell in plasma. The simplest mental picture we can have of this cell is that it is an extremely small flexible bag formed by a continuous membrane and that this tiny sac holds a solution of hemoglobin which does not completely fill the available space. The hemoglobin, of course, must absorb and release oxygen via the membrane whose principal functions are therefore to localize the hemoglobin, so that it does not go into solution in the plasma, and to allow gaseous diffusion. With this picture in mind there is little structural difference, except in scale, between the unbroken yolk of an ordinary hen's egg and a red cell. The thickness and flexibility of the yolk sac, in proportion to its size, is comparable to that of a red cell membrane and the content in both cases is fully fluid; yet if some of the liquid content be withdrawn from the egg yolk sac to render it more flaccid and if it be suspended in a suitable fluid to

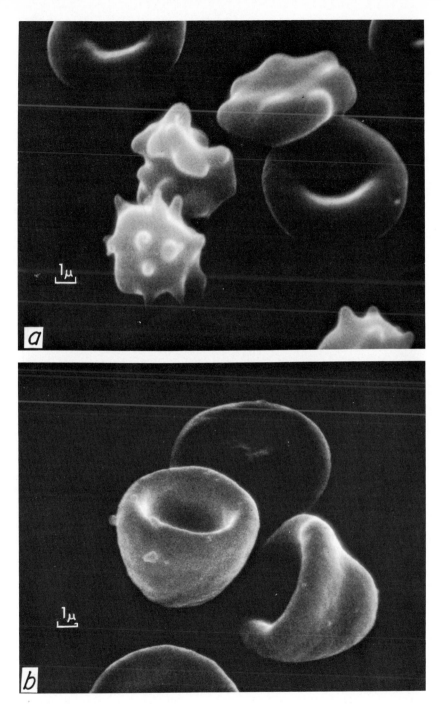

Fig. 1. (*a*) Crenated cells (Echinocytes) with two biconcave cells. (*b*) Cup shaped cell (Stomatocyte) with triconcave cell and two biconcave cells.

represent plasma, it shows no tendency to go into a smooth biconcave shape but goes into a variety of irregular dimpled shapes. The first question to ask therefore is: Why is this so? What essential difference is there between a red cell and the unbroken yolk of an ordinary egg?

Before attempting to answer this question we shall consider another structure which, unlike the egg yolk, does follow a sequence of shapes strongly suggestive of the behavior of the red cell, though only in a two-dimensional sense. This structure is a thin-walled pipe of circular cross section which is made to collapse under external pressure. The cross-sectional profile first becomes ellipsoidal and then biconcave. This effect has been investigated in connection with the collapse of submarine pipes (Kresh, 1977; Southwell, 1913a,b). A convenient means of studying these changes in cross-sectional profile is shown in Fig. 2 where a circular loop of tape made from X-ray film, representing a short length of thin walled elastic pipe, is shown loosely sandwiched between two parallel transparent plastic or glass plates. Such a loop is sufficiently weak for it to collapse with moderate suction applied to the inside of the loop via holes in one of the plates. The loop must be prevented from crossing the suction holes or cutting off the suction when the two sides of the loop finally touch one another. These simple requirements are met by using two suction holes in the lower plate and raising the rim of

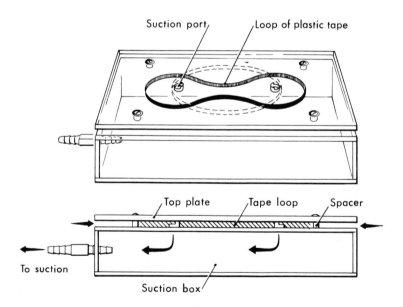

Fig. 2. Two views of transparent chamber and suction box used to demonstrate the change in shape of a circular loop of plastic tape under the influence of a differential pressure change.

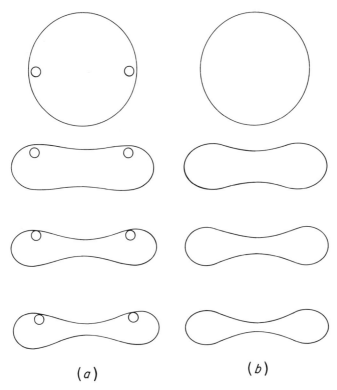

Fig. 3. (*a*) Profiles of plastic loop showing sequential change in shape from circle to biconcave. (*b*) Calculated cross-sectional profiles of red cell from sphere to biconcave disc.

these ports slightly above the surface of the plate. It is a useful apparatus for checking methods of mathematical analysis because the computer-derived shapes can be compared directly with the actual shapes. Fig. 3a shows a series of spontaneously formed loop profiles. Fig. 3b shows a corresponding series of osmotically induced shape changes in a red cell. It is important to note that the long axis of both the loop profile and the red cell profile increases as the shapes become more oblate. It is also important to note that the smoothness and indeed the existence of the loop profile must be solely due to the loop's elastic bending resistance since the forces involved are too small to produce any significant change in loop length and hence to store elastic energy due to stretching. If the loop had been constructed like a bicycle chain so that it had no elastic bending resistance in the plane of the section, it would have had no well-defined shape at all. In the case of the loop of tape the observed increase in length of the long axis of the profile, as the latter becomes more oblate, can occur without increasing the circumferential length of the loop because the profile is a plane figure. If, however, we consider a surface of revolution generated by rotating the profile about its short axis, it is no longer possible for the equatorial diameter to increase in length without increasing the equatorial circumference. This latter requirement cannot be met in any ordinary material without excessive tension because the circumference of the three-dimensional surface is also a loop and the force required to stretch it has to be transmitted from the polar regions to the equatorial region by compression of the intervening material without buckling. Yet this is precisely what the red cell does.

DEFINITION OF TERMS

In order to explain how the red cell can accomplish this remarkable feat it is convenient to use the following terms: *shear resistance, bending resistance, tension, compression, stress* and *strain*. All these terms are commonly used in engineering in connection with the deformation suffered by a solid body when it is acted upon by a system of forces. For the sake of the reader whose specialization lies in a field where these terms are not often encountered in their engineering sense, some definition may be necessary.

Shear

A substance is said to be in shear when a pair of equal and opposite parallel forces, not in the same straight line, act upon it. This arrangement gives rise to a twisting moment, the magnitude of which is equal to the product of one of the forces and the perpendicular distance between them. In Fig. 4a a rectangular piece of solid material is shown being acted upon by a pair of such forces. The shearing effect of these two forces will deform the body so that it takes up the new shape shown in Fig. 4b. If it does not rotate there must be an equal and opposite twisting moment present which, if the piece of material is part of a larger piece, is provided by the reaction from the adjacent material and can be represented by the additional pair of forces shown in Fig. 4c. Since the deformed shape is shown as a rhombus, the two pairs of forces must have equal magnitude; that is, $F_1 = F_2$. Finally, the forces at each end of the diagonal can be resolved into a pair of equal and opposite forces which are in line as shown in Fig. 4d. These forces put the body into what is called simple tension in which there is no twisting effect. This is the kind of tension one would expect in a tendon when the muscle to which it is attached contracts. By the same kind of argument, the original

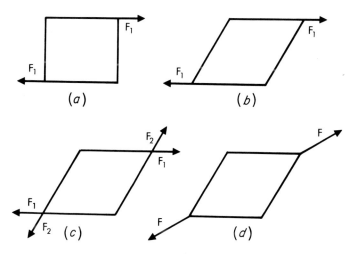

Fig. 4. Representation of shear forces acting on a rectangle of material to show how pure shear can give rise to pure tension and vice versa.

shear condition shown in Fig. 4a could equally well have been represented by two equal and opposite inwardly directed or compressive forces acting in line, and therefore without twisting moment, along the shorter diagonal of the rhombus in Fig. 4d. The surprising result emerges, therefore, that elastic shear deformation, due to a pair of forces which produce a twisting effect in a solid at rest, can be represented as elastic tension or compression with no twisting effect. This explains the somewhat confusing way in which shear, tension and compression are used, apparently interchangeably, in the literature describing the mechanics of membranes.

The above explanation is, of course, oversimplified, but, for those readers who may like to pursue the matter, an excellent rigorous, yet quite readable, mathematical analysis of large elastic deformations has been prepared by Evans and Skalak (1980).

Tension and Compression

When considering the internal forces and deformations within a material, the terms stress and strain are used. Generally, external forces produce a distributed effect within the material upon which they act. Stress refers to the local intensity of that effect. If the material is in tension, the stress is called tensile stress and has the dimensions of force per unit area. In the case of a membrane, however, it is misleading to calculate stress on the basis of the cross-sectional area because in the thickness direction the structure of the membrane is radically different from what it is in the surface tangential plane. Stress is therefore usually replaced by tension or compression meaning force per unit length; the length being measured in the membrane tangential plane and normal to the direction of the force.

This is a special use of the terms tension and compression which would normally mean tensile stress and compressive stress, respectively. There is therefore a troublesome ambiguity in the use of these terms.

Strain

For small deformations, strain is defined as change in length per unit length and is therefore nondimensional. If the relationship between stress (which can be read throughout as tension in the case of membranes) and strain is linear, the ratio, stress divided by strain, is of course constant and is called the *modulus of elasticity* for the particular set of conditions specified. For large elastic deformations such as those encountered in the shear deformation of an easily deformed substance like a rubber band or a piece of biological membrane, the definitions of stress and strain have to be more complicated than those given above because the area (or length if we are considering membrane tension) over which the force acts can no longer be considered the same in the deformed and undeformed states. The reason that strain is also involved in the process of formulating more comprehensive definitions is too complicated to present here but is clearly set out in work previously cited (Evans and Shalak, 1980). It has been shown that if the ratio of the deformed length of a piece of material, in simple elastic tension, to its original unstressed length is called the extension ratio, then for large deformations the strain is a quadratic function of this ratio. For small deformations this reduces to a linear function which agrees with the definitions given above. In either case there is a substantially linear relationship between stress and strain so that the concept of a constant modulus of elasticity is preserved.

Bending Effects

Bending effects are more complicated. Suppose we consider first the properties of a piece of X-ray film which is a typical elastic solid. Fig. 5 shows, diagramatically, an edge-on view of a strip of film lying flat and supported near its ends at A and B. For simplicity, a single concentrated force is shown acting downwards at the center. This results in two upward reaction forces at A and B and the material is deformed so that it takes up a curved shape as shown. This kind of deformation causes a shortening of the

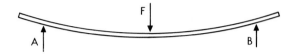

Fig. 5. Simple bending of a flat strip of plastic (edge-on view).

upper surface and a corresponding lengthening of the lower surface. Between these two limiting surfaces there must be a surface which does not change in length. This is called the *neutral surface*. Other layers, or more precisely, laminar elemental surfaces, between the neutral surface and the inner or outer surfaces of the membrane will be lengthened or shortened proportionately to their distance from the neutral surface.

The lengthening or shortening of the laminar elemental surfaces within a piece of material, such as the bent piece of film represented in Fig. 5, is evidence of tension and compression within the material. Thus the ease or difficulty with which the material can be bent is ultimately dependent upon the ease with which the same material can be stretched or compressed, that is, its ability to resist elastic shear deformation. Therefore shear and bending elasticity in an ordinary material are not two independent phenomena which can be treated separately but are different aspects of the same thing. The inability of an egg yolk sac or any other membranous sac of naturally occurring material, other than the red cell membrane, to transform from a spherical shape to a smooth biconcave shape is, as we shall see, primarily due to this interdependence of bending and shear elasticity.

Simple extension, due to tension, produces a net elastic elongation of the material whereas bending does not. In the latter case the neutral surface remains constant in length. The distribution of tension within the thickness of the material is therefore different in the two cases. As a result of this difference, elastic resistance to bending is found to be proportional to the third power of the thickness of the material whereas, elastic resistance to simple elongation is proportional to the first power of the thickness. Thus, in a piece of ordinary isotropic material as thin as the membrane of a red cell, the elastic bending resistance should be vanishingly small compared to the elastic resistance to extension, which we have seen is equivalent to elastic resistance to shear deformation. Therefore, for a membrane in which the elastic properties are completely isotropic, we would have to look for an explanation for the biconcave shape and the ability of the red cell to increase in equatorial diameter, solely on the basis of shear elasticity. This has been attempted both mathematically (Evans, 1973; Fung and Tong, 1968) and experimentally (Fung, 1968) but without success, either because the model fails to show the required change in diameter between the sphered cell and the disc, or because it requires a membrane which does not have the same properties at every point on the surface of the cell. This latter requirement must be met because there is good experimental evidence that the dimples can be relocated. Although they remain in apposition, they can be positioned, at least temporarily, anywhere on the surface of the cell (Bull, 1972; Schmid-Schonbein and Wells, 1969). This is an observation to which we shall refer in more detail later. Therefore, in order to behave as it does, the red cell membrane must be substantially isotropic in the membrane plane, but cannot be isotropic in all three dimensions.

Using the above definitions, we are now in a position to describe the mechanoelastic properties that the red cell membrane must possess to enable it to transform from a sphere to a smooth biconcave disc.

Structural Requirements and Observed Properties

The enclosed volume of the cell must obviously change as the transformation takes place. A sphere has the largest volume for a given surface area of any possible shape, so the biconcave shape must have a lower ratio of volume to surface area than the sphere. It has been found, moreover, that the surface area of the red cell remains constant during this change (Canham & Parkinson, 1970; Evans and LaCelle, 1975). The first requirement of the material is therefore that it should maintain constant surface area under the influence of the stresses involved in normal morphological transformations.

The second requirement is that the equatorial circumference must be able to change. Since the membrane area remains constant this implies that the meridional circumference must change in the opposite sense to the equatorial change. These changes are of the order of 15 to 20% and thus fall into the category of typical large shear deformations of the surface. We have already noted that the red cell membrane is virtually isotropic in the membrane plane so its resting shape, apart from minor memory effects, would be spherical. The osmotic removal of fluid from the inside of a spherical red cell produces a flaccid biconcave cell, which by the definition of flaccidity cannot have any positive internal pressure. So the actual deforming forces acting on the membrane in the biconcave state cannot be tensile, as they are in an inflated balloon or a turgid cell, but must necessarily be compressive. Therefore the elongation of the equator (required to produce the biconcave shape) cannot be due to primary simple tension acting along the equatorial dimension, but must be the secondary response of the material to primary compressive shortening of the meridional dimension. Herein lies the difficulty.

Consider, for example, what would be required to increase the width of a sheet of note paper, or the page on which this is written, by means of a compressive force applied between the top and the bottom edges of the sheet. Obviously the sheet would buckle long before sufficient force could be applied to produce any noticable widening of the page. This would be true even if the page were made of soft rubber, or even of open-celled polyurethane or rubber sponge, unless the material were very thick. We have also noted, from the theory of bending, that increasing the thickness increases the elastic bending resistance at a very much more rapid rate than the elastic shear resistance increases. To avoid buckling, therefore, it is not just a low modulus of shear elasticity which is required, but a high ratio of elastic bending resistance to elastic shear resistance. The same requirement applies to the design of roof trusses and other engineering structures where compression members (called struts) often have to be made thicker than is necessary to carry the load so that they will have sufficient resistance to bending to prevent them from buckling.

The third requirement, therefore, is a high ratio of elastic bending resistance to elastic shear resistance. As we have seen above this is a contradiction in terms unless the material has special properties, because, for a thin homogeneous isotropic membrane, the elastic resistance to bending should be vanishingly small compared to the elastic shear resistance.

The question thus arises: Is it possible to devise a structured material which has the properties of the red cell membrane, and if so what can it tell us about the structure of the membrane? The answer to this question is, yes, such a material can be constructed and there is much to be learned about membranes from considering its structural requirements.

PHYSICAL MODELS

The first published clue to the peculiar properties of the red cell membrane was due to Canham (1970) who showed that a membrane, in which it was assumed that elastic bending resistance was the predominant factor, would have an equilibrium shape similar to that of the red cell. This in itself does not show how bending elasticity can be separated from shear elasticity, but Canham recognized that the lipid bilayer might have this property. This is because a lipid bilayer cannot change its thickness appreciably without radically disturbing its molecular structure even though it is liquid in the membrane plane.

Since the bilayer has a finite and well-defined thickness, curvature must dilate the monolayer on the convex surface and contract the monolayer on the concave surface. The monolayers can resist both effects elastically and so manifest bending resistance even though the liquid nature of the bilayer means that it has no surface shear resistance at all. Dintenfass (1969) also recognized membrane elastic bending resistance as a liquid crystal property. Brailsford and Bull (1973) came independently to the same conclusion as Canham and made what we believe to be the first successful physical model of the red cell membrane. This model decoupled the elastic bending resistance from the elastic shear resistance and when subjected to a small positive difference of pressure between the outside and the inside, was found to transform from a sphere to a biconcave disc, just as the red cell does (Bull, 1972). Fig. 6 shows a later version of the model the surface of which consists entirely of a network of hinged struts. Fig. 7 shows details of its construction.

The principle of these models is that both elastic bending resistance and elastic shear resistance are virtually destroyed in the membrane plane by articulation, but that since the articulation is restricted to the membrane plane by the orientation of the pivots, the bending elasticity in the normal plane is retained. In the earlier model the bending elasticity was supplied by small plastic sleeves which formed part of the simple hinge structure. In the model shown in Fig. 6 the bending elasticity is supplied by the resistance to flexing of the flat strips of plastic which form the struts. Sophisticated mathematical analysis (Jenkins, 1977) shows that pure elastic bending resistance alone would result in a prolate spheroidal shape but it has also been shown that a small amount of elastic shear resistance (such as even the models have) would suppress the prolate form and allow the biconcave form to develop (Brailsford et al., 1976). Thus we now have a demonstrably sufficient reason for the biconcave shape of the red cell but we have not as yet shown that it is a necessary reason.

POSSIBLE SOURCES OF BENDING ELASTICITY

The concept of bending which has been used so far in this account, except for a brief reference to Canham's work, is that of a beam in which the curvature is in a single direction. The red cell membrane, however, is more often than not curved in two mutually perpendicular directions in the membrane plane. This latter type of bending is referred to as the bending of a plate and is more complicated than the bending of a beam. Fortunately the fact that biological membranes are of molecular dimensions reduces the complication somewhat, so we shall attempt to describe, in the simplest possible terms, the various ways in which the peculiar type of bending

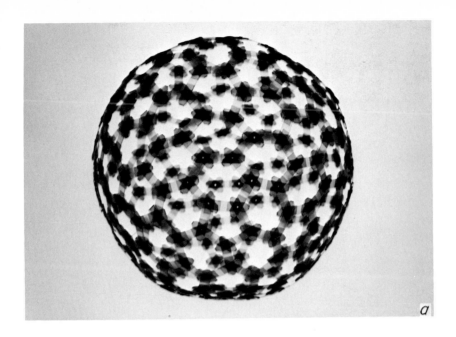

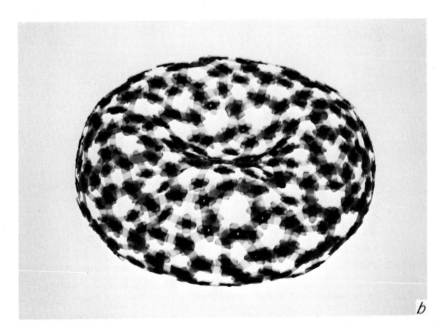

Fig. 6. (*a*) Model simulating red cell in sphered state. (*b*) Oblique view of model in dimpled state. Note increase in equatorial diameter.

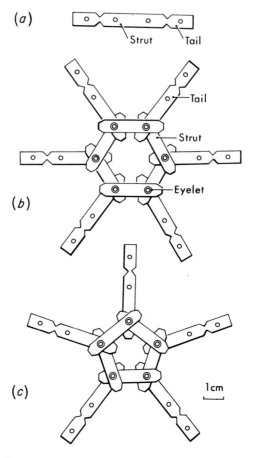

(a)

Strut   Tail

Tail

Strut

Eyelet

(b)

(c)

1 cm

Fig. 7. Details of construction of red cell model. (*a*) Basic constructional element (strut); (*b*) Hexagonal subunit (20 required); (*c*) Pentagonal subunit (12 required). These are positioned at the vertices of an icosahedron. The tails on the struts are turned under when eyeleting to form loops which interfere to restrict the angular movement of the joints.

elasticity required could arise. In order to start, however, some hypothesis of membrane structure is needed and this will be taken to be the Singer–Nicolson model (1972) which consists of a fluid bilayer mosaic of phospholipids and amphipathic proteins. In the red cell an additional layer of spectrin molecules, in the form of a net, is attached to the cytoplasmic surface (Shohet, 1982).

Case I

Let it be assumed that the whole of the bending elasticity resides in the lipid bilayer.

Since the lipid bilayer is fluid in the plane of the membrane there is no problem in fulfilling the requirement of low elastic shear resistance for, by definition, a liquid has none. The problem is to account for the existence of elastic bending resistance. The membrane of a soap bubble is a fully fluid membrane but it does not have any elastic bending strength. Curvature of any membrane of finite thickness must always result in a change in area of the convex surface relative to the concave surface. In the case of the soap bubble, however, bending produces no elastic strain because molecules from the compressed surface can migrate almost instantaneously to the expanded surface and so relieve the strain. In the case of a phospholipid bilayer such migration is resisted by the amphipathic nature of the molecules which have to overcome an energy barrier in order to flip from one monolayer to the other. Diffusion would therefore take a comparatively long period of time. Fig. 8a is a diagramatic representation of a flat symmetrical phospholipid bilayer. Both the polar head groups and the fatty acyl chains are evenly distributed. The surface tension is the same everywhere and the internal pressure is the same everywhere. If we bend the membrane without changing its thickness the molecules must redistribute themselves in one of two ways or a combination of these two ways. Figs. 8b and 8c show the two possible extremes.

In Fig. 8b it is assumed that the polar head groups remain evenly distributed. The acyl chains, however, are attached to the polar heads and therefore must rearrange themselves to accomodate the curvature. The nonuniform distribution of acyl chains constitutes a nonuniform pressure distribution in the fluid interior of the membrane.

If the polar head groups can resist this lateral pressure effect, the free ends of the acyl chains must redistribute so as to restore a uniform pressure distribution and we can say that the inner and outer monolayers have "slipped" relative to one another.

In Fig. 8c it is assumed that the acyl chains remain evenly distributed and that the polar head groups can redistribute. It should be noted that there is no need for rigid attachment between the acyl chains in the two monolayers. All that is necessary is to consider that the dynamic cohesive forces between the fatty acyl chains are similar to those that exist in a bulk quantity of an oil and that the forces involved in maintaining the continuity of the oily layer are sufficient to upset the distribution of the polar head groups. This pro-

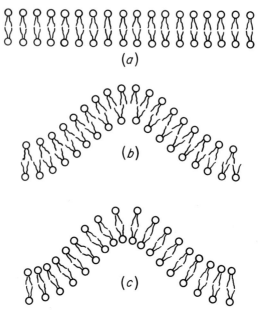

Fig. 8. Diagrammatic representation of a section through a phospholipid bilayer: (*a*) flat resting state; (*b*) bent state in which the polar head groups maintain their uniform distribution; (*c*) bent state in which the acyl chains maintain their uniform distribution.

duces a different kind of elastic strain from that shown in Fig. 8b, although the hydrophobic region is fully fluid in both cases.

The type of bending resistance represented in Fig. 8b is only possible on a closed surface or one in which the edges are restrained. It cannot produce localized elastic bending resistance (Evans, 1974). We have shown mathematically that the nonlocalized type of bending resistance shown in Fig. 8b cannot produce a symmetrical biconcave shape, but that it can produce the cup shaped variant (Brailsford *et al.*, 1980). On the other hand, localized elastic bending resistance resulting from the molecular stress depicted in Fig. 8c, in combination with extremely small amounts of elastic shear resistance, can account for the whole range of biconcave shapes of the red cell (Brailsford *et al.*, 1976).

Although localized elastic bending resistance arising in a lipid bilayer is theoretically capable of producing the biconcave shape, no artificial lipid vesicle that spontaneously adopts the biconcave shape has yet been produced, to our knowledge. Very small vesicles have too small a radius of curvature compared to the thickness of the membrane to expect a biconcave shape and large vesicles are difficult to produce (Boroske *et al.*, 1981). There is evidence, however, for the existence of localized elastic bending resistance in purely lipid bilayers in the very persuasive explanation given by Deuling and Helfrich (1977) for the appearance of myelin shapes. The equations these investigators used only apply to a localized type of bending resistance. The agreement of their results with observation therefore lends support to the concept that elastic bending resistance of this type can originate in the lipid bilayer.

Moreover, the myelin forms found inside and outside aged red cells have no associated protein layer in which the bending resistance might otherwise arise. This being so, an explanation for the absence of biconcavity in large, artificially produced vesicles may be that the elastic bending resistance is not strong enough. A particular arrangement of proteins and electric charges may be needed to induce a strong surface tension to act on the polar head groups and force them together. The existence of such a force in the real membrane is suggested by the experiments of Conrad and Singer (1979) and van Deenen *et al.* (1976) The latter experiments show that certain phospholipases that can hydrolyze monolayers of phospholipids held in a Langmuir's trough at more than about 30 dynes/cm can hydrolyze the membrane of intact erythrocytes, whereas other phospholipases that can only hydrolyze monolayers of phospholipids at less than about 30 dynes/cm are unable to hydrolyze the phospholipids of the erythrocyte membrane. An intrinsic surface tension of about 30 dynes/cm, which is thus suggested, is more than sufficient (in a membrane 10^{-6}cm thick) to produce the elastic bending resistance required to account for the biconcave shape of the red cell.

Case II

Let it be assumed that the whole of the bending resistance arises in the protein skeleton of the membrane.

Although this is an attractive view because it puts no restriction on the fluidity of the lipid bilayer, it is not without its difficulties. The protein skeleton, as its name implies, is considered to have solid properties. That is, it must be able to support elastic shear, in contrast to a liquid which, by definition, cannot support elastic shear. A single molecule of spectrin would be only about 3.5×10^{-7} cm thick, and it does not have the liquid crystal properties of the lipid bilayer. How, then, can it develop a high ratio of bending to shear elastic resistance unless it has a structure equivalent to that of the model shown in Fig. 6? Looseness of structure, such as we associate with a net, will not of itself produce a high ratio of bending to shear elasticity in a thin structure. The spectrin net would have to have its molecules arranged so that they can hinge in the membrane plane but not in the normal plane, so that the bending stiffness of individual spectrin molecules can be transmitted from molecule to molecule throughout the surface without a corresponding increase in surface shear resistance.

It has been suggested, on the basis of the elastic energy required to deform the red cell, that there is a low upper limit to the bending stiffness of the membrane (Evans, 1980). Since the shear resistance must be very much lower than the bending resistance, in order to account for the biconcave shape, and the bending resistance itself is so small, the shear resistance must be extremely small. This has been pointed out in the literature (Fischer *et al.*, 1981), and would imply that the stress–strain relationship cannot be linear down to zero stress, as had been thought from measurements with glass micropipettes at higher stresses (Evans and LaCelle, 1975), because the shear strength extropolated from these measurements would be far too high. There is good evidence for a nonlinear stress–strain relationship from experiments carried out on cells caught on a strand of spider's web and subjected to fluid flow in a specially designed observation chamber (Bull and Brailsford, 1976). If a thin enough web is used, the cells wrap themselves over it and can be stretched by the viscous drag forces induced by the liquid flowing through the chamber. The resulting elongation cannot be measured directly but, because the membrane strongly resists change in area, the part of the cell which is flattened out by contact with the web contracts in exact proportion to the elongation. This contraction is easily observed and can be measured. The validity of these experiments has never received general acceptance, presumably because the results differ so radically from thsoe obtained by the most careful aspiration of red cells into glass micropipettes. However no really convincing refutation has been forthcoming either, so the theoretical need for a nonlinear relationship may yet spark interest in the anomaly.

Case III

Let it be assumed that both the lipid bilayer and the protein skeleton contribute to the bending resistance. This is a very reasonable supposition provided one can accept the concept that while the spectrin molecules can articulate freely in the plane of the membrane they are also able to transmit bending moments in the normal plane. The mental picture of the membrane which then emerges is similar to that of Evans and Hochmuth (1977), in which a spectrin net forms the cytoplasmic base plane of the protein skeleton, with discrete skeletal proteins attached to its outer face. The lipid bilayer, with its free floating amphipathic proteins, covers this outer face and envelops the attached skeletal proteins, some of which penetrate through to the outer surface. The arrangement is depicted in Fig. 9 which is an attempt to show the spacial relationship of the conventionally represented molecules to scale, from the information brought together by Lux (1979).

The hypothesis that the spectrin molecules have attachments to one another, which are the molecular equivalent of the pivots in the model shown in Fig. 6 and thus give rise to anisotropic bending resistance, is included as an unlikely possibility. Without such attachments, however, we have to revert to the position that the spectrin skeleton has no appreciable elastic bending resistance, that is, to Case I. This is because, as we have seen above, if elastic bending resistance exists simultaneously in both the membrane tangential plane and the normal plane it must be vanishingly small compared to the shear resistance.

Problems also arise if we try to envisage a cooperative bending resistance produced by the interaction of the lipid bilayer with the spectrin skeleton. The latter has another property which has not been mentioned so far. The membrane can extend elastically to a remarkable degree. Fig. 10 shows how the red cell can extend to form long filaments, yet recover its initial biconcave shape when the deforming force is removed. During these extraordinary deformations the surface area remains constant. Conservation of surface

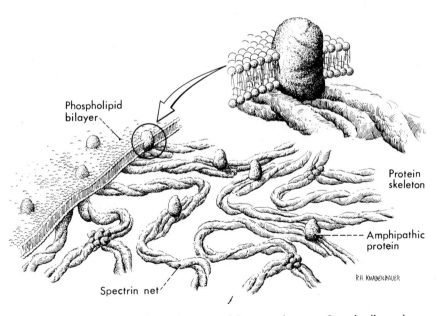

Phospholipid bilayer

Protein skeleton

Amphipathic protein

Spectrin net

R.H. KNABENBAUER

Fig. 9. Diagrammatic spatial representation of the main elements of a red cell membrane showing the interrelationship of the protein skeleton and the lipid bilayer.

area is most likely to be due to the properties of the lipid bilayer and the amphipathic proteins floating in it. If this system is held together by strong surface tension it can act like a two-dimensional liquid having constant surface area. On the other hand, the ability of the continuous protein skeleton to deform to the degree that it must, to account for the extraordinary elastic deformations shown in Fig. 10, would seem to infer that it is a loosely conformed network which can deform in any direction while allowing the lipid bilayer to flow over it.

Suppose, therefore, that a small area of the membrane which is flat in its resting state is deformed into a concave state with its concavity facing inwards. The bending must contract the inner surface and therefore the spectrin net, but if the latter cannot resist area contraction it cannot contribute to the elastic strain energy and will not therefore augment the overall bending resistance. The question thus becomes: Can the spectrin skeleton resist area contraction (and dilation) and at the same time allow enormous shear deformation without change in area? It is difficult to see how this question can be

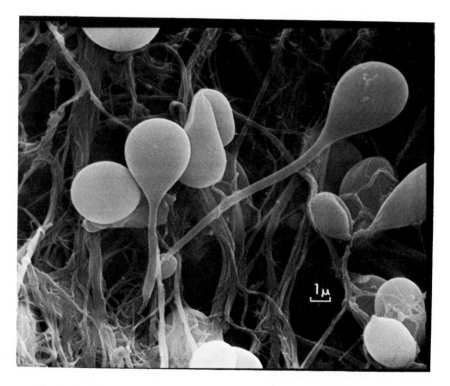

Fig. 10. Red blood cells caught in a fibrin clot and drawn out by liquid flow forces.

answered in the affirmative. Steric interference between the phospholipid polar head groups, together with surface tension, can account for a strong surface of constant surface area and negligible shear resistance. To apply this same argument to the spectrin net would mean that the molecules would have to be pulled together by surface tension (to supply the area stability and dilational strength), and highly convoluted in the membrane plane (to provide the freedom of movement required for large shear deformation). However, once surface tension has been invoked, there is no need to pack the spectrin molecules tightly because the phospholipid can fulfil the constant area requirement without any help from the spectrin.

A more reasonable role for the spectrin skeleton would therefore appear to be that of stabilizing the lipid bilayer and maintaining a proper distribution of intramembranous particles. This does not prevent the spectrin layer from having some form of anisotropic intrinsic bending resistance, but if it does, this resistance is simply added to that offered by the lipid layer (as in Case III). We conclude therefore that localized elastic bending resistance can arise in the lipid bilayer alone, in the protein skeleton alone, or partly in each of these components, but not by interaction between them. Moreover, bending resistance in the skeleton, if present, infers a particular and unusual molecular structure which would decouple the elastic shear resistance in the membrane plane from the elastic bending resistance normal to that plane.

Calculation of Elastic Strain Energy

We can now examine the assumption, which has been made throughout the above discussion that localized elastic bending resistance with very low elastic shear resistance is necessary in order to generate a stable biconcave shape. This assumption has been and still is being challenged by the most able theoreticians (Evans, 1973; Evans and Skalak, 1980; Fung and Tong, 1968) on the very reasonable grounds that there is good evidence for shear resistance but no direct evidence for dominant bending resistance. The presence of the latter would be expected to prevent the membrane from turning sharp corners which it is obviously able to do when attached to a point or when folded over the sharp edge at the entrance to a glass micropipette. Against these observations must be conceded the fact that shear forces alone cannot account for the transformation of a sphere into a biconcave disc: If only shear resistance is present the disc must be the unstressed shape. This is commonly understood in connection with thin objects, like rubber gloves, which are moulded to a particular shape. There is no doubt that a red cell does have a weak tendency to return to a particular biconcave shape in which the dimples have a fixed location on the surface, but this is not to be compared to the strong tendency to form a biconcave shape which persists even though the membrane is "tank-treading" with respect to what appears to be a fixed biconcavity.

This effect was first reported by Schmid-Schönbein and Wells (1969) who put red cells into a strong, dynamic liquid shear field. By means of these and later experiments (Fischer *et al.*, 1978) it was shown unequivocally that the membrane was rotating with a tank-tread motion while leaving the dimples undisturbed. About the same time other experiments were being carried out by Bull (1972) on red cells held by their natural adhesion to glass and deliberately rolled back and forth by a current of fluid induced in a special observation chamber. These experiments revealed the additional informa-tion that while some attachments to the glass can move in the membrane without moving the membrane, other attachments move the whole mem-brane past the dimples without moving the latter. All these experiments clearly demonstrate that the mechanism responsible for the biconcavity is not a localized "set" in the membrane substance, but is a dynamic minimiza-tion of the elastic energy in a two-dimensionally isotropic material. That is, the properties of the membrane material must be the same everywhere on the surface of the cell and the biconcave shape must be continually being formed by a dynamic equilibrating process.

BICONCAVE SHAPE

The most convenient way to calculate the equilibrium shape of the red cell is to calculate the elastic strain energy and to find the shape which has the least energy for a given set of conditions. This can be done by variational calculus or by starting with a mathematical equation which generates a series of cross-sectional profiles that approximate closely to the shapes the cell assumes. Fung and Tong (1968) suggested a suitable equation which has been widely used. Whichever method is used, the bending energy is ex-pressed as a function of the curvature of the surface and some account must therefore be taken of the resting, or unstressed, state of the membrane. Curvature is considered in two orthogonal planes, called the principal planes, which are free from undesirable components of stress. If the curva-ture in these two planes is K_1 and K_2 and the intrinsic or stress free curvature in the same two planes is K_{01} and K_{02} respectively, then the bending energy per unit area due to localized bending resistance is given by

$$\bar{U}_b = M_1 \oint (K_1 + K_2 - K_{01} - K_{02})^2 \cdot dA/A \qquad (1)$$

If the bending resistance is not localized but is derived from the mean curvature, then the energy per unit area is given by

$$\bar{U}_b = M_2 \, [\oint (K_1 + K_2 - K_{01} - K_{02})dA/A]^2 \qquad (2)$$

Where M_1 and M_2 are appropriate constants.

The elastic energy per unit area due to shear can also be calculated from the shape, on the assumption that the shear stress is zero when the cell is either spherical or some particular but arbitrary shape. This energy is then added to the bending energy to give the total elastic strain energy. The shear energy, unlike the bending energy, is not affected by intrinsic precurvature.

If the total strain energy is plotted against cell shape (or rather, some parameter responsible for cell shape) for a particular sphericity, curves such as those shown in Fig. 11 result. Sphericity is defined as the ratio of the cell volume to the volume of a sphere of equal surface area. Only one curve each is shown for localized and nonlocalized bending resistance respectively, corresponding to a single ratio of bending to shear resistance. The localized bending curve, corresponding to equation (1) above, will have a well-defined minimum which will occur at a shape which is unique for the particular ratio of bending to shear resistance chosen and, of course, there will be a unique minimum energy shape for each value of sphericity. However the non-

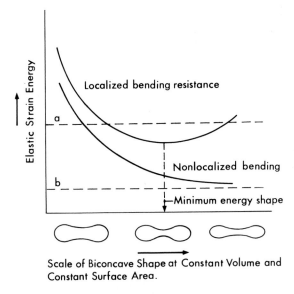

Scale of Biconcave Shape at Constant Volume and Constant Surface Area.

Fig. 11. Diagrammatic representation of change in elastic energy plotted against shape change for the red blood cell. Graph shows that the stability of the biconcave depends upon the type of bending resistance offered by the membrane.

localized bending curve, corresponding to equation (2) above, has no minimum value in the physiological range of shapes. This is true whatever combination of bending resistance, shear resistance or intrinsic precurvature is used. It would seem therefore that the bending resistance responsible for the biconcave shape must be of the localized type.

Experiments have been reported in the literature (Fischer *et al.*, 1981) in which the shear resistance of red cells was manipulated by means of diamide. This agent is thought to cross-link the protein strands of the spectrin and has the effect of progressively diminishing the ability of the cells to deform in their characteristic way. Since it is the shear resistance which is being manipulated, and the bending resistance appears to be unaffected, the necessity for the shear resistance to be small in the normal cell is clearly demonstrated.

Unfortunately it is not possible to deduce from these experiments whether the bending resistance resides in the lipid layer or in the spectrin layer. It is of interest to know whether or not the bending resistance originates in the lipid bilayer. If it does, it would imply that a strong enough surface tension must exist in the naturally occurring red cell membrane to account for its elastic resistance to bending. This has already been discussed and would probably have implications for all biological membranes, since the bending resistance is not then linked specifically with the peculiar properties or presence of a spectrin layer.

OTHER SHAPES

At this juncture it seems appropriate to turn from the biconcave form of the red cell and to consider, briefly, the crenated and cupped shapes which, there is good reason to suppose, are also equilibrium states of a uniform membrane. Considerable interest has been centered in these forms of late because they seemed to agree nicely with the concept that they are caused by differential expansion of one monolayer of the phospholipid bilayer with respect to the other (Sheetz *et al.*, 1976). Thus crenation was thought to be due to expansion of the outer layer and cupping to be due to expansion of the inner layer. Chemically induced bending effects, such as these supposedly acting in the red cell, could therefore be invoked to explain local curvature in other membranes and possibly the spontaneous formation and separation of vesicles. This simple and attractive hypothesis has, however, run into difficulty when careful calculations are made of the changes in surface area which must occur when the shape transformations take place.

Calculations of the differential change in area between the inner and outer surfaces of a hollow shell of constant thickness are comparatively easy to make, once the shape has been determined. Clearly the area of the outer surface of a spherical shell is greater than the area of the inner surface. If the shell is not spherical the difference in area can be calculated by deriving an expression for a small generalized element of the surface and integrating over the whole surface. If the area of the element is dA and the change in the outer surface with respect to the inner surface is $d(dA)$ then the change in area is given approximately by

$$d(dA) = h(K_1 + K_2)\, dA \tag{3}$$

The mean change in area per unit area for the whole surface is therefore

$$\delta A/A = \oint h(K_1 + K_2)\, dA/A \tag{4}$$

Where h is the thickness of the shell and K_1 and K_2 are the principal curvatures of the surface. The approximation is very good when the radius of curvature of the surface is large compared with the thickness of the membrane. This is generally true for biological membranes. When the cell is in the spherical state the outer surface of the membrane is greater in area than its inner surface by about 0.6%. The difference in area increases by about 1.5% to become 0.609% when the cell is in the normal biconcave shape. This does not mean that expansion of the outer surface will automatically produce a biconcave shape unless that shape happens to be a minimum energy form, but it does mean that a transformation from a sphere to a biconcave shape results in an increase in the outside area with respect to the inner area of the membrane.

Transformation of a portion of the surface of a biconcave cell to a crenated shape reveals the interesting result that the amount of change in surface area depends upon the initial curvature of the surface. Thus a crenation starting from a flat or concave region, such as the dimple, always requires an increase in the outer surface area. Crenation starting from a strongly positively curved region, such as the rim of the biconcave cell, at first requires a decrease in surface area changing to an increase in area as the crenation becomes larger. Fig. 12 shows the required change in surface area as crenation develops from uncrenated surfaces of different degrees of curvature. Therefore it appears that if crenation were simply the result of a chemically induced increase in the area of the outer surface with respect to the inner surface of the membrane, it would always start on a flat or concave portion of the cell and never on the rim. This, however, is contrary to observation, for crenation always starts on the rim and never in the dimple. We can conclude therefore that negative curvature is required to start the process of crenation.

The question naturally arises: How then can the process proceed if the

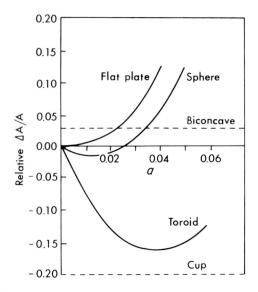

Fig. 12. Relative change in outer surface area per unit area to produce a crenation of semi-height a. The height of the crenation is normalized against the equatorial radius of the cell. The three curves correspond to three kinds of surface from which the crenation is assumed to rise.

opposite kind of curvature is required to bring it to completion? Negative curvature will favor the formation of the base of a crenation where the profile is curved in the opposite direction to the curvature of a sphere. The apex of the crenation, however, is always positively curved, therefore the material in this region (which in its unstressed state would be negatively curved due to the action of the chemical agent causing the crenation) is severely deformed into the opposite state of curvature. It has been shown that this degree of deformation is sufficient to disrupt the outer layer of the membrane and so relieve the stress (Brailsford *et al.*, 1980). The elastic energy released at the tip of the crenation is thus available to enable the base of the crenation to grow due to its natural tendency to become more negatively curved. Sufficient attention does not seem to have been given to the membrane disrupting effect of sharp curvature. The two cases of extremely sharp curvature, cited earlier, where a cell is attached to another body at a single point, and where a cell membrane passes over the sharp edge at the entrance to a glass micropipette, could be circumstances where breakdown of the membrane, due to the small radius of curvature, is the reason for the apparent absence of bending resistance. Of course, the word disruption is not meant to convey the impression that a hole appears in one layer of the membrane but rather that there is an abrupt change in the organization of the molecules. Even localized "slippage" as discussed earlier would radically modify the distribution of bending energy.

It has been found that the cup shape corresponds to a decrease in the outer surface area with respect to the inner surface, as expected, but that it is not then the lowest energy form if the membrane can support localized bending. The cup shape, however, does show the possibility of being a minimum energy equilibrium form if the membrane is characterized by nonlocalized bending resistance (Brailsford *et al.*, 1980).

Conclusion

The foregoing discussion has only dealt with the mechanoelastic properties of the membrane in so far as they affect the morphology of the stationary red cell. Consequently we have not been concerned with viscous effects which limit the rate at which deformation can take place. These are of primary importance in the rapidly growing branch of biology known as biorheology, reference to which is available in work already cited (Evans and Skalak, 1980), but the foundation for a proper understanding of the dynamic behavior of red cells, as they flow through the blood vessels, is still an accurate understanding of their elastic properties under static conditions.

The bulk of the evidence available at present indicates that localized bending resistance is a major shape-generating factor for the biconcave and crenated forms of the red cell. There is some indication, however, that this gives way to nonlocalized bending in the cup shaped form. Chemically induced intrinsic curvature of the membrane also plays an important role. The interesting proposition emerges that crenation may require negative intrinsic curvature and localized bending resistance, the biconcave shape may require zero or positive intrinsic curvature with localized bending resistance, while the cup shape may require zero or negative intrinsic curvature with nonlocalized bending resistance.

The source of the localized bending resistance is not easy to determine because it could be in the lipid bilayer, or the spectrin dominated skeleton, or partly in both, but it is unlikely to be the whole membrane acting cooperatively as a trilaminar structure. There is good support for the view that the localized bending resistance arises solely in the lipid bilayer. If this is so, surface tension effects, probably mediated by the amphipathic proteins and sugar moieties present in the natural membrane, would seem to be essential in order to give it sufficient magnitude. Obviously although these complicated requirements need more study and may be peculiar to the red cell membrane, they are indicative of changes and stress conditions which can occur in other biological membranes, but would not be suspected or measureable were it not for the peculiar requirements and morphological behavior of the red cell.

Acknowledgments

The author wishes to thank Dr. Brian S. Bull, Chairman of the Department of Pathology and Laboratory Medicine, School of Medicine, Loma Linda University, for his personal interest in this project and his many helpful suggestions.

References

Bessis, M. (1974). "Corpuscles: Atlas of Red Blood Cell Shapes." Springer-Verlag, Berlin and New York.
Boroske, E., Elwenspoek, M., and Helfrich, W. (1981). *Biophys. J.* **34,** 95–108.
Brailsford, J. D., and Bull, B. S. (1973). *J. Theor. Biol.* **39,** 325–332.
Brailsford, J. D., Korpman, R. A., and Bull, B. S. (1976). *J. Theor. Biol.* **60,** 131–145.
Brailsford, J. D., Korpman, R. A., and Bull, B. S. (1980). *J. Theor. Biol.* **86,** 513–546.
Bull, B. S. (1972). *Nouv. Rev. Fr. Hematol.* **12** (6), 835–844.
Bull, B. S., and Brailsford, J. D. (1976). *Blood* **48** (5), 663–667.
Canham, P. B. (1970). *J. Theor. Biol.* **26,** 61–81.
Canham, P. B., and Parkinson, D. R. (1970). *Can. J. Physiol. Pharmacol.* **48,** 369–376.
Conrad, M. J., and Singer, S. J., (1979). *Proc. Nat. Acad. Sci. USA* **76,** 5202–5206.
Deuling, H. J., and Helfrich, W. (1977). *Blood Cells* **3,** 713–720.
Dintenfass, L. (1969). "Molecular Crystals and Liquid Crystals," Vol. 8, pp. 101–139. Gordon and Breach, New York.
Evans, E. A. (1973). *Biophys. J.* **13,** 926.
Evans, E. A. (1974). *Biophys. J.* **14,** 923–931.
Evans, E. A. (1980). *Biophys. J.* **30,** 265–284.
Evans, E. A., and Hochmuth, R. M. (1977). *J. Membrane Biol.* **30,** 351–362.
Evans, E. A., and LaCelle, P. L. (1975). *Blood* **45,** 29.
Evans, E. A., and Skalak, R. (1980). "Mechanics and Thermodynamics of Biomembranes." CRC Press, Boca Roton, Florida.
Fischer, T. M., Stohr-Liesen, M. and Schmid-Schönbein, H. (1978). *Science* **202,** 892–896.
Fischer, T. M., Haest, C. W. M., Stohr-Liesen, M. Schmid-Schonbein, H., and Skalak, R. (1981). *Biophys. J.* **34,** 409–422.
Fung, Y. C. (1968). *Fed. Proc.* **25,** 1761–1772.
Fung, Y. C., and Tong, P. (1968). *Biophys. J.* **8,** 175–198.

Jenkins, J. T., (1977). *J. Math. Biol.* **4**, 149–169.
Kresh, E. (1977). *Bull. Math. Biol.* **39**, 679–691.
Lux, S. H. (1979). *Nature (London)* **281**, 426–429.
Ponder, E. (1948). "Hemolysis and Related Phenomena." Grune and Stratton, New York.
Schmid-Schönbein, H., and Wells, R. (1969). *Science* **165**, 288–291.
Sheetz, M. P., Painter, R. G., and Singer, S. J. (1976). *J. Cell Biol.* **70**, 193–203.
Shohet, S. B. (1982). *New Engl. J. Med.* **306**, 1170–1171.
Singer, S. J., and Nicolson, G. L. (1972). *Science* **175**, 720–731.
Southwell, R. V. (1913a). *Philos. Mag.* **25**, 687–698.
Southwell, R. V. (1913b). *Philos. Mag.* **26**, 502–511.
Van Deenen, L. L. M. *et al.* (1976). "The Structural Basis of Membrane Function" (Y. Hatefi and I. Djavadi-Ohaniance, eds.), pp. 21–38. Academic, New York.

Index

A

Absorption difference spectroscopy, 225
Acanthamoeba sp., 249
Acetylcholine receptors, 29
Acholeplasma laidlawii, 76, 247, 251, 269, 277
Acidic phospholipids (APL), 237, 239
ADP–ATP translocase, 119
Adriamycin, 60
Air drying, negative membrane image, 189
Alfalfa leaf lipid classes, 279
All-trans configuration (membrane lipids), 6
Aminopyrine, 207
Amoeba proteus, 269
Anesthetic potency, 77
Anesthetics, 21, 77
Annealed bilayers, 9
Annular lipids, 26, 76
Arrhenius discontinuity, 26
Asymmetry, membrane, 3, 57
ATP hydrolysis, 265, 266, 267
ATP synthase, 112–114
  basepiece, 113
  elementary particle, 112
  headpiece, F_1-ATPase, 112
  proton gradient, 114

B

Bacillus stearnothermophilus, 32
Bending effects, 298, 299
Bending elasticity, 302
Bending resistance, 296, 312
Benzphetamine, 207, 219, 222
Benzphetamine N-demethylation, 217, 218, 219, 222, 226

Benzphetamine N-hydroxylation, 216
Bilayer configuration, 24, 40, 45, 48, 172
  cholesterol, 48
  glycolipids, 48
  phosphospholipids, 45, 48
Biconcave shape, 291, 292, 312
Bilayer curvature, 313, 317
Bilayer–nonbilayer trigger, 47–73
  calcium effects, 48
  cardiolipin, 69
  cytochrome C, 69
  gramacidin, 59
  phase temperatures, 47
  pH effects, 54, 55
  temperature, 73
Bilayer stabilization, 53–60
  adriamycin, 60
  glycophorin, 59
  phosphatidylcholine, 57
  poly (L-lysine), 60
  rhodopsin, 59
  sphingomyelin, 57
Bilayer thickness, 107
Birefringence, positive, negative, and form, 122
Blebbing off, membranes, 56–57
Boundary lipid, 26, 76
Bovine red blood cells, 240
Brain lipid changes with age, 278–279
2-Bromo-2-chloro-1,1,1-trifluoroethane, 229

C

C. lipolytica, 267
Ca^{2+} effects, 58
Calcium ATPase, 204, 265, 272
Calcium, negative membrane image, 194

Capping/patching, 28
Carbon tetrachloride, 229
Carboxypeptidase A, 88
Cardiolipin (CL), 17, 48, 49, 52–54, 59, 63,
    70, 237, 239, 248, 281
Catecholamine release, 65
Ca^{2+} trigger, 133, 134
Cell membrane codes, 248
Ceramide aminoethylphosphonate, 237
Ceramide polyhexosides, 283–285
Cerebroside, 17, 237
Chemiosmotic hypothesis, 115
Chlorella sorokiniana, 277
2-Chloro-1,1-difluoroethylene, 229
2-Chloro-1,1,1-trifluoroethane, 229
1-Chloro-2,2,2-trifluoroethane, 229
1-Chloro-2,2,2-trifluoroethyl radical, 230
Chloroplast
    air-dried, 189, 191
    development, 192, 194
    envelope, 175
    low denaturation embedding, 188
    negative membrane image, 176, 188, 189,
        191–196
Cholate dialysis technique, 206
Cholesterol, 17, 21, 22, 48, 144, 145, 166,
    244, 279
    ATPase activity, 145
    fluidity effect, 144
    packing, 283–285
    phospholipid/cholesterol ratios, 245, 246
    protein interaction, 66
    RBC shape, 145
Chromaffin granules, 66, 67
Cluster–cluster interaction, 4
Cluster formation, 204
Cochleate domains, 54
Colchicine, 29
Compartmentation, membrane, 71
Cone shaped lipids, 3, 71–77
Cooperative unit site, 13
    grain boundary, 14
    isoenergetic phases, 14
    line defect, 14
Cooperativity, 26
Crenation (RBC), 315
Criteria for membrane images, 92
Critical micellar concentration (CMC), 43
Cryoprotection
    cryoultramicrotomy, 182
    dimethyl sulfoxide (DMSO), 177

glycerol, 177
intramembranous particles, 177
membrane images, 180
Cryoultramicrotomy, negative membrane
    images, 176
    technique, 182
Crystal lattice defects, 4, 5
Cubic phase, 46
Cumene hydroperoxide, 216
Cychohexane, 207
Cyclopropane ring, 230
Cytochalasin B, 29
Cytochrome bc_1, 110–112
Cytochrome b_5, 221–229
    lipid requirement, 223–225
Cytochrome c, 59, 68, 69, 111
Cytochrome oxidase, 107, 109, 111, 112
    cytochrome c interaction, 111
Cytochrome P-450, 201–206, 211–222,
    226–230
    lipid interactions, 209–215, 220, 221, 228
Cytochrome P-450 reductase
    conditions of reconstitution, 205–207
    uncoupling, 216

D

Dark-field EM, 97, 188
Delta (Δ^n) fatty acid chain codes, 248–250
Dense-band image
    erythrocyte ghosts, 152
    proteins, 152
Detergent–phospholipid dispersions, 204
Diacylphosphatidylcholesterol, 22
Dielaidoylphosphatidylcholine (DEPC), 16
Digalactosyldiglycerides (DGPG), 237–239,
    249, 279
Dilauroylphosphatidylethanolamine (DLPE),
    73
Dimethyl adipimidate, 161, 162
Dimethyl suberimidate, 161, 162
Dimyristoylphosphatidic acid (DMPA), 55,
    209–212
Dimyristoylphosphatydlethanolamine
    (DMPE), 73
Dimyristoylphosphatidylcholine (DMPC), 7,
    8, 10, 16, 181, 209–211
Dioleoylphosphatidylcholine (DOPC), 16,
    18, 46, 50, 230, 231, 272, 273
Dioleoylphosphatidylethanolamine (DOPE),
    18, 43, 50, 73

Dioleoylphosphatidylserine (DOPS), 55
Dipalmitoylphosphatidylcholine (DPPC), 11
Diphosphatidylglycerol, *see* Cardiolipin
Disk membrane function, 133–134
  Ca^{2+} trigger, 133
  energy transduction, 134
  signal transmission, 134
Disk membranes, 123, 129, 130
  function, 133
  isolation, 131, 132
  particle density and size, 131–133
  plasma membrane interaction, 135
Distearoylphosphatidylcholine (DSPC), 16
DNA
  mitochondrial, 110
  nuclear, 110
Domains (membrane)
  boundaries, 8
  cytochrome, 114
  respiratory chain, 113
  size, 18
Drosophila, 275

E

E. coli, 25, 59, 240, 247, 251, 264, 268
Echinocytes, 293
Egg PA, 210, 211
Egg PC, 41, 209, 212–214
Egg PE, 211, 213
Egg PS, 53, 67
Elastic bending resistance/elastic shear
  resistance ratio, 301
Elastic shear deformation, 297
Elastic strain energy, 305, 311–313
Electron coupling, 205
Electron microscopy
  low-temperature fixation, 91
  methodology, 84, 89
Electron transfer, 216–220, 215
Electrostatic interaction, 225
Embedding agents for electron microscopy,
  91
Endocytosis, 60
Endoplasmic reticulum, 201
Energy transduction, 134
Enthalpy of transition (ΔH), 11
Erythrocyte, *see* Red blood cell
Essential fatty acid deficiency, 248
Eutectic mixtures, 14, 15
Exocytosis, 60–67

catecholamine release, 65
chromaffin granules, 65
model, 66, 67
soya PE, PS, PL, 67

F

F_1 ATPase, 89
F_1 complex, 113
Fatty acid-chain codes, 247–251
Fatty acid-chain length equivalents, 250
Fatty acid packing, 247
Fatty acid replacement families, 237
Fertilization, 60
3T3 Fibroblasts, 29
Fixation criteria, 85
Flash-induced transient dichroism, 167
Flash photolysis, 161
Flavin–porphyrin interaction, 220
Flip-flop (lipids), 3, 71
Fluid mosaic membrane model, 121–122,
  139, 144, 145, 175, 185
Fluorescence photobleaching recovery
  (FPR), 167
Fluorescence polarization, 273, 274
Formaldehyde, 207, 219, 222
Found to calculated ratio (F/C), 253–285
Fracture face complementarity, 124
Free energy, 15
Free radicals, 229, 230
Freeze-drying, 164–183
  globular membrane structure, 178
  low-denaturation technique, 187
  negative membrane image, 164, 176–180
  technique, 177, 178
Freeze-etching, 129, 175, 177
Freeze-fixation, 176–177
Freeze-fracture plane, 101–105, 139
  globular protein, 103
  hydrogen bonding, 103
  interatomic bonding, 103
  particulate surface, 104
  smooth surface, 105
Freeze-fracture technique, 44, 103–107,
  116, 151, 152, 159, 166, 175, 177
  crista membranes, 107
  cross fracture, 116
  glutaraldehyde, 159
  limit of resolution, 103
  OsO_4, 151, 152
  plastic deformation, 107

surface fracture, 116
Freeze-sectioning (cryoultramicrotomy)
    negative membrane images, 183
Freeze substitution
    lipid extraction, 179
    negative membrane images, 176,
        179–183, 195
    technique, 179, 182
Fusion, membrane, 61, 65, 71
Fusogens, 61

G

Ganglioside packing, 283–285
Gauche configuration (conformer), 6, 10, 13,
    17, 23, 27
Gauche-trans configuration, 17
2 gl kink, 6
Globular membrane structure
    air drying, 188
    freeze-sectioning, 183
    glutaraldehyde, 188
    negative membrane image, 178
    thylakoids, 189
Globular proteins, 103, 172
Glutaraldehyde
    globular membrane structure, 188
    protein interaction, 156
Glutaraldehyde–urea
    negative membrane images, 176
    technique, 183–184
Glutathione, 229
Glycerol monoleate (GMO), 61, 62, 63
Glycophorin, 59
Grain(s), 5, 9
Grain boundary, 5, 6, 10, 14
Gramacidin, 59
Graphic analysis, 252–257

H

Halobacterium halobium, 84
Halothane, 229
Hexagonal lipid packing, 3, 45
Hexagonal (H_{II}) phase, 43, 44, 46, 48,
    50–52, 54, 59, 61, 68, 72, 215, 216
Hexagonal (H_{II}) phase induction, 48–60
    ATP depletion, 57
    Ba^{2+}, 52
    Ca^{2+}, 52–55
    cardiolipin, 52, 53, 59

cholesterol, 48
cytochrome *c*, 59
gramacidin, 59
inverted micelles, 51
lipid asymmetry, 57
lipidic particles, 50
Hexobarbital, 207
Human aorta, 239
Human brain lipids, 242
Human red blood cells, 246, 247
Hydrogen bonding, 103
Hydrogen peroxide production, 205
Hydrophobic interaction, 2, 144, 271
Hysteresis, 7

I

Imidates, 165
Inert dehydration
    negative membrane images, 186
    technique, 185, 186
Inner mitochondrial membrane, 116–119
Integral membrane proteins, 74, 144, 165,
    166
    lipid binding, 154, 155
Interatomic bonds, 103
Intracrystal space, 115
Intramembrane particles, 124, 139, 153
    OsO_4, 151, 152
    proteins, 150
    redistribution, 177
Inverted cylinders, 51
Inverted micelles, 51
Ion permeability, 21
Isoenergetic states, 14
Isothermal modulation of membrane lipids,
    52–60
Isothermal phase transition, 21–23, 71
Isotropic motional averaging, 45

K

Kink isomers, 11, 12, 13

L

Lateral compressibility, 13
Lateral diffusion (lipids and proteins), 28
Lateral domains, 25
Lateral mobility, 205
Lateral organization in biomembranes, 23

Lateral phase separation, 3, 15, 17, 20–22, 60, 209–212
Ligand binding, 28
Ligand–receptor complex, 28
  movement, 29
Line defects, 4, 5, 14
Lipid class replacements, 239
Lipid clustering, 20
Lipid composition
  alfalfa, 239
  aorta, human, 239
  brain, human, 242
  E. coli, 240
  lung, animal, 270
  lung, human, 270
  red blood cells, 243
  Semiliki forrest virus, 243
  sindbis virus, 243
Lipid domains, freeze-fracture, 24
Lipid extraction (during preparation for electron microscopy), 176
  freeze-drying, 178
  freeze-substitution, 179
  low-denaturation embedding, 187
  methacrylate, 179
  negative membrane images, 179
Lipid influence on enzyme activity, 203
Lipidic particles, 50
Lipid packing
  bilayer configuration, 42
  cholesterol, 22, 23
  hexagonal (H_{II}) phase, 43, 45
  linear array, 22, 23
  micellar phase, 43
  nonrandom distribution, 24, 25
  trans configuration, 6
  visualization techniques, 44
Lipid–protein interaction, 207
Lipid retention
  air drying, 188
  dense-band image, 152
Lipid shapes, 71, 77
Liquid–crystalline phase transition, 7
Liquid–liquid immiscibility, 18
Liver mitochondria, 113
Liver necrosis, 229
LM fibroblasts, 276
Localized bending resistance, 312, 313
Log plots in graphic analysis, 252–285
Low-denaturation embedding, 113, 115, 116, 124

lipid extraction, 187
negative membrane image, 187
technique, 187
Lysobisphosphatidic acid (LBPA), 237
Lysophosphatidylcholine (LPC), 73

M

M. sporium, 266
M. xanthus, 268
Magnetic circular dichroism, 217, 219, 225
Main transition, 10
Membrane asymmetry, 3, 57
Membrane domains, 4, 8, 24
Membrane fusion, 60–65, 71, 215
Membrane image
  dense band, 142, 153, 158–161
  dense fibrillar band, 163, 165
  trilamellar, 147–150, 152, 158, 159, 165, 175
  unit membrane, 147, 172
Membrane-imaging criteria, 92
Membrane lipids, isothermal modulation, 52–60
Membrane-lipid variability, 247
Membrane-packing principles, 238–252
Membrane permeability barrier, 67, 68
Membrane proteins
  globular shape, 86
  loss due to OsO_4, 156
  OsO_4, 150
  peptide-chain folds, 86
Membrane receptors, 28
Methacrylate embedding technique, 184, 188
Micelles, 202, 204
Mitochondria
  freeze drying, 177
  membrane construction, 186
  negative images, 94–96, 98, 99, 100, 102, 177, 182, 191
Mitochondrial membranes
  cristae, 109, 175
  globular, 172
  intracrystal space, 115
  mass density, 188
  polar–nonpolar surfaces, 109
  protein–lipid ratio, 172
  protein motion, 109
Mixed function oxidases, 204
Modulus of elasticity, 298

Modulus of shear elasticity, 301
Monogalactosyldiglycerides (MGDG),
    237–239, 249, 279
Monolayer coupling, 305
Monotectic phases, 14
Monoxygenase, 205
Mouse LM cells, 248
Mouse lymphocyte, 29

N

N-acyl PE (NAPE), 237
NADH-cytochrome b_5 reductase, 221, 222,
    228, 229
NADH dehydrogenase, 114
NADPH-cytochrome P-450 reductase,
    202–206, 216–222, 226–229
Negative bilayer curvature, 313–317
Negative images, 94–100, 102, 171–192
Negative staining, 100
Neuroblastoma cells, 29
Neutrophils, 29
Nonaqueous fixation, 182
Norcardia leishmanii, 249

O

OsO_4, 115
    protein loss, 153, 157
Outer mitochondrial membrane, 119–121
    bilayer arrangement, 121
Oxidative phosphorylation, 114–115
    cytochrome chain domains, 114

P

Packing constraints, 8, 9, 13, 22
Packing principles of lipids in membrane
    compartments, 243–252
Partition coefficient, 77
Patching/capping, 28
Peripheral membrane proteins, 113, 144
Phase boundaries, 3, 22
Pβ′ phase, 7, 12, 18
Phase separation, 3, 15, 17, 20–22, 60,
    209–212
    cation-induced, 20
    cholesterol, 21, 22
Phase transition, 7, 11–13
Phosphatidic acid (PA), 17, 20, 70, 206–209,
    236, 239

Phosphatidylcholine (PC), 17, 20, 22, 45, 48,
    53, 54, 67, 203, 206–209, 213–215, 230,
    236, 239, 242, 247–250, 274, 276, 280
Phosphatidylethanolamine (PE), 17, 41, 46,
    48, 54, 58, 63, 67, 203, 206, 208, 209,
    213, 214, 236, 239, 248, 249, 276, 278
Phosphatidylglycerol (PG), 48, 49, 237
Phosphatidylinositol (PI), 20, 49, 63, 236,
    239, 279, 282
Phosphatidylserine (PS), 17, 20, 42–49, 58,
    62, 63
Phospholipase, 13
Phospholipid–cholesterol, 23
Phospholipid exchange, 2, 13, 213–215
Phospholipid packing, 13, 15, 22, 243–252
Phospholipid shapes, 72, 76
Photoactivatable agents, 165, 166
Photoreceptor cells, 122–140
Photoreceptor membrane, interpretation of
    freeze fracture, 128–130
Planar bilayers, 202
Plate tectonics, 2
Point defects, 4, 5
Polarization optical analysis, 122–123
    disk membranes, 123, 129, 130
    form birefringence, 123
    negative birefringence, 122
    positive birefringence, 122
    rhodopsin bleaching, 123
Polyglutaraldehyde
    negative membrane images, 176, 184, 185
    technique, 183
Polykaryocytes, 60
Poly (L-lysine), 60
Pore proteins, 164, 165
Potassium permanganate, 115
Protein aggregates, 121
Protein binding sites, 27
Protein denaturation, 175, 185
    freeze-drying, 178
    glutaraldehyde, 159, 188
    negative membrane image, 196
    OsO_4, 147, 188, 189
    protection by tannic acid, 189
Protein, extraction from membrane, 149,
    153
    with OsO_4, 153, 163
Protein–lipid interaction, 201
Protein–lipid ratios, 146, 185, 206
Protein motion, 109
Protein–protein interaction, 109

Proton gradient, 114, 115
Proton translocation, 114

R

R. capsulata, 266
Rabbit sperm membranes, 248
Range variations in biological systems, 263
Rat testis membranes, 248
RBC membrane model, 309
RBC proteins, 153, 154, 161
  removal by OsO₄, 152, 154
RBC shape
  cholesterol, 145
  fibrin clot, 310
  hexagonal subunits, 304
  icosahedron, 304
  model, 303
  sphere-biconcave disk, 295
  toroid, 316
Receptor recycling, 30
Receptors, 28
Red blood cell (RBC), 25, 29, 239, 240, 246,
  247
Residual acidic phospholipids (RAPL), 237,
  238, 240, 242, 278
Respiratory chain, 110
Retinal, 129, 130, 131
Rhodopsin, 59, 123, 130–134
Rhodopsin bleaching, 123
Rhombic phase, 46
Rippled (membrane) domain, 8
Rod outer segment plasma membrane,
  134–139
  particle distribution, 135
  protein molecule motility, 138
  thickness, 135
Rotational diffusion, 204

S

Sarcoplasmic reticulum vesicles, 267
Shear (membrane parameter), 269, 297
Shear resistance, 296
Signal transmission, 134
Single (membrane) domain, 4
Skeletal muscle microsomes, 265
Slope changes in biological relationships,
  260
Sodium dithionate, 216

Sodium–potassium ATPase, 264, 265
Solid–liquid immiscibility, 18
Solid or gel phase, 7
Soya PC, PE, PS, 53, 67
Spectrin, 153, 309–311
Sphingomyelin (SPH), 17, 22, 41, 45, 46,
  55, 57, 67, 280
Stearoyl–coenzyme A desaturase, 221
Stomatocytes, 293
Strain (membrane parameter), 296, 298
Stress–strain relationship, 308
Submitochondrial particles, 119
Sulfatide (Sulf), 237, 242, 278
Sulfocholine, 247
Sulfolipids (SL), 237
Sums analysis, 238, 239, 241
Superoxide anion radical, 216, 219

T

Tannic acid
  fixative, 189
  glutaraldehyde, 159
  mordant, 189, 197
  negative image, 191, 196
Tannin
  fixative, 194
  mordant, 195
  negative membrane image, 194
Temperature effects on enzyme activity, 207
Tension/compression, 296–298
Tetrahymena pyriformis, 25, 32, 249
Thin-layer chromatography (TLC), 237
Thylakoid membrane
  globular structure, 172
  protein–lipid ratio, 172
T_m, 11–13
Total polar lipid (TPoL), 278, 279, 282
Transbilayer exchange, 3
Transbilayer transport, 66–69
Trans configuration (lipid packing), 6, 17
Trans–gauche, 31
Trans–gauche conformation, free energy
  change, 27
Tricarboxylic acid cycle enzymes, 113
Trilamellar membrane image, 145–183
  erythrocyte, 149
  freeze-sectioning, 183
  OsO₄ fixation, 147, 149, 164
  protein loss, 149
  tannic acid fixation, 165

Tripartite (membrane) image, 187
Twisting movement, 296

U

Ubiquinone, 114
Unit membrane image, 143, 146, 172
  trilamellar, 153

V

Van der Waals interaction, 221
Vesicle fusion, 215
Viscosity of gases, 261, 262

W

Water density, 263
Water-soluble epoxy
  "inert" dehydration, 186
  lipid retention, 183
  low-denaturation technique, 187
  methacrylate, 186
  negative images, 176
Wedge shaped lipids, 3, 71–77

X

X-ray crystallography, 130
X-ray diffraction, 123, 145, 146